Oxford Case Histories

Oxford Case Histories

Series Editors

Sarah Pendlebury and Peter Rothwell

Published:

Neurological Case Histories (Sarah Pendlebury, Philip Anslow, and Peter Rothwell)

Oxford Case Histories in Cardiology (Rajkumar Rajendram, Javed Ehtisham, and Colin Forfar)

Oxford Case Histories in Gastroenterology and Hepatology (Alissa Walsh, Otto Buchel, Jane Collier, and Simon Travis)

Oxford Case Histories in Respiratory Medicine (John Stradling, Andrew Stanton, Najib Rahman, Annabel Nickol, and Helen Davies)

Oxford Case Histories in Rheumatology (Joel David, Anne Miller, Anushka Soni, and Lyn Williamson)

Oxford Case Histories in TIA and Stroke (Sarah Pendlebury, Ursula Schulz, Aneil Malhotra, and Peter Rothwell)

Oxford Case Histories in Neurosurgery (Harutomo Hasegawa, Matthew Crocker, and Pawan Singh Minhas)

Oxford Case Histories in Neurosurgery

Harutomo Hasegawa
Specialty Registrar in Neurosurgery, London Deanery, UK

Matthew Crocker
Consultant Neurosurgeon, Atkinson Morley Wing,
St. George's Hospital, London, UK

Pawan Singh Minhas
Consultant Neurosurgeon, Atkinson Morley Wing,
St. George's Hospital, London, UK

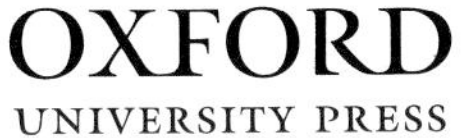

OXFORD
UNIVERSITY PRESS

Great Clarendon Street, Oxford OX2 6DP
United Kingdom

Oxford University Press is a department of the University of Oxford. It furthers the University's objective of excellence in research, scholarship, and education by publishing worldwide. Oxford is a registered trade mark of Oxford University Press in the UK and in certain other countries

First published 2013

British Library Cataloguing in Publication Data
Data available

ISBN 978–0–19–959983–7

Printed and bound by
CPI Group (UK) Ltd, Croydon, CR0 4YY

A note from the series editors

Case histories have always had an important role in medical education, but most published material has been directed at undergraduates or residents. The Oxford Case Histories series aims to provide more complex case-based learning for clinicians in specialist training and consultants, with a view to aiding preparation for entry- and exit-level specialty examinations or revalidation.

Each case book follows the same format with approximately 50 cases, each comprising a brief clinical history and investigations, followed by questions on differential diagnosis and management, and detailed answers with discussion.

At the end of each book, cases are listed by mode of presentation, aetiology, and diagnosis. We are grateful to our colleagues in the various medical specialties for their enthusiasm and hard work in making the series possible.

Sarah Pendlebury and Peter Rothwell

Acknowledgements

We would like to thank Anthony Pereira and Phil Rich for their helpful comments in reviewing the manuscript and Oxford University Press for their care and attention throughout the publishing process. We would also like to thank Steve Connor for Fig. 62.1, Mihai Danciut for Figs. 21.5 and 47.3, James Laban for Fig. 55.1, and Donal Walsh for his help in preparing cases 18 and 23. We are grateful to our teachers in neurosurgery, and to our patients whom we were privileged to treat.

Foreword

Safe, successful care of patients requires both a sound knowledge base and the skill to apply it effectively. In neurosurgery there is no shortage of didactic, factual accounts to support the systematic study of disciplines such as neuroanatomy, neurophysiology, neuropathology, neuroimaging and how abnormalities are expressed and managed in various clinical conditions. Unfortunately these subjects have a reputation for being difficult, complicated, even mysterious, leaving doctors within, or those liaising with neurosurgery, experiencing hesitancy and insecurity in the face of the complexities of the care of a patient. An antidote to this situation is now available through this compendium of presentations which convey how the key information relevant to a range of clinical problems can be selected and used to achieve timely, effective decision-making and treatment.

The emphasis is on learning from vividly described case histories portraying the presentation, investigation and management of individual patients suffering from a wide breadth of clinical problems. The flow of information mirrors clinical experience. The successive sets of questions that are posed and then answered throughout each case engage, stimulate and inform the reader and convey how knowledge and understanding are applied to the clinical situation of real-world cases. This problem-based learning approach is familiar to modern students and graduates but until now there has been little written material to support case-based learning as part of private study. This is increasingly relevant to the emphasis on scenario and patient-based questions in speciality training exit examinations.

The principle of placing the patient at the centre of learning fits well with the philosophy of key figures in the original emergence of neurosurgery as a separate discipline. While a resident in general surgery, Harvey Cushing was stimulated and encouraged to specialise in neurosurgery by Sir William Osler, then professor of medicine in Baltimore, later Regius Professor in Oxford. In his Pulitzer prize-winning biography of Osler, Cushing paid tribute to how his mentor had made clinical teaching the foundation of modern medical education, as expressed in his dictum 'He who studies medicine without books sails an uncharted sea, but he who studies medicine without patients does not go to sea at all'.

Standard texts retain a place in neurosurgical education but it is through the study of individual patients that the skills necessary for confident and competent clinical diagnosis and management are gained. The wealth of information conveyed so memorably by the patient stories assembled by Messrs Hasegawa, Crocker and Minhas will powerfully promote these abilities in undergraduates, trainees and qualified specialists, whether in neurosurgery or in specialties interfacing with it, and hence the quality of care they give to their patients.

Sir Graham Teasdale
FRCS, FRCP, F Med Sci, FRSE
Emeritus Professor of Neurosurgery, University of Glasgow
Past President of the Society of British Neurological Surgeons and of the Royal College of Physicians and Surgeons of Glasgow

Preface

This book is intended for medical students, for junior doctors working within neurosurgery or looking after potential neurosurgical patients in a wide range of specialities, and for other allied healthcare professionals. So often, when learning medicine, it is immensely helpful to remember a particular patient in order to fix in one's mind how they presented and the clinical features that were apparent. We have tried to cover a comprehensive syllabus in neurosurgery by describing case histories. Each is based on a real patient whom at least one of the authors has cared for. We have attempted to keep the details authentic and include discussions about the difficulties of diagnosis and choices in management that present regularly. We hope that this will better equip the reader to manage neurosurgical patients with confidence in the future.

We hope that the book can be used at a number of different levels: the neurosurgically unaccustomed reader might wish to skim through the details to become familiar with the main clinical features and imaging for a particular diagnosis. Those more involved in looking after neurosurgical patients may gain from a more in-depth study of individual case histories to appreciate the options that were available, the complications that may have arisen, and other issues. The problem-based learning approach also fits in well with this format.

Finally, learning never stops in clinical practice. We are eager to hear readers' opinions regarding the book with regard to how effectively the message comes across, as well as if they have seen various conditions that have been managed differently to the options we have presented. Thank you in advance for your helpful comments.

Harutomo Hasegawa
Matthew Crocker
Pawan Singh Minhas
London, February 2013

Contents

Abbreviations *viii*

Section 1. Cranial trauma *1*

Cases 1–8 *3*

Section 2. Spinal trauma *67*

Cases 9–16 *69*

Section 3. Vascular neurosurgery *117*

Cases 17–28 *119*

Section 4. Neuro-oncology *213*

Cases 29–45 *215*

Section 5. Spinal neurosurgery *319*

Cases 46–52 *321*

Section 6. Paediatric neurosurgery and hydrocephalus *355*

Cases 53–61 *357*

Section 7. Miscellaneous *405*

Cases 62–67 *407*

List of cases by diagnosis *439*

List of cases by principal clinical features at presentation *441*

List of cases by aetiological mechanism *442*

Index *443*

Abbreviations

ACA	anterior cerebral artery
ACD	anterior cervical discectomy
ACom	anterior communicating artery
ADC	apparent diffusion coefficient
ADH	antidiuretic hormone
AF	atrial fibrillation
AAGBI	Association of Anaesthetists of Great Britain and Ireland
AICA	anterior inferior cerebellar artery
AP	anteroposterior
ASIA	American Spinal Injury Association
ATLS	Advanced Trauma Life Support
ATP	adenosine triphosphate
AVM	arteriovenous malformation
bd	twice daily
BIH	benign intracranial hypertension
bpm	beats per minute
CBF	cerebral blood flow
CPP	cerebral perfusion pressure
CRP	C-reactive protein
CSF	cerebrospinal fluid
CSW	cerebral salt wasting
CT	computed tomography
CTA	CT angiography/angiogram
CTS	carpal tunnel syndrome
CVP	central venous pressure
CVR	cerebral vascular resistance
DAI	diffuse axonal injury
DBS	deep brain stimulation
DCI	delayed cerebral ischaemia
DDAVP	1-deamino-8D-arginine vasopressin
DI	diabetes insipidus
DIND	delayed ischaemic neurological deficit
DNET	dysembryoplastic neuroepithelial tumour
DVLA	Driver and Vehicle Licensing Agency
DVT	deep vein thrombosis
DWI	diffusion-weighted imaging
E	eye-opening (GCS)
EC	extracranial
ECF	extracellular fluid
ENT	ear, nose, and throat
ETV	endoscopic third ventriculostomy
EVD	external ventricular drain
FLAIR	fluid attenuated inversion recovery
GCS	Glasgow Coma Scale/Score
GP	general practitioner
GPi	globus pallidus internus
HIV	human immunodeficiency virus
IC	intracranial
ICA	internal carotid artery
ICH	intracranial haemorrhage
ICP	intracranial pressure
ICU	intensive care unit
IGF-1	insulin-like growth factor 1
IIH	idiopathic intracranial hypertension
INR	international normalized ratio
ISAT	International Subarachnoid Aneurysm Trial
L	litre
LP	lumbar puncture
M	motor response (GCS)
MAP	mean arterial pressure
MCA	middle cerebral artery
MEP	motor evoked potential
mg	milligram
MIP	maximum intensity projection
mL	millilitre
MRA	magnetic resonance angiography

MRC	Medical Research Council
MRI	magnetic resonance imaging/image
MRS	magnetic resonance spectroscopy
ng	nasogastric
NICE	National Institute for Health and Clinical Excellence
NPH	normal pressure hydrocephalus
PCA	posterior cerebral artery
PCom	posterior communicating artery
PCV	procarbazine–lomustine (CCNU)–vincristine
PE	pulmonary embolism
PET	positron emission tomography
PICA	posterior inferior cerebellar artery
PNET	primitive neuroectodermal tumour
po	by mouth
RCT	randomized controlled trial
RTA	road traffic accident
SAH	subarachnoid haemorrhage
SCA	superior cerebellar artery
SIADH	syndrome of inappropriate ADH secretion
SSEP	somatosensory evoked potential
STN	subthalamic nucleus
TB	tuberculosis
TIA	transient ischaemic attack
V	verbal response (GCS)
VP	ventriculoperitoneal
VTE	venous thromboembolism
WHO	World Health Organization

Section 1

Cranial trauma

Case 1

A 78-year-old man was admitted to hospital with a 2 week history of progressive confusion and unsteadiness. His medical history included parkinsonism and a metallic mitral valve replacement. On examination his GCS was 14/15 (E4, V4, M6) (see 'Glasgow Coma Scale and Score', p. 196), and he had left-sided weakness. He was taking warfarin, and the INR was 3.8.

Questions

1. What is the differential diagnosis?
2. A CT scan of the brain is performed (Fig. 1.1). Describe the appearances.

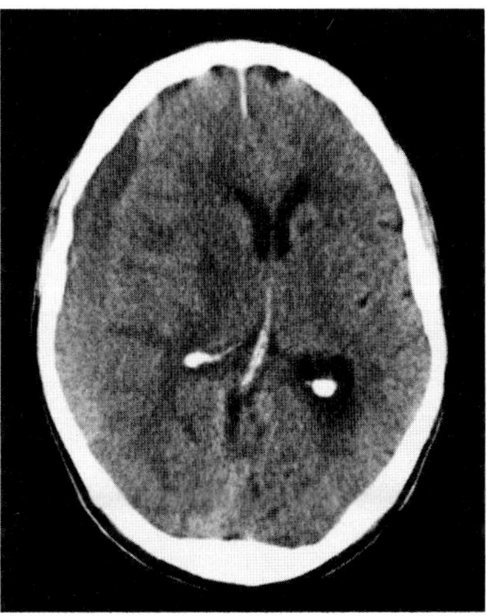

Fig. 1.1

Answers

1. What is the differential diagnosis?

Progressive confusion and gait disturbance with a left hemiparesis point to a right hemisphere lesion. The differential diagnosis includes cerebral infarction or haemorrhage, subdural haematoma, and a neoplastic lesion. The time course of the symptoms is central to distinguishing them: intracerebral haemorrhage or stroke typically presents with sudden-onset symptoms; progressive symptoms suggest a slowly enlarging mass such as a tumour or chronic subdural haematoma.

2. A CT scan of the brain is performed (Fig. 1.1). Describe the appearances (Fig. 1.2).

There is an extra-axial crescent shaped fluid collection over the right cerebral convexity (A, B) indicating a chronic subdural haematoma (Fig. 1.2). The patient is scanned supine. There is layering according to density, with a hypodense fluid supernatant (A) above hyperdense thrombus or cellular precipitant (B). This appearance could be due to a single episode of haemorrhage or rebleeding into a chronic collection. There is midline shift (C) with obliteration of cerebral sulci and the trigone (not seen, D) on the right.

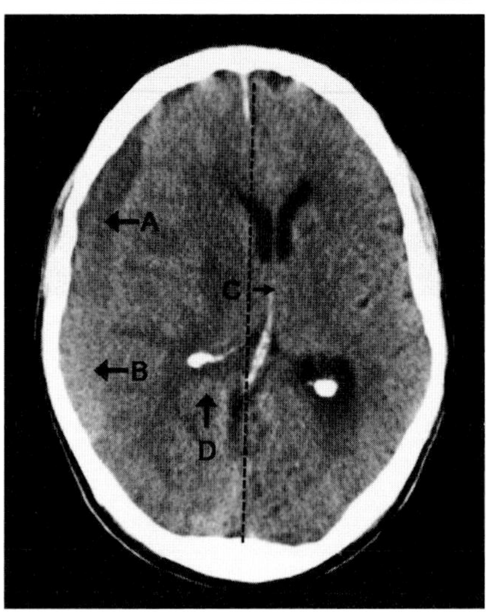

Fig. 1.2

Questions

3. What is the pathophysiology of chronic subdural haematomas?
4. What are the initial considerations in the management of this case?
5. What is the urgency of surgery? When should surgery be performed if the patient presents in the middle of the night?
6. What are the surgical options?
7. What are the complications of surgery?
8. The wife of the patient expresses her concern about plans for surgery. She tells you that her husband was never keen on surgery and that he would not have liked to survive with neurological impairment. She does not want you to perform the operation.
   (a) How would you approach this conversation and what points would you cover in the discussion?
   (b) What is the legal position of the family's views on a patient's treatment?
9. The subdural haematoma is evacuated with burrholes, and the patient makes a good recovery. How should his anticoagulation be managed postoperatively?

Answers

3. What is the pathophysiology of chronic subdural haematomas?

Chronic subdural haematomas are typically caused by tearing of dural bridging veins. Cerebral atrophy (e.g. in the elderly or in alcoholic patients) causes increased tension on these veins, predisposing them to tearing. The trauma causing the initial bleed can be sufficiently mild to be absent from the history, even in retrospect, in over 50% of patients. A local inflammatory reaction follows the haemorrhage and results in the formation of a haematoma cavity with membranes within it. The clot liquefies over time and this collection may expand. The processes that mediate this are poorly understood, but may include recurrent microbleeds from dural capillaries and haematoma membranes, secretion of fluid from haematoma membranes, and osmotic fluid shifts into the haematoma cavity.

4. What are the initial considerations in the management of this case?

The initial consideration is whether the patient should be managed operatively or conservatively. Operative management is appropriate in the presence of a neurological deficit or severe and persistent headache. In either case the INR requires normalization and blood tests, including serum sodium and clotting, should be performed.

5. What is the urgency of surgery? When should surgery be performed if the patient presents in the middle of the night?

Surgery should be performed as soon as possible, but the practicalities of operating overnight require consideration if the patient presents in the middle of the night. Surgery should be considered overnight if symptoms have progressed rapidly or if the haematoma is large (e.g. with significant midline shift and contralateral ventricular enlargement from encystment). However, if deterioration has occurred over several days or weeks, it would be reasonable to wait until the morning.

6. What are the surgical options?

There are several options for chronic subdural haematomas. Burrhole drainage is the most common. There are specific indications for performing a craniotomy, such as the presence of subdural membranes and recurrent episodes (see 'Surgery for chronic subdural haematomas', p. 8 and 'Varieties of chronic subdural haematomas', p. 9).

7. What are the complications of surgery?

Seizures, intracranial haematoma, pneumocephalus, and infection (including subdural empyema). Patients should also be advised of the risk of recurrence (up to 30%) and risk to life with a general anaesthetic, especially in a condition affecting an almost exclusively elderly population.

8. The wife of the patient expresses her concern about plans for surgery. She tells you that her husband was never keen on surgery and that he would not have liked to survive with neurological impairment. She does not want you to perform the operation.

a) How would you approach this conversation and what points would you cover in the discussion?

The patient's present condition and his prognosis with and without surgery should be carefully communicated to the family. If this is done effectively and there is a clear case for intervention, it is unusual for the family to disagree with the proposed treatment. The existence of advance directives or a legal guardian (an individual who is legally authorized to make decisions on behalf of the patient) should also be determined.

b) What is the legal position of the family's views on a patient's treatment?

If a patient lacks capacity to consent for treatment, in the UK the doctor is required to make a decision in the patient's best interests. The views of the family will inform this decision but they (or any other individual) cannot consent on behalf of the patient. Therefore a discussion with the family is essential before proceeding to surgery (although this should not delay life-threatening surgery). If there is any doubt about advance directives or legal guardians, the doctor should make a decision in the patient's best interests based on available information (for further guidance on patient autonomy and consent see *Good Medical Practice*, General Medical Council, UK).

9. The subdural haematoma is evacuated with burrholes, and the patient makes a good recovery. How should his anticoagulation be managed postoperatively?

The risk of further intracranial bleeding must be balanced against the risk from systemic embolization from a metallic heart valve. In general, the latter risk is greater and anticoagulation should be recommenced early, although observational studies have shown that stopping anticoagulation perioperatively for up to 2 weeks in patients with mechanical heart valves is safe. In this patient a CT scan was performed 48 hours after surgery to exclude ongoing haemorrhage. This was negative and he was restarted on warfarin (see 'Anticoagulation in neurosurgery', p. 11).

Further reading

General Medical Council (UK) (2011). *Good Medical Practice.* Available online at: http://www.gmc-uk.org/static/documents/content/GMP_0910.pdf (accessed 27 February 2011).

Haines DE, Harkey HL, Al-Mefty O (1993). The 'subdural' space: a new look at an outdated concept. *Neurosurgery*; **32**: 111–20.

Wilberger JE (2000). Pathophysiology of evolution and recurrence of chronic subdural hematoma. *Neurosurg Clin N Am*; **11**: 435–8.

Yamashima T, Yamamoto S (1985). The origin of inner membranes in chronic subdural hematomas. *Acta Neuropathol*; **67**: 219–25.

Surgery for chronic subdural haematomas

Chronic subdural haematomas are a very common neurosurgical condition but remain challenging to treat for various reasons.

- They are frequently due to multiple bleeds and hence have membranes causing compartmentalization or 'loculation' of the haematoma, making it harder to drain via a single hole.
- They usually occur in elderly people with multiple comorbidities.
- The brains of elderly people are slower to re-expand and fill the subdural space after the haematoma is evacuated. Therefore there is a large space between the brain and the skull which continues to stretch the bridging veins and has a tendency to fill with venous blood, causing re-accumulation of the haematoma.
- They are more common in patients on anticoagulation. If there is a compelling reason for anticoagulation (e.g. mechanical heart valve), there is justifiable anxiety about temporary withdrawal of anticoagulation.

Various surgical options are available and a balance is required between minimizing discomfort (performing the operation under local anaesthesia) and minimizing risk of recurrence (which may require a larger operation). The options (in increasing order of magnitude) are as follows.

1. Twist drill craniostomy: this can be done under local anaesthetic, even on the ward. A small-diameter drill bit is used, similar to that used to place an ICP monitor, and the burrhole drilled without direct vision. The skin is closed over the burrhole without formal irrigation in the hope that a completely liquefied haematoma will be absorbed into the galea. This is less invasive than all the other options and probably less effective.
2. Burrhole drainage: this can also be performed under local anaesthetic with or without sedation in a suitable patient, but an anaesthetist should be available in case the need for urgent general anaesthesia arises. It must be performed in the operating theatre. The burrholes allow formal irrigation of the clot either in and out of a single burrhole or through two burrholes. The burrholes are left open and the haematoma cavity again communicates with the subgaleal space. High-quality evidence supports a period of postoperative drainage using a soft subdural catheter for 2 days (Santarius *et al.* 2009).
3. Craniotomy: this is usually reserved for re-collected subdural haematomas or those with loculations that cannot be managed using burrholes alone. A modest craniotomy will allow direct visualization of the subdural space and the opportunity to divide or excise the membranes that form compartments within the haematoma cavity. This typically requires general anaesthesia.

Decisions to be made in the postoperative period include the following.

- When to allow the patient to sit up and mobilize: theoretically maintaining the patient supine will reduce venous return and encourage the brain to re-expand and obliterate the subdural space. This is probably associated with a lower risk of recurrence (Abouzari *et al.* 2007).
- When to restart anticoagulation (see 'Anticoagulation in neurosurgery', p. 11).

Varieties of chronic subdural haematomas

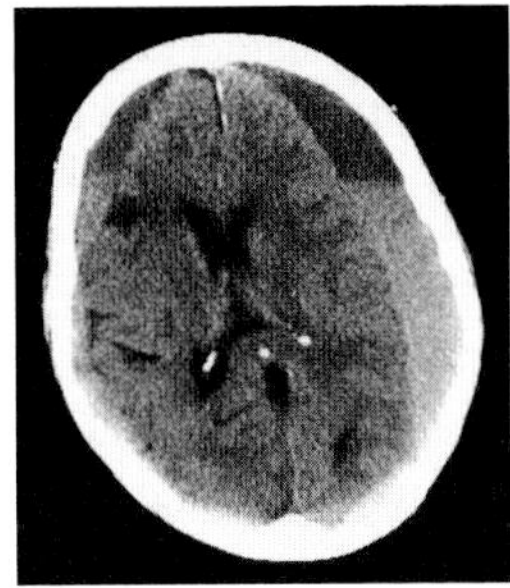

Fig. 1.3

This 86-year-old man (Fig. 1.3) has bilateral chronic subdural haematomas. Bilateral subdural haematomas may exert considerable pressure on the brain. There is midline shift to the right as the larger haematoma on the left exerts more pressure than the smaller collection on the right. There is greater sulcal effacement on the left under the larger collection. As a consequence of the mass effect there is often also vertical shift of the brain which is harder to appreciate on axial images. Bilateral burrholes are required to manage this condition. If only one side is evacuated, more midline shift will result from the unopposed haematoma on the other side.

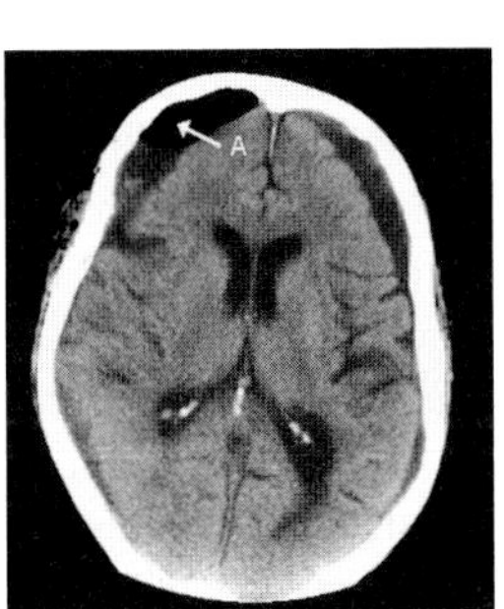

Fig. 1.4

The patient returns to hospital one week after drainage of the subdural haematomas due to increasing drowsiness. The scan (Fig. 1.4) shows bilateral subdural collections and some air over the right frontal lobe (A). There is less mass effect and the midline shift has resolved. The question is whether the residual collections are responsible for the symptoms. In this case the patient is clinically worse but the scan looks better. Therefore other causes for the drowsiness should be considered before surgery to re-evacuate the residual collections is contemplated. This patient had hyponatraemia and he improved when this was corrected. The term 'recurrent chronic subdural haematoma' is often used when a patient who has had a chronic subdural haematoma drained returns with a scan showing persisting subdural collections. This could represent a new episode of subdural haemorrhage, re-accumulation of fluid secreted by membranes, or simply saline wash used to irrigate the subdural cavity in the previous operation. A postoperative subdural collection could also be infected, presenting with sepsis with worsening headache or neurological deficit.

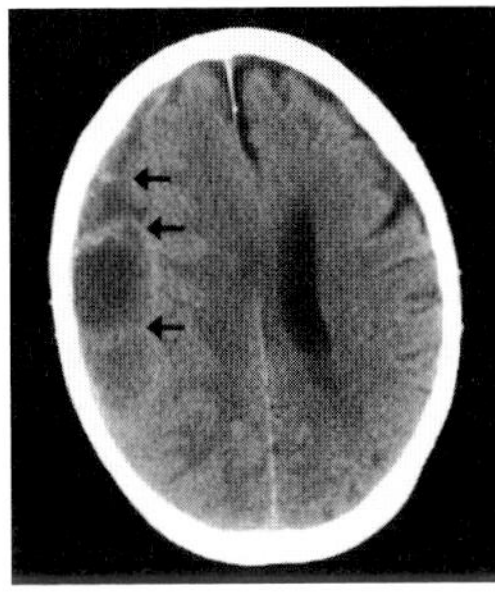

Fig. 1.5

The chronic subdural haematoma in this 87-year-old man contains septations within the collection (Fig. 1.5: arrows) representing membranes. There is mass effect on the right hemisphere causing effacement of sulci. The right lateral ventricle is displaced downwards out of the imaging plane of this slice, indicating downward brain herniation. Little midline shift is evident as this image is at the level of the falx (the bright line in the mid-sagittal plane) which restrains brain herniation apart from adjacent to the left lateral ventricle where subfalcine herniation of the medial right frontal lobe

(continued)

Varieties of chronic subdural haematomas *(continued)*

is apparent. Burrholes are unlikely to be successful because it will not be possible to access all the subdural compartments formed by the membranes. A larger (>2.5cm diameter) burrhole or a craniotomy enables the membranes to be accessed and divided, and will offer the best chance of improvement.

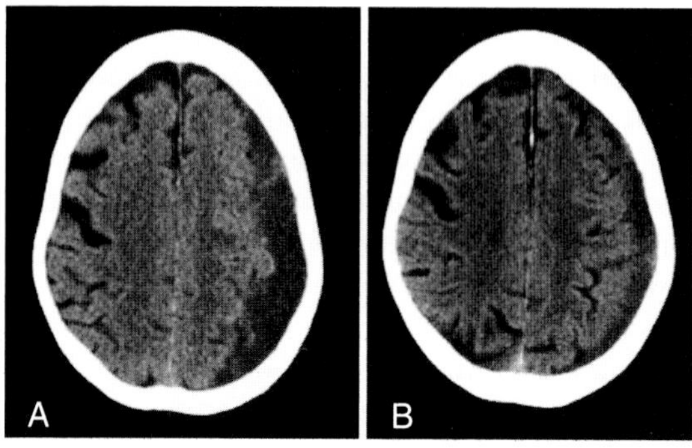

Fig. 1.6

This 74-year-old woman (Fig. 1.6) presented with headaches but without any neurological deficits. She has a left-sided chronic subdural haematoma with mass effect (note the effacement of sulci on the left) but no midline shift (Fig. 1.6(A)). Surgery in such a situation is unlikely to make her better. However, it could be argued that she may deteriorate if untreated because of expansion of the haematoma. Some surgeons may operate but it would also be reasonable to manage her conservatively. A small dose of dexamethasone (2mg bd for 10 days) will tend to settle the headache and even a mild neurological deficit somewhat faster. Its mechanism of action is unknown, but it is thought to stabilize the chronic subdural membrane and have a protective effect on the cerebral cortex. She was managed conservatively and her CT scan one week later (Fig. 1.6(B)) shows reduction in the size of the haematoma and less mass effect (the sulci are now visible in the left hemisphere).

Anticoagulation in neurosurgery

An increasing number of patients are anticoagulated. Common indications are prevention of cardiovascular disease, prevention of stroke in atrial fibrillation and prosthetic heart valves, and treatment of venous thromboembolism (DVT and PE). Here we discuss the perioperative management of anticoagulation in neurosurgical patients.

Reversal of anticoagulation

Elective patients

Antiplatelet therapy and warfarin should be stopped a few days before surgery. Warfarin bridging can be performed if the thromboembolic risk is particularly high: patients are admitted to hospital a few days before surgery and commenced on heparin while warfarin is stopped. Full anticoagulation can continue until several hours before surgery (typically 6 hours for unfractionated heparin and 12 hours for low molecular weight heparin). Elective surgery should be postponed if the acute event necessitating anticoagulation is recent, as the thromboembolic risk is particularly high and surgery will increase the risk further.

Emergency patients

Patients requiring emergency surgery and those with intracranial haemorrhage (ICH) require rapid and complete reversal of anticoagulation.

Warfarin

Intravenous vitamin K and prothrombin complex should be given.

Antiplatelets

Aspirin irreversibly blocks platelet function for the life of the platelet (approximately 10 days). Restoration of platelet function depends on the synthesis of new platelets. The number of new functional platelets can be estimated (10% of platelets are replenished per day; hence if the platelet count is 250×10^9/L, 25×10^9 new platelets will be produced per day). A platelet transfusion can be given if a patient is deemed to have insufficient functional platelets. One pool of platelets will raise the platelet count by approximately 50×10^9 platelets. Clopidogrel has stronger antiplatelet activity and two pools of platelets may be given (Beshay *et al.* 2010). The role of platelet transfusions in conservatively managed intracerebral haemorrhage is unclear (Morgenstern *et al.* 2010).

Postoperative issues

Venous thromboembolism (VTE) prophylaxis

The incidence of VTE in neurosurgical patients is high and many are asymptomatic (Iorio and Agnelli 2000). A recent meta-analysis showed that low-dose

(continued)

Anticoagulation in neurosurgery *(continued)*

heparin reduced the risk of VTE but with a slight increase in haemorrhagic events (9.1% absolute risk reduction in VTE; 0.7% absolute risk increase in ICH) (Hamilton *et al.* 2011). NICE (2010) advises mechanical prophylaxis for neurosurgical patients at increased risk of VTE with postoperative heparin (usually commenced 12–24 hours postoperatively) if the risk of major bleeding is low. If the presentation is with cranial or spinal haemorrhage, heparin prophylaxis is not recommended until the lesion is secured or the condition is stable (Morgenstern *et al.* 2010; NICE 2010).

Recommencement of anticoagulation

Anticoagulation should be restarted as soon as the risk of haemorrhage from a particular condition has passed. Retrospective studies show that withholding warfarin for up to 2 weeks is safe in patients with prosthetic heart valves (Romualdi *et al.* 2009).

Intracranial haemorrhage (ICH)

All anticoagulants (including antiplatelet agents) increase the risk of ICH. The majority are intracerebral and subdural haematomas. Population estimates for the absolute risk of ICH on anticoagulants are 0.2–0.3%/year for aspirin, 0.3–0.4%/year for aspirin plus clopidogrel, and 0.3–1%/year for warfarin (vs. 0.15%/year in the general population aged 70) (Hart *et al.* 2005). The individual risk varies considerably depending on age, comorbidities, intensity of anticoagulation, and lifestyle.

When an anticoagulated patient survives an ICH, a decision is required on whether it should be continued. This decision is based on the risk of recurrent ICH, the risk of thromboembolism (Table 1.1) and the overall neurological status of the patient. One systematic review found an aggregate recurrence rate for ICH without anticoagulation of 2.3%/year (Bailey *et al.* 2001). In one study, anticoagulation increased the risk of recurrent ICH three-fold (Vermeer *et al.* 2002). The individual risk of recurrent ICH (influenced by age, comorbidities, mobility, lifestyle, and anticoagulant use) requires careful consideration and needs to be balanced against the thromboembolic risk derived from cardiovascular risk stratification. Antiplatelet agents are safer than warfarin and have been recommended for patients at a relatively low risk of thromboembolism and a higher risk of ICH, or in those with very poor neurological function (Furie *et al.* 2011). If warfarin is to be continued, a CT scan may be helpful to exclude a persistent or postoperative haematoma. Some guidelines (e.g. Furie *et al.* 2011) suggest that all anticoagulants, including antiplatelet drugs, should be withheld for at least 1–2 weeks following ICH (including intracerebral, subdural, and subarachnoid haemorrhage) although individual practices vary according to experience and the perceived balance of risks and benefits.

Table 1.1 Thromboembolic risk without anticoagulation

Condition	Risk of thromboembolic complications off warfarin (%/year)	Notes
Metallic heart valve (Mok *et al.* 1985; Cannegieter *et al.* 1994)	4–12	Increased risk in mitral valves, ball-cage valves, increasing age, comorbidities (e.g. atrial fibrillation, left ventricular dysfunction)
Atrial fibrillation (Gage *et al.* 2001)	1.9–18.2	Increased risk with additional comorbidities (congestive heart failure, hypertension, age ≥75, diabetes, previous stroke)
DVT/PE (Kearon and Hirsh 1997)	15	40% in first month, 10% in next 2 months after initial event Risk increased 100-fold in postoperative period

References

Abouzari M, Rashidi A, Rezaii J, *et al.* (2007). The role of postoperative patient posture in the recurrence of traumatic chronic subdural hematoma after burr-hole surgery. *Neurosurgery* 2007; **61**: 794–7.

Bailey RD, Hart RG, Benavente O, Pearce LA (2001). Recurrent brain hemorrhage is more frequent than ischemic stroke after intracranial hemorrhage. *Neurology*; **56**: 773–7.

Beshay JE, Morgan HM, Madden C, Yu W, Sarode R (2010). Emergency reversal of anticoagulation and antiplatelet therapies in neurosurgical patients. *J Neurosurg*; **112**: 307–18.

Cannegieter SC, Rosendaal FR, Briet E (1994). Thromboembolic and bleeding complications in patients with mechanical heart valve prosthesis. *Circulation*; **89**: 635–41.

Furie KL, Kasner SE, Adams RJ, *et al.* (2011). Guidelines for the prevention of stroke in patients with stroke or transient ischemic attack: a guideline for healthcare professionals from the American Heart Association/American Stroke Association. *Stroke*; **42**: 227–76.

Gage BF, Waterman AD, Shannon W, *et al.* (2001). Validation of clinical classification schemes for predicting stroke: results from the National Registry of Atrial Fibrillation. *JAMA*; **285**: 2864–70.

Hamilton MG, Yee WH, Hull RD, Ghali WA (2011). Venous thromboembolism prophylaxis in patients undergoing cranial neurosurgery: a systematic review and meta-analysis. *Neurosurgery*; **68**: 571–81.

Hart RG, Boop BS, Anderson DC (1995). Oral anticoagulants and intracranial hemorrhage: Facts and hypotheses. *Stroke*; **26**: 1471–7.

Hart RG, Tonarelli SB, Pearce LA (2005). Avoiding central nervous system bleeding during antithrombotic therapy: recent data and ideas. *Stroke*; **36**: 1588–93.

Iorio A, Agnelli G (2000). Low molecular weight and unfractionated heparin for prevention of venous thromboembolism in neurosurgery. *Ann Int Med*; **160**: 2327–32.

Kearon C, Hirsh J (1997). Management of anticoagulation before and after surgery. *N Engl J Med*; **336**:1506–11.

Mok CK, Boey J, Wang R, *et al.* (1985). Warfarin versus dipyridamole-aspirin and pentoxifyllineaspirin for the prevention of prosthetic heart valve thromboembolism: a prospective clinical trial. *Circulation*; **72**: 1059–63.

Morgenstern LB, Hemphill C, Anderson C, *et al.* (2010). Guidelines for the management of spontaneous intracerebral hemorrhage. A guideline for healthcare professionals from the American Heart Association/American Stroke Association. *Stroke*; **41**: 2108–29.

NICE (2010). *Venous thromboembolism—reducing the risk. NICE Guideline CG92.* Available online at: http://www.nice.org.uk/nicemedia/live/12695/47920/47920.pdf (accessed 24 April 2011).

Romualdi E, Micieli E, Ageno W, Squizzato A (2009). Oral anticoagulant therapy in patients with mechanical heart valve and intracranial haemorrhage. *Thromb Haemost*; **101**: 290–7.

Santarius T, Kirkpatrick PJ, Ganesan D, *et al.* (2009). Use of drains versus no drains after burr-hole evacuation of chronic subdural haematoma: a randomised controlled trial. *Lancet*; **374**: 1067–73.

Vermeer SE, Algra A, Franke CL, Koudstaal PJ, Rinkel GJE (2002). Long-term prognosis after recovery from primary intracerebral hemorrhage. *Neurology*; **59**: 205–9.

Case 2

You are the neurosurgeon on call and receive a referral concerning a 20-year-old man who is admitted to the local emergency department following a road traffic accident. He was the front-seat passenger in a car travelling at approximately 70km/hour when it skidded and hit a stationary car head on. He was not wearing a seatbelt and his head hit the windscreen. According to the ambulance crew his GCS was 3 at the scene and his pupils were equal and reacting. On arrival in the local emergency department he is intubated and ventilated and his cervical spine is immobilized with a collar and blocks. His GCS is 3 and his pupils are both 5mm in diameter. The right pupil constricts to light but the left does not.

Questions

1. What are the priorities in the management of this patient?
2. Explain the mechanism of action of mannitol.
3. The CT scan of the head is shown in Fig. 2.1. Describe the appearances on the scan.
4. Explain why this is not an extradural haematoma.
5. Both pupils become reactive after mannitol and the GCS improves to 7/15 (E1, V2, M4). He flexes to pain with the left arm but no movement is seen on the right side of the body. How is his motor deficit explained?
6. What is the definitive management of this case?
7. What practical steps need to be taken to transfer the patient to your hospital for urgent surgery?
8. The intensive care unit is full. What are the options?
9. An intensive care bed is made available and you contact the local hospital to advise them of the need for urgent transfer. You are then informed that the patient has become hypotensive (75/40mmHg). How will this affect your decision to transfer the patient?

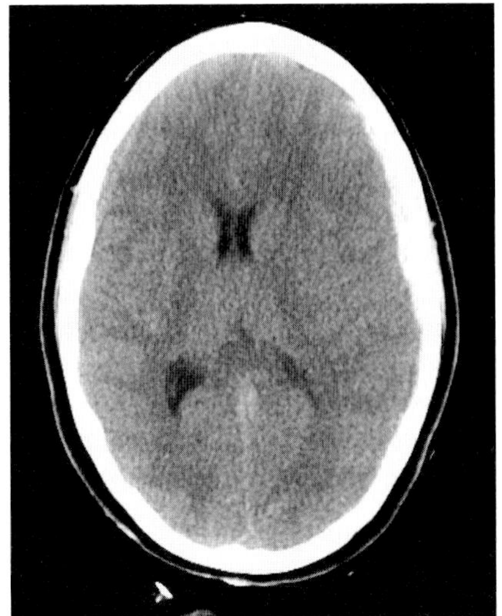

Fig. 2.1

Answers

1. What are the priorities in the management of this patient?

He has sustained a high-impact head injury and the priority is a rapid primary survey followed by a CT scan of the head and cervical spine. He has a dilated unreactive pupil on one side, suggesting asymmetric mass effect, and mannitol should be administered. Hypertonic saline can also be initiated. The cervical spine should be cleared promptly as wearing a tight hard collar may further increase intracranial pressure by reducing venous return. For similar reasons, unless the thoracolumbar spine is injured, the entire bed should be tilted head up 30°. He should also be mildly hyperventilated (PCO_2 4–4.5kPa).

2. Explain the mechanism of action of mannitol.

Mannitol is an organic compound originally extracted from secretions from the flowering ash, a deciduous tree. It is a hyperosmolar substance and reduces intracranial pressure by establishing an osmotic gradient across the blood brain barrier, which it does not cross, hence moving water out of the brain. There is also evidence that it reduces red cell viscosity and within autoregulating regions of the brain improved cerebral blood flow can be accompanied by reduced cerebral blood volume and hence reduced intracranial pressures.

3. The CT scan of the head is shown in Fig. 2.1. Describe the appearances on the scan (Fig. 2.2).

There is a thin hyperdense extra-axial collection overlying the left hemisphere indicating an acute subdural haematoma (A). This is exerting mass effect,

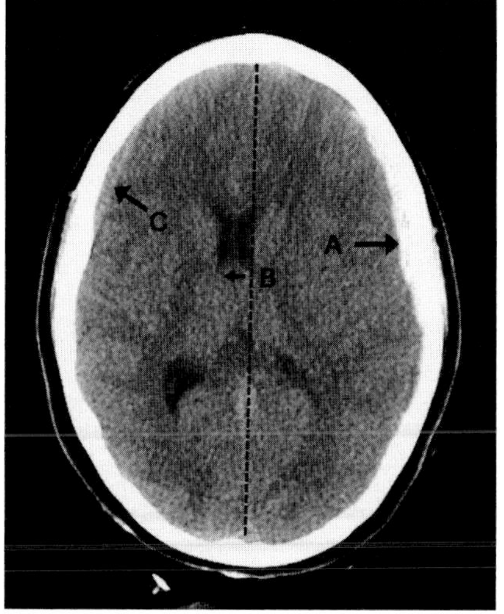

Fig. 2.2

demonstrated by the shift of the midline to the right (B). Small subdural haematomas can easily be missed but the presence of midline shift should prompt a search for the responsible lesion. There is some beam-hardening artefact in the superficial right frontal region (C) which might be mistaken for a small right-sided haematoma.

4. Explain why this is unlikely to be an extradural haematoma.

The clinical presentation is more in keeping with an acute subdural haematoma. Subdural haematomas are caused by high-energy injuries which frequently result in coma from the outset. There is a higher incidence of underlying brain injury than with extradural haematomas and a worse prognosis overall. There may occasionally be a 'lucid interval', although this is more often seen with extradural haematomas. Radiologically, extradural haematomas appear biconvex (as the haematoma tends not to cross suture lines) whereas subdural haematomas are concave (as the blood spreads evenly over the brain). Depending on the location, subdural haematomas may occasionally appear biconvex but extradural haematomas are seldom concave (see 'Structure of the meninges', p. 23).

5. Both pupils become reactive after mannitol and the GCS improves to 7/15 (E1, V2, M4). He flexes to pain with the left arm but no movement is seen on the right side of the body. How is his motor deficit explained?

The patient has a right hemiparesis due to a mass effect from the left hemisphere resulting in compression of the left cerebral peduncle. The pyramidal tract fibres which traverse this area cross over in the medulla oblongata; hence compression of the left cerebral peduncle causes a right hemiparesis. It is not cortical compression which causes the hemiparesis. If this was the case one would expect structures other than the arm and leg to be affected.

6. What is the definitive management of this case?

The patient requires an urgent craniotomy and evacuation of the haematoma. The timing of surgery in acute subdural haematomas is critical in determining survival and functional recovery (mortality of 30% if surgery takes place within 4 hours of injury but 90% after 4 hours).

7. What practical steps need to be taken to transfer the patient to your hospital for urgent surgery?

The intensive care unit should be consulted to check bed availability, after which the referring hospital should be advised to transfer the patient (possibly directly to theatre) without delay. The anaesthetic and theatre staff should be informed to prepare the operating theatre. The senior neurosurgeon responsible for admissions (the consultant in the UK) should also be notified.

8. The intensive care unit is full. What are the options?

One option would be to redirect the patient to the next nearest neurosurgical unit, but this may result in further delay. Another option would be to transfer the patient directly to the operating theatre so that the search for an intensive care bed (possibly at another hospital) can be made while the patient is having surgery. This is not ideal for postoperative care but it may be outweighed by the need for urgent surgery in some circumstances. If the patient is to be transferred out to another hospital postoperatively, a CT scan may be performed before transfer to check postoperative appearances in order to reassure the transferring team. In London the Emergency Bed Service run by the London Ambulance Service NHS Trust is a city-wide service that will identify a vacant intensive care bed amongst the neurosurgical centres in the city.

9. An intensive care bed is made available and you contact the local hospital to advise them of the need for urgent transfer. You are then informed that the patient has become hypotensive (75/40mmHg). How will this affect your decision to transfer the patient?

Although urgent neurosurgery is required for a life-threatening condition, transferring a haemodynamically unstable patient risks cardiorespiratory arrest and the patient should not be transferred until the anaesthetist at the local hospital is satisfied that he is fit for inter-hospital transfer (see the AAGBI guidelines for inter-hospital transfer).

The patient eventually arrives and undergoes a craniectomy and evacuation of the subdural haematoma. The postoperative scan is shown in Fig. 2.3. The midline shift has resolved. The bone flap has been left out to allow for postoperative brain swelling and an intraparenchymal intracranial pressure monitor has been placed in the left frontal lobe (A). The patient should have a cranioplasty at a later date (usually 3–4 months) to cover the cranial defect if the recovery is satisfactory.

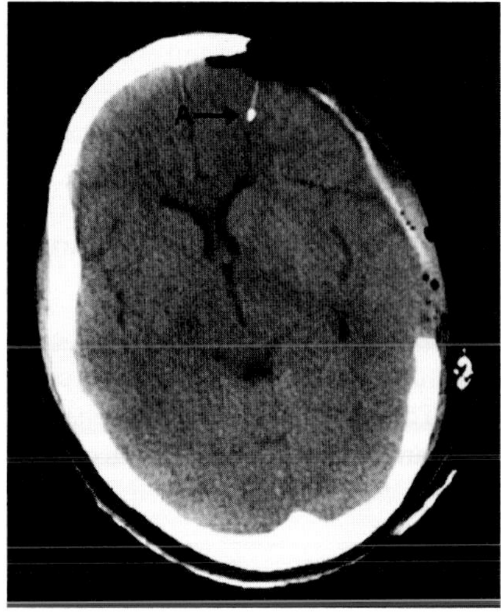

Fig. 2.3

Questions

10. What factors determine when the patient should be extubated?
11. When should acute subdural haematomas be managed conservatively?

Answers

10. What factors determine when the patient should be extubated?

This is an important postoperative decision and depends on whether the patient is likely to achieve a sufficiently conscious state to maintain his airway when woken—this also implies that the intracranial pressure must be acceptable. A variety of factors inform this assessment, including the premorbid state, the nature of the injury, and the effect of surgery. It is desirable to wake patients as soon as possible to reduce the risk of ventilator-associated complications. In this case, the patient is radiologically 'cured' but his preoperative state was dire. Some clinicians would opt to wean sedation and attempt to wake the patient soon after the operation, whilst others may opt to keep the patient sedated for a period to monitor the trend in intracranial pressure before weaning sedation.

11. When should acute subdural haematomas be managed conservatively?

An operation is generally required in the presence of a neurological deficit, a large haematoma, or significant mass effect. Patients with small acute subdural haematomas without neurological deficits may be managed conservatively. Elderly patients may also be managed conservatively if the neurological deficit is relatively mild. This is because acute subdural haematomas typically require a large craniotomy for the haematoma to be evacuated, an operation which is poorly tolerated by the elderly. If the haematoma is left to turn 'chronic' (after a few days to weeks), the liquefied chronic subdural haematoma can be washed out through burrholes, a much smaller operation which may even be performed under local anaesthetic. Conservative management consists of regular neurological observations and monitoring serum sodium. A CT scan should be repeated if there is any neurological deterioration or symptoms of raised intracranial pressure caused by an expanding haematoma.

The CT scans shown in Fig. 2.4 are from a 62-year-old woman who fell off a horse and sustained a right-sided acute subdural haematoma (Fig. 2.4(A)). There is mass effect but the patient was well with headaches only. She was admitted to hospital and observed on the ward. Five days later she developed nausea, and the scan was repeated (Fig. 2.4(B)). Note that the subdural haematoma has enlarged in size and is now of lower density as the thrombus is being degraded. There is some residual dense blood posteriorly. There is more severe midline shift. The right lateral ventricle is now compressed and contralateral hydrocephalus has developed (distortion of the foramen of Monro by the midline shift obstructs the left lateral ventricle which has enlarged, exacerbating the overall mass effect on the brain). The chronic subdural haematoma was evacuated through burrholes and the patient made an excellent recovery.

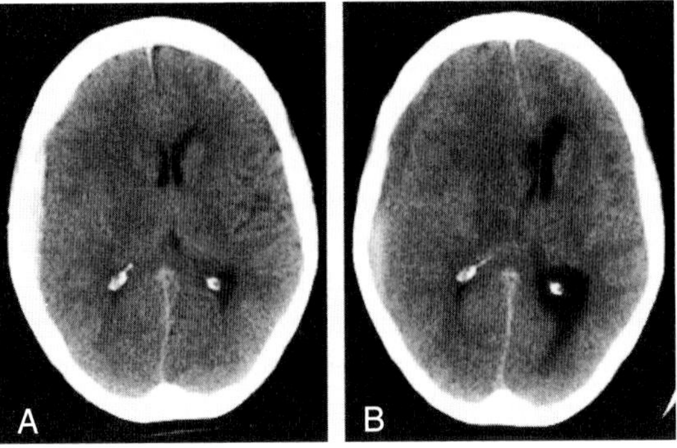

Fig. 2.4

Further reading

AAGBI (2009). *Safety Guideline: Interhospital Transfer*. Available online at: http://www.aagbi.org/publications/guidelines/docs/interhospital09.pdf (accessed 1 April 2011).

Seelig JM, Becker DP, Miller JD, *et al.* (1981). Traumatic acute subdural hematoma: major mortality reduction in comatose patients treated within four hours. *JAMA*; **304**: 1511–18.

Structure of the meninges

Familiarity with the meninges is integral to understanding neurosurgical pathology. The three layers of the meninges are, from outer to inner, the dura mater, the arachnoid, and the pia.

Dura mater

The dura is composed of tough connective tissue and consists of two layers, an outer periosteal layer which is the periosteum of the skull and an inner meningeal layer. The two layers separate in defined locations to form the intracranial venous sinuses. Fig. 2.5(a) shows the formation of the superior sagittal sinus. The falx cerebri, tentorium cerebelli, falx cerebelli, and diaphragma sellae are double folds of dura that form partitions within the cranium (Fig. 2.5(b)). The periosteal dura is continuous with the periosteum of the skull through the cranial foraminae and foramen magnum. At the foramen magnum, the meningeal dura continues down the spinal canal as the thecal sac. The dura is firmly adherent to bone at the convexity suture lines. For this reason extradural haematomas which form between the bone and the periosteal dura do not usually cross suture lines. The exception is at the sagittal suture, where a haematoma crossing the midline can only be extradural (Fig. 2.5(a)). The dura is firmly attached to the base of the skull and a fracture here has the propensity to tear the dura, resulting in a CSF leak.

(continued)

Structure of the meninges *(continued)*

Arachnoid

The arachnoid is a thin avascular membrane covered with mesothelial cells. It adheres to the inner aspect of the meningeal dura. The subarachnoid space below it contains CSF. Major blood vessels and nerves traverse the subarachnoid space. Some spaces are larger than others, and the expanded subarachnoid spaces are called cisterns (Fig. 2.5(c)). The term 'basal cisterns' refers to the subarachnoid cisterns around the brainstem. Effacement of the basal cisterns occurs in raised intracranial pressure and is a bad prognostic sign.

Pia

The pia is a thin membrane composed of mesodermal cells. It is closely adherent to the brain and invaginates into fissures and sulci.

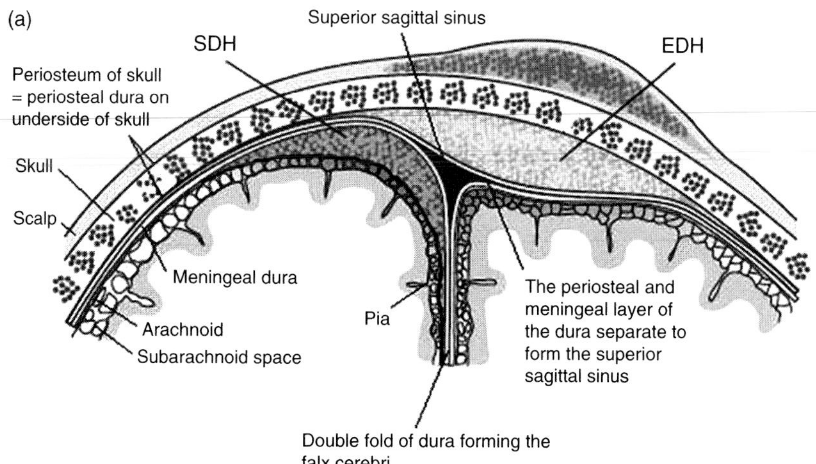

Fig. 2.5 (a) The meninges, formation of the venous sinuses and the location of subdural and extradural haematomas. Reproduced and modified with permission from Drake, R *et al.*, *Gray's Anatomy for Students*. © Elsevier 2005, and Gean AD. *Imaging of Head Trauma*. © Lippincott, Williams & Wilkins, 1994.

(continued)

Structure of the meninges *(continued)*

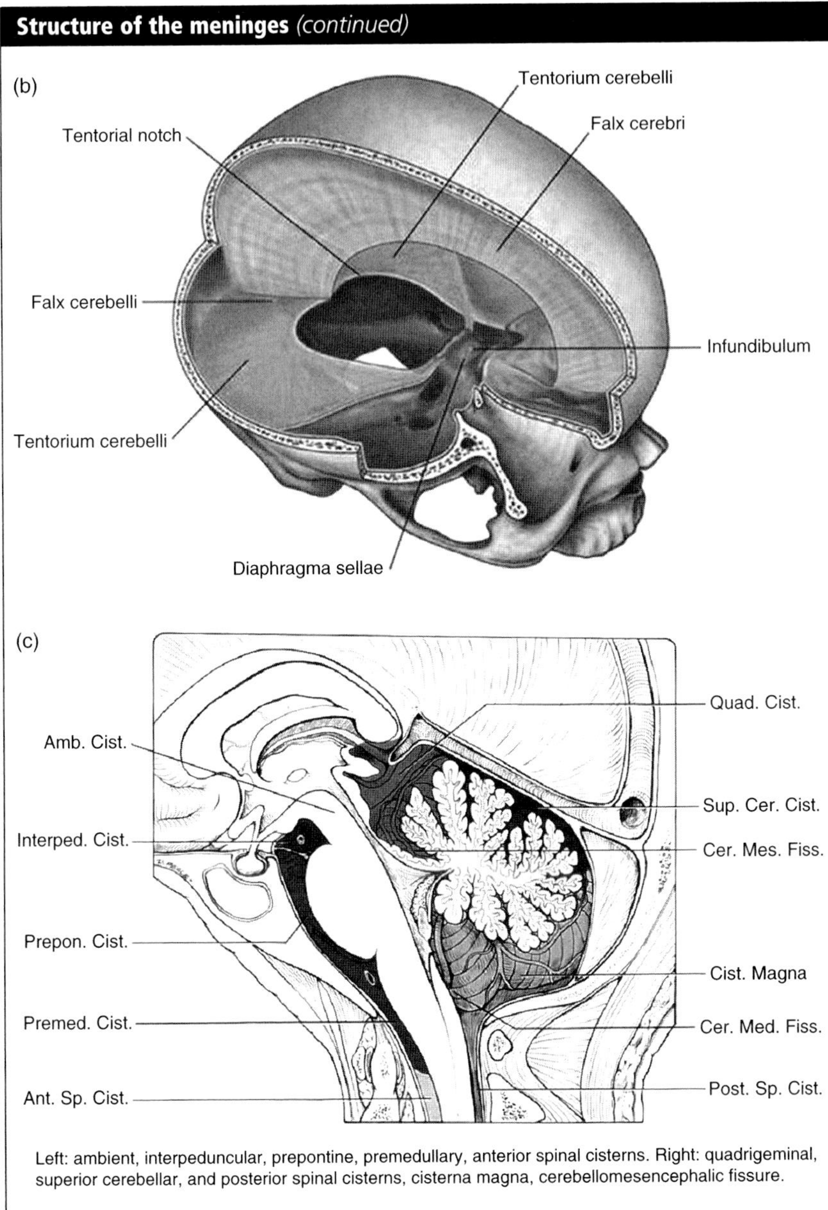

Left: ambient, interpeduncular, prepontine, premedullary, anterior spinal cisterns. Right: quadrigeminal, superior cerebellar, and posterior spinal cisterns, cisterna magna, cerebellomesencephalic fissure.

Fig. 2.5 (b) Dural partitions of the cranial cavity. Reproduced and modified with permission from Drake, R *et al.*, *Gray's Anatomy for Students*. © Elsevier 2005. (c) Subarachnoid cisterns. Reproduced with permission from Rhoton, The posterior fossa cisterns, *Neurosurgery*, **47**(3), Lippincott, Williams & Wilkins, 2000.

Case 3

An 18-year-old man attends the emergency department 30 minutes after being hit on the head with a champagne bottle at a party. There was no loss of consciousness. He had vomited several times and complains of a severe headache over the left side of his head. On examination, his GCS is 15/15, his pupils are equal and reactive, and there are no focal neurological deficits.

Questions

1. Are there any evidence-based guidelines on whether this patient requires a CT scan of the brain?
2. The CT scan is performed (Fig. 3.1). Describe the findings.

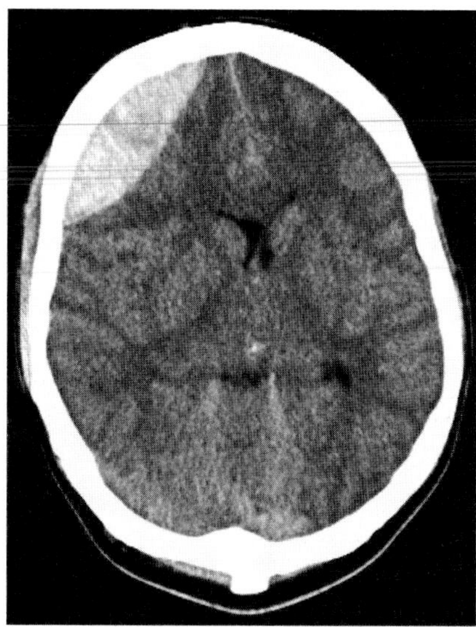

Fig. 3.1

Answers

1. Are there any evidence-based guidelines on whether this patient requires a CT scan of the brain?

An immediate CT brain scan is recommended by NICE (2007) if any of the following factors are present following a head injury:

- GCS <13 at initial assessment in emergency department or <15 two hours after injury
- focal neurological deficit
- seizure
- suspected open or depressed skull fracture
- vomiting more than once in an adult
- amnesia more than 30 minutes before incident
- loss of consciousness or any amnesia in the presence of the following: age over 65, coagulopathy, dangerous mechanism of injury.

This patient merits a scan as he has vomited more than once.

2. The CT scan is performed (Fig. 3.1). Describe the findings.

There is an extra-axial biconvex high-density lesion overlying the right frontal lobe, typical of an extradural haematoma. There is a midline shift with distortion of the ventricles. There is a scalp haematoma on the right.

Questions

3. Explain why extradural haematomas typically appear biconvex.
4. The rupture of which vessels usually leads to an extradural haematoma?
5. What is the management of this case?
6. The patient works as a delivery driver and asks if his licence will be affected. How would you answer his question?

Answers

3. Explain why extradural haematomas typically appear biconvex.

The periosteal layer of the dura mater is tightly bound to the skull and folds into the cranial sutures. An extradural haematoma lies between the bone and the periosteal dura. As it enlarges, it strips the dura from the bone but is restrained at the sutures and hence appears convex. Enlargement typically does not traverse suture lines (see 'Structure of the meninges', p. 23).

4. The rupture of which vessels usually leads to an extradural haematoma?

Extradural haematomas are usually caused by arterial bleeding, classically from the middle meningeal artery. They can also be caused by bleeding from an overlying skull fracture (these tend to be smaller) or from venous haemorrhage if the dura is breached over a venous sinus.

5. What is the management of this case?

Extradural haematomas can be managed operatively or conservatively. An expanding extradural haematoma can cause rapid neurological deterioration, and immediate surgery is indicated if there is significant or ongoing neurological deficit. Conservative management may be suitable if the haematoma is small and the patient is neurologically intact. In this case, the haematoma is large but the patient is neurologically intact. The risks of surgery must be balanced against the risk of deterioration from conservative management. Further factors to consider in this case are the mass effect and midline shift. In addition it is highly likely that arterial haemorrhage (rather than venous or fracture haemorrhage) is the underlying cause of this extradural haematoma because of its large size and location. Arterial bleeding will not stop due to tamponade of the haematoma (unlike venous or fracture site bleeding), and for these reasons this patient should undergo urgent surgery consisting of a craniotomy and evacuation of the haematoma.

His postoperative CT scan (Fig. 3.2) shows complete evacuation of the haematoma and resolution of the midline shift. There is a small area of low density at the right frontal pole indicating a contusion (arrow).

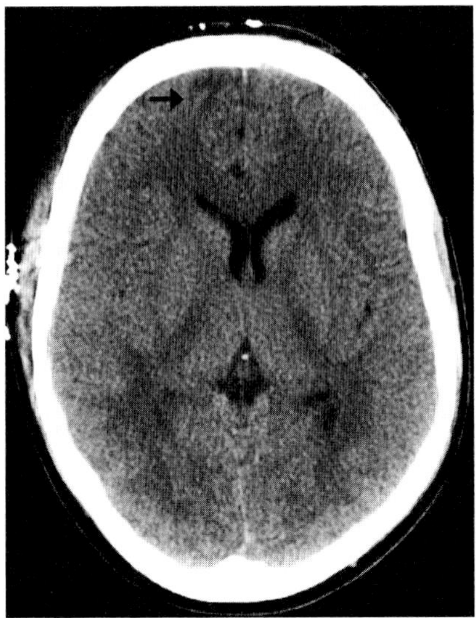

Fig. 3.2

6. The patient works as a delivery driver and asks if his licence will be affected. How would you answer his question?

Patients are required by law to report their medical condition to the DVLA, and the doctor must encourage patients to do this. A document specifying the driving restrictions for specific neurosurgical conditions is available on the DVLA website. A significant head injury usually requires 6–12 months off driving for group 1 entitlement but may result in refusal or revocation of a group 2 licence. The patient should be advised to contact the DVLA for further advice.

Questions

7. A 54-year-old man sustained a head injury in a bicycle accident. On arrival, his GCS is 13/15 (E4, V4, M5) and he is agitated and combative. A CT scan is performed, and is shown in Fig. 3.3. What does it show?
8. What are the options for management?

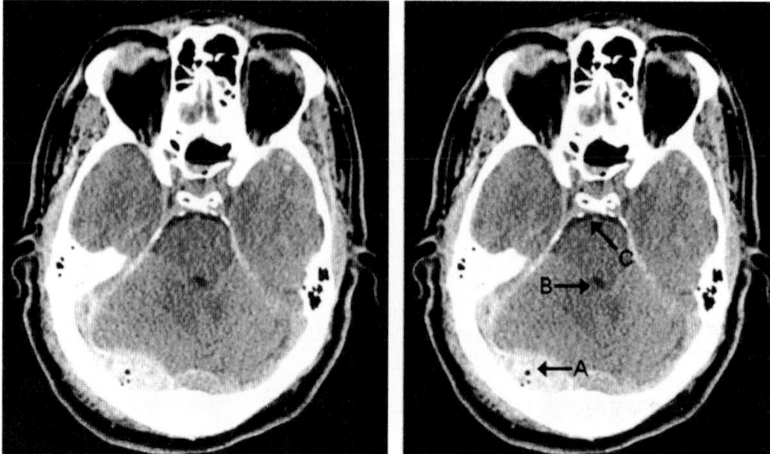

Fig. 3.3

Answers

7. A 54-year-old man sustained a head injury in a bicycle accident. On arrival, his GCS is 13/15 (E4, V4, M5), and he is agitated and combative. A CT scan is performed, and is shown in Fig. 3.3. What does it show?

There is a posterior fossa extradural haematoma (A). Locules of air are present within the haematoma, and there is opacification of the right mastoid air cells. This is due to a fracture through the occipital bone extending into the petrous temporal bone (not shown). There is some mass effect with compression of the fourth ventricle (B) and partial effacement of the prepontine cistern (C).

8. What are the options for management?

The options are operative or conservative. The major risk of surgery in this case is heavy haemorrhage from the transverse sinus, from which this venous extradural haematoma has probably arisen. The risk of conservative management is brainstem compression from an enlarging haematoma. As the neurological deficit is relatively mild, it would be reasonable to opt for conservative management with close neurological observation. Venous extradural haematomas are less likely to enlarge than their arterial counterparts as the bleeding is under relatively lower pressure and is tamponaded by anatomical structures, principally the dura. Very close observation is required as rapid cardiorespiratory deterioration can occur with posterior fossa extradural haematomas as a result of brainstem compression without neurological deterioration. Many surgeons would advocate an early repeat CT scan to ensure that the haematoma is not enlarging, especially if the first scan was within 4 hours of the initial injury. Surgery would be indicated if there is further neurological deterioration. This patient was managed conservatively with a good outcome.

Questions

9. A 62-year-old woman presents to the emergency department. Last night, when intoxicated, she fell down a full flight of stairs at home but does not remember exactly how she fell and whether she hit her head. She has developed a worsening headache, and her husband called an ambulance as she appeared confused the next morning. On arrival she is confused and drowsy, only eye opening to pain. She goes for a CT scan (Fig. 3.4); on returning from the radiology department she is no longer obeying commands. What does the CT show?
10. How would you manage the patient, and what concerns would you have?

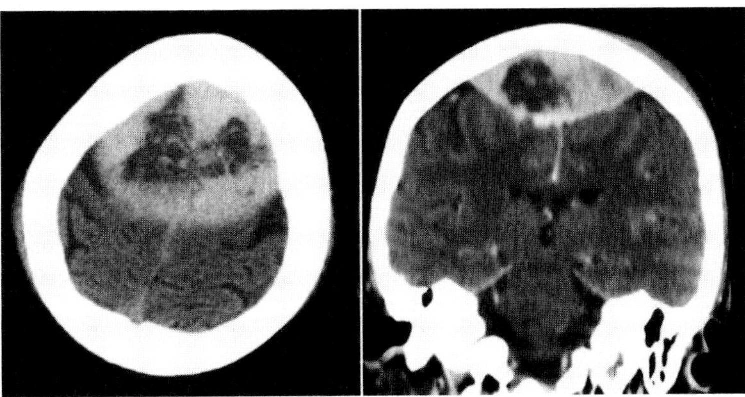

Fig. 3.4 With kind permission from Springer Science+Business Media: *Acta Neurochir* (Wien). 2011 Sep; **153**(9): 1819–20. © Springer 2011.

Answers

9. A 62-year-old woman presents to the emergency department. Last night, when intoxicated, she fell down a full flight of stairs at home but does not remember exactly how she fell and whether she hit her head. She has developed a worsening headache, and her husband called an ambulance as she appeared confused the next morning. On arrival she is confused and drowsy, only eye opening to pain. She goes for a CT scan (Fig. 3.4); on returning from the radiology department she is no longer obeying commands. What does the CT show?

The axial view (left) shows a midline mass which is both hyper- and hypodense (compared with brain). Its exact nature is difficult to appreciate on this image alone but in the setting of acute trauma it is likely to represent blood, with the mixed density of the clot indicating solid and liquid components and therefore active haemorrhage. The coronal view (right) demonstrates a haematoma crossing the midline which is therefore an extradural haematoma (see 'Structure of the meninges', p. 23). Given its location, the aetiology is likely to be a torn sagittal sinus caused by an associated skull fracture. The venous aetiology of the haematoma would also account for the slightly delayed (12 hours or more) presentation of the patient rather than the more rapid deterioration associated with the classic arterial extradural haematoma.

10. How would you manage the patient, and what concerns would you have?

Conservative management is generally preferred for a torn sagittal sinus because extension is unlikely due to low-pressure venous blood and the considerable risk of haemorrhage intraoperatively, but surgery is indicated in this case because of her deteriorating neurological state. In the process of evacuating the haematoma the torn sinus is likely to be encountered and cannot simply be stopped with bipolar coagulation as is the case with the dural arteries. The torn sinus must be repaired or at least tamponaded to prevent further bleeding whilst maintaining its patency. In addition, an open major venous sinus during surgery risks negative venous pressure (if the opening is appreciably higher than the right atrium, as is usually the case in cranial surgery) and consequently air being 'sucked in' to the open sinus, causing an air embolism. Therefore surgery should be urgent but carefully planned, with blood available for transfusion, an experienced anaesthetist aware of this specific issue, and senior surgical support as appropriate.

This patient's haematoma was evacuated through bilateral craniotomies which left a midline strip of bone over the sagittal sinus (which was indeed torn and the source of the bleeding). The dura was stitched up to the bone to tamponade the dura against haemostatic material which was left *in situ*. There was no air embolism but there was an intraoperative blood loss of 1500mL. The postoperative CT scan (Fig. 3.5) shows the bilateral craniotomies and the skull fracture, which are more clearly seen on bone windowing. The patient made an uncomplicated and full recovery.

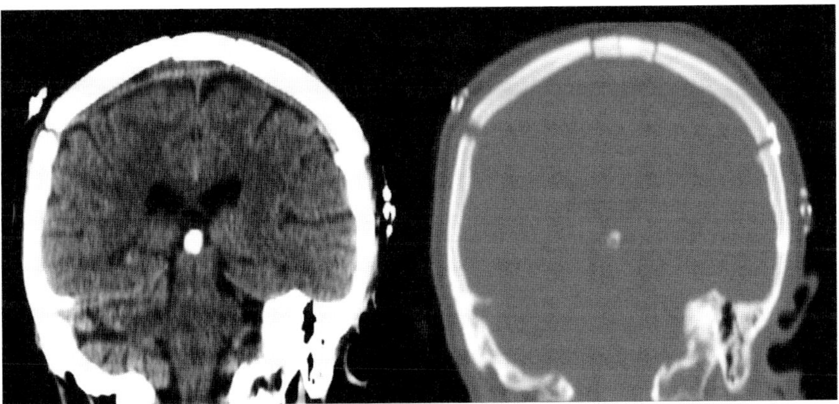

Fig. 3.5 With kind permission from Springer Science+Business Media: *Acta Neurochir* (Wien). 2011 Sep; **153**(9): 1819–20. © Springer 2011.

Further reading

Bor-Seng-Shu E, Aguiar PH, de Almeida LRJ, *et al.* (2004). Epidural hematomas of the posterior cranial fossa. *Neurosurg Focus*; **16**: 1–4.

DVLA (2011). *At a Glance Guide to the Current Medical Standards of Fitness to Drive.* Swansea: DVLA. Available online at: http://www.dft.gov.uk/dvla/medical/ataglance.aspx (accessed 1 April 2011).

NICE (2007). *NICE Guideline CG56. Head Injury.* CG56. Available online at: http://www.nice.org.uk/CG056 (accessed 13 March 2011).

Ozer FD, Yurt AL, Sucu HK, *et al.* (2005). Depressed fractures over cranial venous sinus. *J Emerg Med*; **29**: 137–9.

Yilmazlar S, Kocaeli H, Dogan S, *et al.* (2005). Traumatic epidural haematomas of nonarterial origin: analysis of 30 consecutive cases. *Acta Neurochir (Wien)*; **147**: 1241–8.

Case 4

A 58-year-old man was admitted after falling down a flight of concrete steps whilst drinking alcohol. On admission to the emergency department he smelt strongly of alcohol and complained of headache and neck pain. He was agitated and was attempting to climb off his trolley. He was disorientated but obeying commands (GCS E4, V4, M6), and his pupils were equal and reactive.

Questions

1. What are the priorities in the management of this patient?
2. How should his agitation be managed?
3. When is intubation indicated in a patient with a reduced level of consciousness?
4. The CT scan is shown in Fig. 4.1. Describe the findings on the scan.
5. How should this patient be managed?
6. One day after admission, he is no longer disorientated and feels well. He has no focal neurological deficits. He asks how long he needs to stay in hospital and whether any more tests are required. How would you answer his question?
7. The patient has a blood test prior to discharge (6 days into his admission) and his sodium level is 116mmol/L. He is alert and orientated.
   (a) What are the risks associated with hyponatraemia?
   (b) What is the likely diagnosis, and which investigations are required?
   (c) The results of the above investigations are as follows: plasma osmolality 265mmol/kg, urine osmolality 218mmol/kg, urine sodium 40mmol/L. He is clinically euvolaemic. How should he be managed?

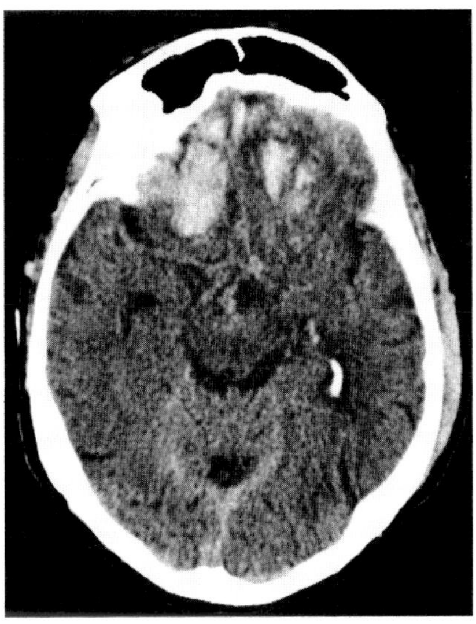

Fig. 4.1

Answers

1. What are the priorities in the management of this patient?

A rapid primary survey (airway with cervical spine immobilization, breathing, circulation) is required, followed by a CT scan of the brain to look for intracranial pathology. In trauma, the neck is frequently imaged at the same time to exclude cervical spine injuries. He will need a secondary survey in due course to ensure that no other injury has been missed.

2. How should his agitation be managed?

Patients with head injuries may be agitated for many reasons. The use of sedatives masks neurological deterioration and is not recommended in the acute setting. Specialist nurses are required to manage agitated patients with head injuries. Treating simple causes of agitation often proves effective (e.g. analgesia for pain, immobilizing/reducing a limb fracture, a urinary catheter for a full bladder). A small dose of promazine is often helpful in controlling agitation without adversely affecting the conscious state. Removal of the collar and blocks may help if the cervical spine is cleared.

3. When is intubation indicated in a patient with a reduced level of consciousness?

Intubation is indicated if the patient is unable to maintain their airway (and therefore is at risk of airway obstruction or aspiration) or if agitation renders essential supportive therapy (e.g. oxygen, intravenous fluids) or diagnostic investigations (CT scan) impossible. The decision must be made on an individual basis: a post-ictal patient with a GCS of 7/15 may not need intubation, whereas a patient with a GCS of 13/15 who is combative and needing a CT scan does.

4. The CT scan is shown in Fig. 4.1. Describe the findings on the scan (Fig. 4.2).

There are extensive bifrontal contusions (A). The hypodense areas surrounding the blood (B) are indicative of oedema. Traumatic subarachnoid haemorrhage is also present (C).

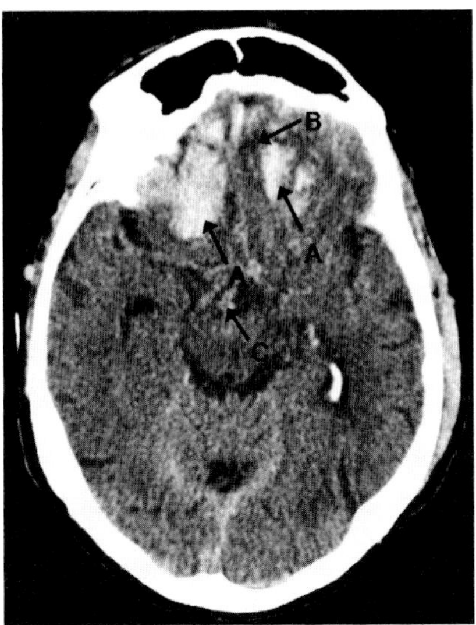

Fig. 4.2

5. How should this patient be managed?

This patient requires admission to the neurosurgical unit for close observation. Sodium levels, clotting, and liver function should be checked, the latter in view of the history of alcohol use. Anticonvulsants are recommended for one week after severe traumatic brain injuries and then discontinued if there has not been a seizure (see 'Anticonvulsants in neurosurgery', p. 40).

6. One day after admission, he is no longer disorientated and feels well. He has no focal neurological deficits. He asks how long he needs to stay in hospital and whether any more tests are required. How would you answer his question?

The scan shows sizeable contusions with surrounding oedema. Cerebral oedema around evolving contusions is maximal 24–48 hours after the injury, but can also manifest several days after the injury and lead to neurological decline. A further period of hospital observation would be recommended for this patient (typically a few days). He should have a repeat CT scan and his serum electrolytes should be tested prior to discharge.

7. The patient has a blood test prior to discharge (6 days into his admission) and his sodium level is 116mmol/L. He is alert and orientated.

(a) What are the risks associated with hyponatraemia?

Altered mental state, seizures, cerebral oedema, and death.

(b) What is the likely diagnosis, and which investigations are required?

Hyponatraemia in neurosurgery is commonly due to the syndrome of inappropriate ADH secretion (SIADH) or cerebral salt wasting (CSW). Plasma osmolality, urine osmolality, and urine sodium concentration should be checked to exclude other causes of hyponatraemia. A clinical assessment of the extracellular volume status of the patient should be made to determine if the diagnosis is more likely to be SIADH (euvolaemic or hypervolaemic) or CSW (hypovolaemic).

(c) The results of the above investigations are as follows: plasma osmolality 265mmol/kg, urine osmolality 218mmol/kg, urine sodium 40mmol/L. He is clinically euvolaemic. How should he be managed?

The management of a hyponatraemic patient with a clinical picture consistent with both SIADH and CSW is controversial. This patient was managed with fluid restriction in the high-dependency unit and his sodium level normalized over a period of 72 hours (see 'Hyponatraemia in neurosurgery', p. 38).

Further reading

Rahman M, Friedman WA (2009). Hyponatremia in neurosurgical patients: clinical guidelines development. *Neurosurgery*; **65**: 925–36.

Hyponatraemia in neurosurgery

Initial tests in a hyponatraemic neurosurgical patient should include plasma osmolality, urine osmolality, and urine sodium concentration to determine the cause of hyponatraemia (Fig. 4.3). SIADH and CSW are common in neurosurgery. Both are characterized by low plasma osmolality, high urine osmolality, and high urine sodium concentration. Assessment of the extracellular volume (ECV) status may be helpful in distinguishing between them, although this is not always reliable. A patient with CSW is expected to be dehydrated whereas a patient with SIADH will be expected to be euvolaemic or hypervolaemic, but most patients do not lie on the clinical extremes. SIADH is relatively more common in head injuries and CSW in subarachnoid haemorrhage, although both can occur in either diagnosis. Another common cause of hyponatraemia is cortisol deficiency following pituitary surgery.

Management is guided by the magnitude of hyponatraemia, the underlying diagnosis, and clinical symptoms of hyponatraemia. If the patient is symptomatic, immediate salt and water replacement with intravenous hypertonic saline is required. If the patient is asymptomatic and/or the hyponatraemia is relatively mild, either salt and water replacement or fluid restriction can be trialled, although fluid restriction is not advised in subarachnoid haemorrhage as it may precipitate cerebral ischaemia. Whichever approach is adopted, the sodium concentration should not be raised abruptly (typically not more than 8mmol/L in 24 hours) in order to avoid central pontine myelinolysis. An endocrinology opinion should be considered.

(continued)

Hyponatraemia in neurosurgery *(continued)*

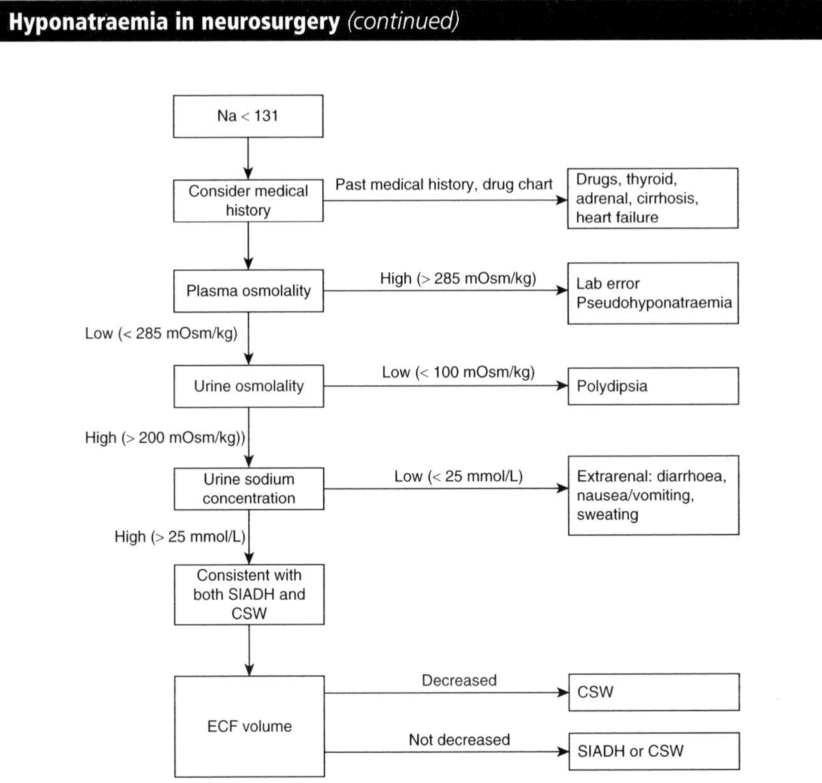

Fig. 4.3 Diagnostic approach to hyponatraemia in neurosurgery.

Syndrome of inappropriate ADH secretion (SIADH)

The hypothalamic osmoreceptors detect changes in plasma osmolality and in response secrete antidiuretic hormone (ADH). ADH alters the water permeability of the collecting ducts in the kidney. More ADH results in more aquaporins in the kidney collecting ducts, leading to increased water reabsorption independent of sodium reabsorption. In SIADH there is excess water reabsorption, leading to a low-volume concentrated urine and relatively increased plasma volume. The plasma sodium and osmolality are low (due to dilution), and urine osmolality is high. Total urinary sodium excretion is normal but the urine sodium concentration is increased due to the low urine volume. Treatment is to limit or decrease the plasma volume with fluid restriction or diuretics. If the patient is symptomatic, the priority is to increase the plasma sodium level, and intravenous salt supplementation is indicated (this outweighs the increase in plasma volume due to the sodium infusion).

(continued)

Hyponatraemia in neurosurgery *(continued)*

Cerebral salt wasting (CSW)

Although the pathophysiology of this condition is not completely understood, it is thought to result from impaired sodium reabsorption in the kidney leading to net sodium loss and therefore water loss. This leads to hyponatraemia with low plasma osmolality and high (or normal) urine osmolality. It is of particular concern following subarachnoid haemorrhage, and in conjunction with cerebral arterial vasospasm is a major cause of delayed neurological deterioration after the haemorrhage. The patient is clinically dehydrated and treatment is with aggressive salt and fluid supplementation. Fludrocortisone increases sodium and water retention in the kidney and is often used to manage this condition.

Anticonvulsants in neurosurgery

Common clinical questions are:

- Are anticonvulsants indicated?
- Which one should be used?
- How long should it be continued?
- Do levels need to be monitored and if so when?
- What action is required if levels are sub-therapeutic?

Most of the literature concerns particular groups of patients and/or drugs or includes a diverse group of patients and/or drugs, so applying the conclusions to individual patients is difficult. This is clearly reflected in the case of brain tumours (see below). Some published guidance is summarized in Table 4.1. Patients with a central nervous system lesion who have a seizure satisfy the diagnosis of epilepsy and should be managed as such.

Table 4.1 Anticonvulsant use in neurosurgery

Condition	Seizure risk	Setting	Guidance
Brain tumour	Depends on tumour type and location: up to 100% for DNETs, 75% for low-grade astrocytomas, 50–60% for high-grade astrocytomas.[1]	Prophylaxis	See below
		Treatment after seizure	Treat as epilepsy. Non-enzyme inducers (e.g. levetiracetam) do not affect the efficacy of corticosteroids and chemotherapy and may be preferred.[1] Continue for as long as tumour is present; may taper after resection.

(continued)

Anticonvulsants in neurosurgery *(continued)*

Table 4.1 *(continued)* Anticonvulsant use in neurosurgery

Condition	Seizure risk	Setting	Guidance
Traumatic brain injury	Depends on severity. 15% with severe TBI. Risk increased (>20%) in penetrating injury, depressed skull fracture, early seizure, subdural haematoma.[2]	Prophylaxis	Phenytoin for 1 week prevents early (<7 days) seizures although this has no effect on outcome.[3]
		Treatment after seizure	Treat as epilepsy. No specific guidance exists for traumatic brain injury.[2]
Subarachnoid haemorrhage	5–8%[4]	Prophylaxis	Generally not recommended[5,6] as prophylactic phenytoin use has been associated with worse outcomes although newer drugs have not been fully assessed.
		Treatment after seizure	Treat as per epilepsy, with drug other than phenytoin.[6]
Spontaneous intracerebral haemorrhage	2.7–17%[7]	Prophylaxis	Not recommended, as prophylactic anticonvulsants (mostly phenytoin) have been associated with worse outcomes.[7]
		Treatment after seizure	Treat as epilepsy.[7]
Fitting neurosurgical patient: acute treatment			The seizure should be terminated with a benzodiazepine following which an anticonvulsant should be instituted. The drug of choice is one which attains a therapeutic effect rapidly and can be given intravenously if swallowing is not possible. The traditional choice is phenytoin, but levetiracetam and sodium valproate (neither of which require serum-level monitoring)

(continued)

Anticonvulsants in neurosurgery *(continued)*

Table 4.1 *(continued)* Anticonvulsant use in neurosurgery

Condition	Seizure risk	Setting	Guidance
			are alternatives. If phenytoin is used in the acute situation an initial level can be taken after 1 hour to determine the subsequent dose or need for reloading. An alternative drug should be instituted if long-term therapy is indicated in order to avoid the side effects of phenytoin.

DNET, dysembryoplastic neuroepithelial tumour.

[1] Rossetti and Stupp 2010

[2] Temkin 2009

[3] Brain Trauma Association 2007

[4] Rosengart *et al.* 2007

[5] Bederson *et al.* 2009

[6] Rabinstein *et al.* 2010

[7] Morgenstern *et al.* 2010

Seizure prophylaxis in brain tumours

Meta-analyses (Glantz *et al.* 2000; Sirven *et al.* 2004; Tremont-Lukats *et al.* 2008) based on four randomized studies (see Table 4.2) and a cohort study (Forsyth 2003) do not recommend seizure prophylaxis in patients with brain tumours because of lack of efficacy and morbidity from medication side effects, but this conclusion has limitations. First, the randomized studies include a wide variety of tumours and non-neoplastic pathologies and do not apply to an individual patient whose seizure risk should be assessed individually based on the type and location of the tumour. Secondly, the anticonvulsants studied were limited to phenytoin, phenobarbital, and sodium valproate. Thirdly, many patients (up to 67%) had subtherapeutic drug levels at the time of seizure. Therefore decisions about prophylactic anticonvulsant treatment in patients with brain tumours must be tailored to the individual and not based solely on recommendations from meta-analyses.

(continued)

Anticonvulsants in neurosurgery *(continued)*

Table 4.2 Randomized studies of seizure prophylaxis in brain tumours

Study	Diagnosis (no. of subjects)	Anticonvulsant used	Percentage sub-therapeutic at time of seizure	Percentage side effects in drug group	Median follow-up
Glantz *et al.* (1996) (RCT, *n* = 74)	Metastasis (57) NHL (2) GBM (9) Other (6)	Sodium valproate	23%	5%	7 months
Franceschetti *et al.* (1990) (RCT, *n* = 63)	Meningioma (27) GBM (23) Metastasis (13)	Phenytoin Phenobarbitone	67%	10%	6–12 months
Lee *et al.* (1989) (RCT, *n* = 80 for tumours, *n* =374 for whole study)	Meningioma (50) Glioma (30) Aneurysm (41) ICH (18) AVM (12) Metastasis (5) Head trauma (210) Others (8)	Phenytoin	50%	Not indicated	1.5 days
North *et al.* (1983) (RCT, n=81 for tumours, n=281 for whole study)	Meningioma (19) Metastasis (13) Glioma (32) Sellar tumour (17) Aneurysm (55) Head trauma (100) VP shunt (25) Other (20)	Phenytoin	Not indicated	Not indicated	Not indicated
Forsyth *et al.* (2003) (cohort study, *n* = 100, including 28 infratentorial)	GBM (28) Low-grade glioma (3) Anaplastic glioma (9) Metastasis (60)	Phenytoin Phenobarbital	47% non-compliant at predetermined test time (not at time of seizure)	13%	5.4 months

RCT, randomized controlled trial; NHL, non-Hodgkin lymphoma; GBM, glioblastoma multiforme; ICH, intracranial haemorrhage; AVM, arteriovenous malformation; VP, ventriculoperitoneal.

References

Bederson JB, Connolly Jr S, Hunt Batjer H, *et al.* (2009). Guidelines for the management of aneurysmal subarachnoid hemorrhage. A Statement for Healthcare Professionals from a Special Writing Group of the Stroke Council, American Heart Association. *Stroke*; **40**: 994–1025.

Brain Trauma Association (2007). *Guidelines for the Management of Severe Traumatic Brain Injury* (3rd edn). Available online at: https://www.braintrauma.org/coma-guidelines/btf-guidelines/ (accessed 1 April 2011).

Forsyth PA, Weaver S, Fulton D, *et al.* (2003). Prophylactic anticonvulsants in patients with brain tumour. *Can J Neurol Sci*; **30**: 106–12.

Franceschetti S, Binelli S, Casazza M, *et al.* (1990). Influence of surgery and antiepileptic drugs on seizures symptomatic of cerebral tumours. *Acta Neurochir (Wien)*; **103**: 47–51.

Glantz MJ, Cole BF, Friedbert MH, *et al.* (1996). A randomized, blinded, placebo-controlled trial of divalproex sodium prophylaxis in adults with newly diagnosed brain tumours. *Neurology*; **46**: 985–91.

Glantz MJ, Cole BF, Forsyth PA, *et al.* (2000). Practice parameter: anticonvulsant prophylaxis in patients with newly diagnosed brain tumours. Report of the Quality Standards Subcommittee of the American Academy of Neurology. *Neurology*; **54**: 1886–93.

Lee ST, Lui TN, Chang CN, *et al.* (1989). Prophylactic anticonvulsants for prevention of immediate and early postcraniotomy seizures. *Surg Neurol*; **31**: 361–4.

Morgenstern LB, Hemphill C, Anderson C, *et al.* (2010). Guidelines for the management of spontaneous intracerebral hemorrhage. A guideline for healthcare professionals from the American Heart Association/American Stroke Association. *Stroke*; **41**: 2108–29.

North JB, Penhall RK, Hanieh A, Frewin DB, Taylor WB (1983). Phenytoin and postoperative epilepsy: a double-blind study. *J Neurosurg*; **58**: 672–7.

Rabinstein AA, Lanzino G, Wijdicks EFM (2010). Multidisciplinary management and emerging therapeutic strategies in subarachnoid haemorrhage. *Lancet Neurol* 2010; **9**: 504–19.

Rosengart AJ, Huo D, Tolentino J, *et al.* (2007). Outcome of patients with subarachnoid hemorrhage treated with antiepileptic drugs. *J Neurosurg*; **107**: 253–60.

Rossetti AO, Stupp R (2010). Epilepsy in brain tumour patients. *Curr Opin Neurol*; **23**: 603–9.

Sirven JI, Wingerchuck DM, Drazkowski JF, *et al.* (2004). Seizure prophylaxis in patients with brain tumours: a meta-analysis. *Mayo Clin Proc*; **79**: 1489–94.

Temkin NR (2009). Preventing and treating posttraumatic seizures: the human experience. *Epilepsia*; **50** (Suppl 2): 10–13.

Tremont-Lukats IW, Ratilal BO, Armstrong T, Gilbert MR (2008). Antiepileptic drugs for preventing seizures in patients with brain tumours. *Cochrane Database Syst Rev* 2008; **16**: CD004424.

Case 5

A 27-year-old woman is admitted to hospital after being found collapsed in the bathroom. She had been drinking large quantities of alcohol earlier in the day. Her GCS was 12/15 (E4, V2, M6) at the scene and her pupils were equal and reactive. When she arrived in the emergency department, she was obeying commands but was confused and agitated (GCS E4, V4, M6). There was blood-stained discharge in the left ear. Her blood pressure was 120/60mmHg, her pulse was 85bpm, and oxygen saturation was 100%. Arterial blood gases showed a pH of 7.23, PO_2 10.3, PCO_2 4.5, bicarbonate 15, and base excess –7. She was intubated for a CT scan (Fig. 5.1).

Questions

1. Describe the abnormalities on the scan. Where and how should this patient be managed?
2. In the context of head injury, what is the significance of having blood-stained discharge from the ear or nose?
3. The patient arrives on the neurointensive care unit 2 hours after admission to hospital. What considerations should be made regarding (a) weaning sedation with a view to extubation, (b) insertion of an ICP monitor, and (c) blood pressure management?
4. What is likely to happen to the intracranial pressure of this patient over the next 24 hours?

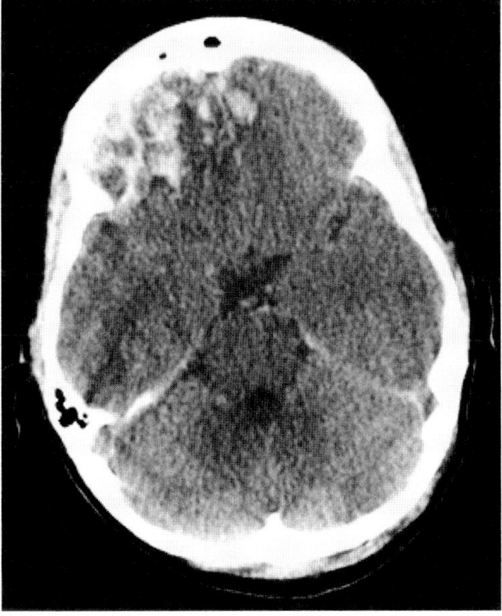

Fig. 5.1

Answers

1. Describe the abnormalities on the scan. Where and how should this patient be managed?

There are extensive bifrontal contusions, worse on the right, with extension into the temporal lobe. This scan is radiologically more severe than in Case 4 (it appears 'tighter') because of the absence of sulcal spaces. This is a severe head injury which should be managed on the neurointensive care unit. This will involve continued mechanical ventilation, sedation, and control of physiological parameters (oxygenation, blood pressure, fluid, and acid–base balance). Close attention should be paid to the patient's sodium balance because of the risk of hyponatraemia (see 'Hyponatraemia in neurosurgery', p. 38).

2. In the context of head injury, what is the significance of having blood-stained discharge from the ear or nose?

Discharge from the ear (otorrhoea) or nose (rhinorrhoea) following a head injury may represent a CSF leak associated with a base of skull fracture. This may be evident on the CT bone windows, although a fracture is not always apparent radiologically (see 'Base of skull fractures', p. 50).

3. The patient arrives on the neurointensive care unit 2 hours after admission to hospital. What considerations should be made regarding (a) weaning sedation with a view to extubation, (b) insertion of an ICP monitor, and (c) blood pressure management?

(a) For patients with a mild or moderate head injury (GCS >8 pre-intubation), sedation may be lightened to assess the patient's neurological status and, if tolerated, the patient can be extubated. In severe head injury (GCS <8) or when the patient's physiological parameters are not stable or if the intracranial pressure is likely to be significantly raised (based on the clinical history or radiological appearances), the patient can be kept ventilated and sedated for optimum control of ICP.

(b) An ICP monitor is required in a patient with potentially raised ICP in whom accurate neurological examination is not possible (e.g. an intubated patient). A patient with a severe head injury who remains intubated usually requires an ICP monitor. Measuring the ICP also allows the cerebral perfusion pressure to be estimated so that the blood pressure to be optimized (see below).

(c) The goal in traumatic brain injury should be to maintain an adequate cerebral perfusion pressure, aiming for a *minimum* of 60mmHg (see 'Cerebral blood flow and autoregulation', p. 50).

Although this patient's admission GCS was 14/15, she had a radiologically severe head injury. This pattern of contusional injury is easily underestimated radiologically as there will be little midline shift (it is bilateral and subfrontal). However, it should be expected to swell and therefore she was kept intubated. An ICP monitor was placed with initial pressure 17mmHg, and she was managed medically in the first instance.

4. What is likely to happen to the intracranial pressure of this patient over the next 24 hours?

Brain oedema following traumatic brain injury worsens 24–48 hours after the head injury, so the ICP is likely to rise during this period.

Questions

5. Her ICP rises to 30mmHg five hours later and a CT scan is repeated (Fig. 5.2). What does it show?
6. List the ways in which the intracranial pressure can be controlled in an intensive care unit.

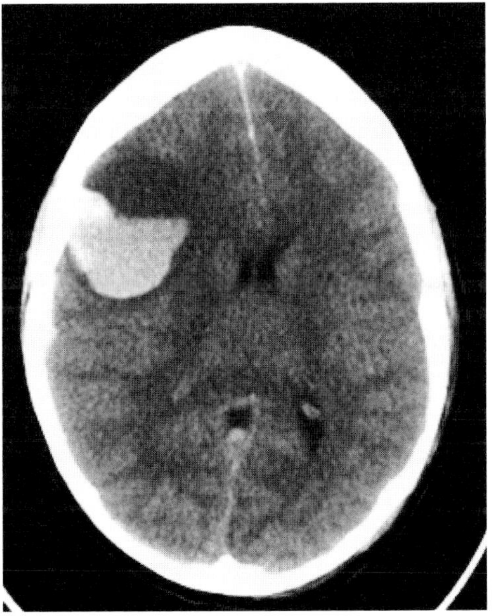

Fig. 5.2

Answers

5. Her ICP rises to 30mmHg five hours later and a CT scan is repeated. What does it show?

A haematoma has formed in the right frontal lobe. There is some surrounding oedema and mass effect with midline shift and effacement of the left lateral ventricle.

6. List the ways in which the intracranial pressure can be controlled in an intensive care unit.

- Sedation and paralysis.
- Hyperventilation. A moderately low CO_2 level causes cerebral vasoconstriction. Hence ICP is reduced, but the risk of cerebral ischaemia is increased. Hyperventilation is only recommended as a temporary measure in situations where the ICP rises acutely.
- Head elevation (30°) (increases venous return to heart and therefore reduces ICP).
- Osmotic therapy. Hypertonic saline or mannitol can be given in bolus doses as a temporary measure. Osmotic therapy is only effective in areas of the brain with intact blood–brain barriers (i.e. normal brain) and does not affect pathological brain oedema. Furthermore, the ICP rises when osmotic therapy is withdrawn. It should therefore be used sparingly.
- Temperature control (<37.5°C) with paracetamol, external cooling, and treatment of infections.
- Treating and preventing seizures.
- Barbiturate coma with thiopental.
- Drainage of CSF or decompressive craniectomy.

Question

7. The patient undergoes a craniectomy and evacuation of the haematoma. Postoperatively, the ICP readings are around 18, and a scan is repeated (Fig. 5.3). What does the scan show, and how should the patient be managed now?

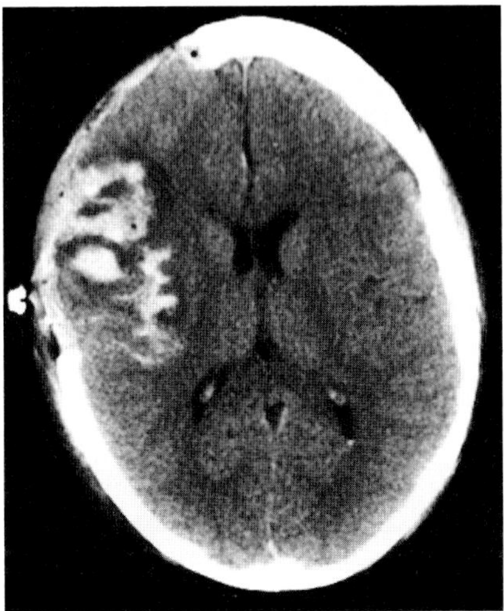

Fig. 5.3

Answer

7. The patient undergoes a craniectomy and evacuation of the haematoma. Postoperatively, the ICP readings are around 18, and a scan is repeated (Fig. 5.3). What does the scan show, and how should the patient be managed now?

There is a craniectomy providing a decompressive effect as shown by the brain herniating through the bony defect. The haematoma has been evacuated, although some acute blood remains, and the midline shift has resolved. The next step would be to progressively wean the measures instituted for ICP control and see if the patient tolerates it (i.e. see if the ICP does not rise), with the aim of having the patient off sedation and extubated.

Further reading

Brain Trauma Association (2007). *Guidelines for the Management of Severe Traumatic Brain Injury* (3rd edn). Available online at: https://www.braintrauma.org/coma-guidelines/btf-guidelines/ (accessed 1 April 2011).

Cerebral blood flow and autoregulation

The brain requires a constant blood flow. Requirements vary for different parts of the brain from 20mL/g/min for white matter to 100mL/g/min for grey matter. Cerebral blood flow (CBF) is related to the cerebral vascular resistance (CVR) and cerebral perfusion pressure (CPP), and therefore the mean arterial pressure (MAP) and the ICP, by the following formula:

$$CBF = CPP/CVR$$

where $CPP = MAP - ICP$.

In a healthy brain, autoregulation maintains a constant cerebral blood flow over a range of cerebral perfusion pressures by altering the vascular resistance. In head injury, autoregulation is impaired so that cerebral blood flow correlates more with cerebral perfusion pressure. Population studies have shown an adverse outcome in head injury for CPP <60mmHg. Therefore, if the ICP is known, the mean arterial pressure can be titrated to achieve a CPP >60mmHg.

Base of skull fractures

The dura is firmly adherent to the base of the skull, more so than on the convexity. For this reason fractures can cause dural tears relatively easily, leading to a CSF leak. Fluid in the middle ear discharges through the nose via the Eustachian tube or through the ear via a perforated tympanic membrane. If the tympanic membrane is intact, fluid behind it may be evident on otoscopy. Other signs of a base of skull fracture include Battle's sign (bruise behind the ear) and raccoon eyes (periorbital

(continued)

Base of skull fractures *(continued)*

bruising) in the absence of orbital trauma. These signs may take several hours to develop. When a skull base fracture is suspected clinically the CT bone windows should be examined. The presence of intracranial air (pneumocephalus) indicates that the intracranial cavity has been breached and is also consistent with a base of skull fracture.

The management of a patient with a base of skull fracture involves monitoring for complications: CSF fistula, meningitis, cerebral abscess, and neurological injury (particularly of the facial and vestibulocochlear nerves in the petrous temporal bone). If there is a CSF leak, the patient should stay in hospital until it stops. Persistent CSF leaks may require surgical repair. There is no class 1 evidence for antibiotic prophylaxis in skull base fractures with or without a CSF leak, although practices vary. Pneumovax should be given for the prevention of meningitis. An ENT opinion should be sought for hearing and the integrity of the tympanic membrane to be examined.

There are reports of nasogastric tubes entering the brain in the context of skull base fractures. This is considered to be due to a thin or broken cribriform plate. This has sometimes led to the advice that nasogastric tubes should not be used in the presence of a basal skull fracture, but this is irrelevant if the fracture site is known and is remote from the ethmoid bone.

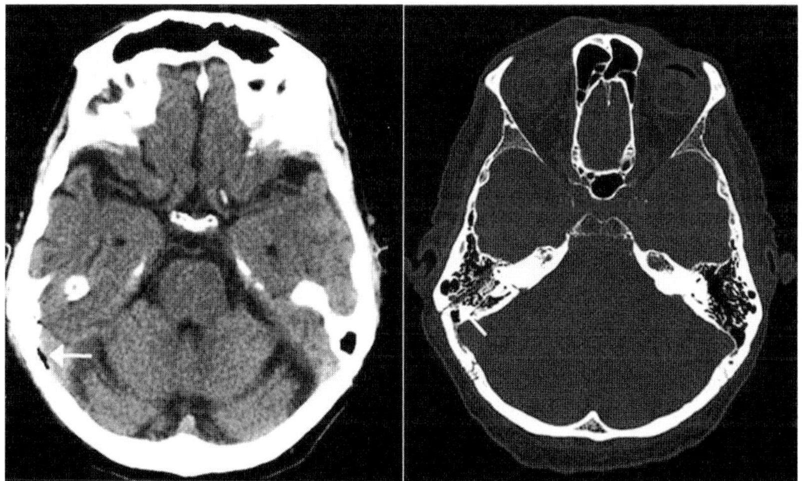

Fig. 5.4 Base of skull fracture. There is pneumocephalus (arrow, left image) indicating breach of the intracranial compartment. A longitudinal fracture through the right petrous temporal bone is seen on the bone window (arrow, right image). The mastoid air cells are partially opacified on the right, indicating fluid (CSF or blood) in the middle ear cavity.

Further reading

Ratilal B, Costa J, Sampaio C (2006). Antibiotic prophylaxis for preventing meningitis in patients with basilar skull fractures. *Cochrane Database Syst Rev*; **25**: CD004884.

Case 6

A 15-year-old boy is referred from the emergency department. He fell off his bicycle during his paper round and landed on the right side of his head in a pile of bricks by the side of the road. He was found to be 'dazed' by some passers-by who called an ambulance. By the time he was formally assessed he was alert and very slightly confused, but this has since improved in the department and he is orientated and has no focal deficit. He has a graze to his right temporal region which is swollen and very tender.

Questions

1. What is the role of skull X-rays for this patient?
2. A CT scan is performed (Fig. 6.1). What does it show?
3. How should the patient be managed?

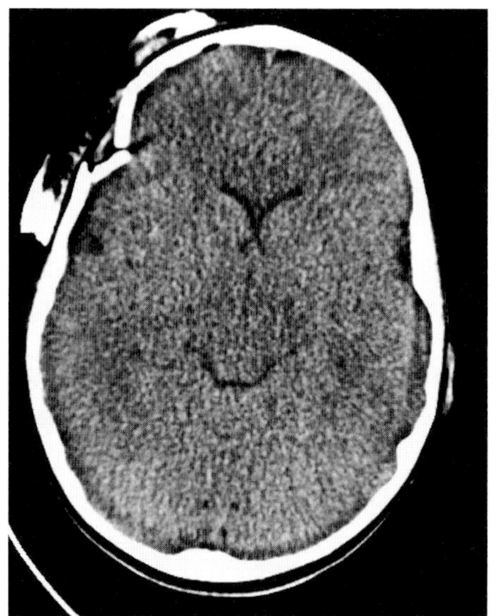

Fig. 6.1

Answers

1. What is the role of skull X-rays for this patient?

Skull X-rays are of little clinical value for this patient. Historically they were used to triage patients for CT scan: head-injured patients with neurological symptoms and a skull fracture on X-ray are far more likely to have intracranial pathology than those without a fracture on X-ray. The widespread access to CT makes it the first line investigation today. Skull X-rays still have a role in children, as per NICE guidance (NICE 2007), as part of a skeletal survey in suspected non-accidental injury.

2. A CT scan is performed (Fig. 6.1). What does it show?

There is a right frontotemporal skull fracture. The fracture is comminuted and the fragments are indented towards the brain. There is no evidence of underlying subdural or extradural haematoma, or contusional injury.

3. How should the patient be managed?

The patient is well and does not have intracranial pathology necessitating surgery. As such, surgery for the depressed fracture may be offered to elevate it and restore the contour of the skull as closely as possible. The decision to operate or not is multifactorial but the key aspects are summarized in Table 6.1.

On examination there is a contaminated graze over the swelling. It is difficult to tell if the fracture is open through this graze where there is some skin loss. However, the fracture is appreciably depressed and is in a location where it may be evident in the future if left alone. The decision is made to elevate the fracture, and this takes place shortly afterwards.

Table 6.1 Factors for and against surgery in depressed skull fractures

Factor	For surgery	Against surgery
Cosmesis	Cosmetically important area (forehead)	Very young (will remodel) or cosmetically less important area (parietal)
Contamination	Open wound communicating with fracture; obvious contamination (e.g. with mud)	Closed fracture
Location	Convexity; away from venous sinuses	Posterior fossa or midline; near venous sinuses
Severity	Fracture depressed more than one table width of the skull in that area	Fracture minimally depressed
Dural laceration	Suspected dural laceration due to bone fragment in child <6 years old (risk of growing skull fracture if dura not closed)	Minimally depressed fracture or older patient (i.e. skull has stopped growing)
Neurological deficit	Progressive or severe fixed deficit attributable to underlying cortical compression	No deficit or minimal fixed deficit

Question

4. Would management be different if the depressed skull fracture was over a venous sinus?

Answer

4. Would management be different if the depressed skull fracture was over a venous sinus?

The surgical risk of exploring skull fractures that may be associated with underlying venous sinus injury is much greater due to the risk of haemorrhage. Therefore caution should be exercised in the decision to operate, with much less concern over cosmetic issues and a greater role for antibiotics and skin debridement only for compound fractures.

Further reading

Curry DJ, Frim DM (1999). Delayed repair of open depressed skull fracture. *Pediatr Neurosurg*; **31**: 294–7.

Garniak A, Feivel M, Hertz M, Tadmor R (1986). Skull X-rays in head trauma: are they still necessary? A review of 1000 cases. *Eur J Radiol*; **6**: 89–91.

Hung KL, Liao HT, Huang JS (2005). Rational management of simple depressed skull fractures in infants. *J Neurosurg*; **103** (Suppl 1); 69–72.

Le Feuvre D, Taylor A, Peter JC (2004). Compound depressed skull fractures involving a venous sinus. *Surg Neurol*; **62**: 121–5.

NICE (2007). *Head Injury. NICE Guideline CG56*. Available online at: http://www.nice.org.uk/CG056 (accessed 13 March 2011).

Case 7

A 53-year-old man is admitted from home where he was found by a neighbour. He has a history of a subarachnoid haemorrhage and surgery to clip the aneurysm. After the event he was well and discharged home, but he was left with personality changes and mood swings and subsequently lost his job. His personal life became more difficult and he became depressed. He has recently been considering suicide, and on this occasion had tried to kill himself with a nail gun and fired one nail into the medial aspect of his left eye. He was found alert, with a headache, talking, and orientated.

On examination there is a small puncture wound in the medial corner of the left eye. Movements of the eye are restricted but he does not complain of diplopia and has no perception of light in the left eye. A CT scan is performed (scout lateral and AP, and axial views) (Fig. 7.1).

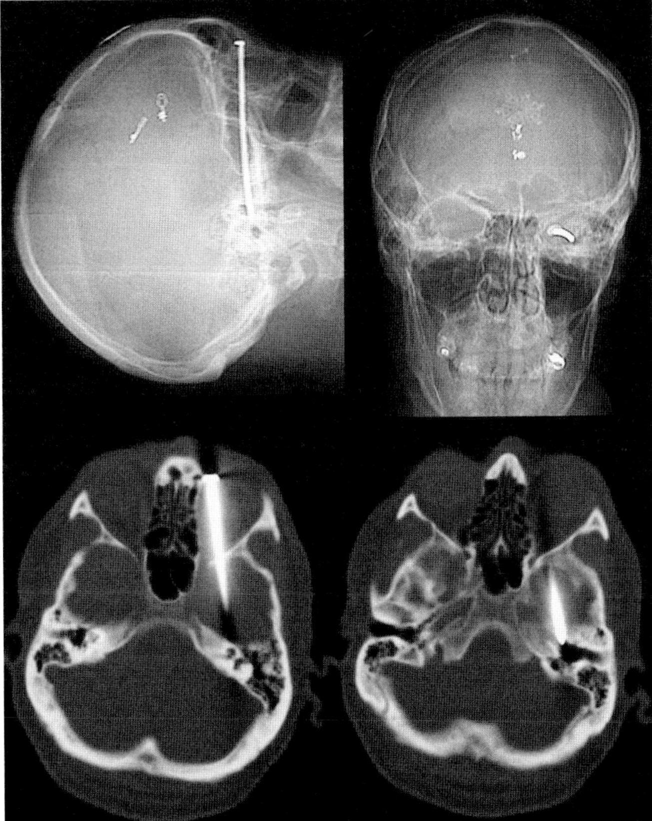

Fig. 7.1

Questions

1. Where is the nail and what are the potential complications associated with it?
2. What are the options for removal of the nail if vascular injury is suspected?

Answers

1. Where is the nail and what are the potential complications associated with it?

The scout views (Fig. 7.2) show the nail (A) and two aneurysm clips (B) and craniotomy fixation devices (C). The nail is seen on the bone windows of the axial scans running posteriorly through the orbital apex into the middle cranial fossa. The tip abuts the left petrous apex.

Nail gun injuries are low-energy injuries that damage structures they traverse but are not associated with major volumes of tissue damage. They are rarely fatal unless they directly damage a critical structure such as a major artery. On the other hand, high-velocity injuries such as those from bullets create a blast wave and cavitation of the brain behind them and are associated with major volumes of tissue damage.

This man has restricted eye movements but no double vision. On examination he had no left direct or consensual light reflex (a light shone into the left eye did not cause the left or right pupils to constrict). This implies complete failure of the left optic nerve owing to transection by the nail.

Other complications of penetrating injuries include epilepsy, CSF leak, and infection, including abscess formation along the tract. These are managed expectantly apart from infection, for which a course of prophylactic antibiotics is necessary. Vascular injury causing haemorrhage after removal or damage to the wall of a vessel not causing haemorrhage but formation of a false aneurysm can be suspected from the course of the nail.

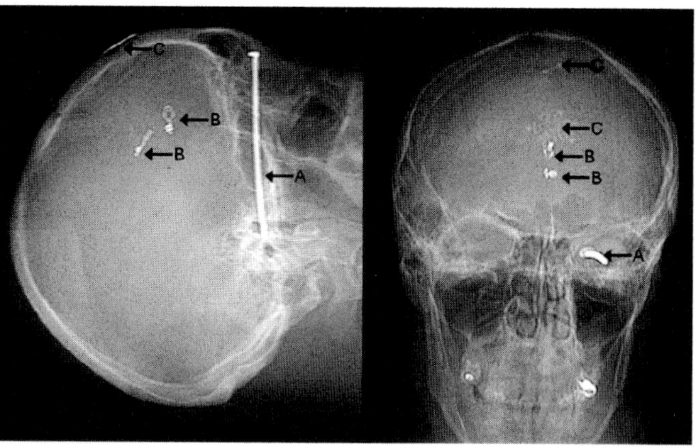

Fig. 7.2

2. What are the options for removal of the nail if vascular injury is suspected?

Angiography should be performed if vascular injury is suspected. If haemorrhage were anticipated during removal due to proximity to an artery the options are as follows.

1. Removal of the nail with exposure of the whole tract to deal with bleeding under direct vision. This would require a major exposure for this patient.
2. Removal of the nail with open surgical proximal control of the implicated artery (e.g. in the neck). This would be problematic because of cross-flow in the circle of Willis.
3. Removal with radiological control of the feeding artery using a balloon catheter or covered stent ready to be deployed to cover the site of vessel rupture.

Because of the low risk of intracranial vascular injury this patient's nail was removed through a skin incision in the medial aspect of the eye. He awoke without any new deficits although he remained blind in the left eye. He was given a two-week course of antibiotics and a one-week course of phenytoin for seizure prophylaxis.

Case 8

A 32-year-old man is admitted to the emergency department following a car accident. He was the unrestrained front-seat passenger in a car which hit a tree at around 50mph. The driver was declared dead at the scene. The patient was attended by the helicopter service but transported 5 miles to the hospital by ambulance. At the scene he was maintaining his own airway with oxygen saturations of 93% on 15L of supplementary oxygen via face mask. He had bilateral air entry in his chest with evidence of severe bruising to the chest wall anteriorly. His pulse was 110bpm and blood pressure was 100/62mmHg. He was localizing with both arms and making occasional words but only opening his eyes to painful stimulus. He appeared to be in severe discomfort when being moved onto the stretcher, and pressure on his anterior superior iliac spines caused him severe pain.

Questions

1. How should the patient be managed in the emergency department?
2. The chest and pelvis X-rays (Fig. 8.1) are performed during the first 20 minutes. What do they show and how should his management proceed?

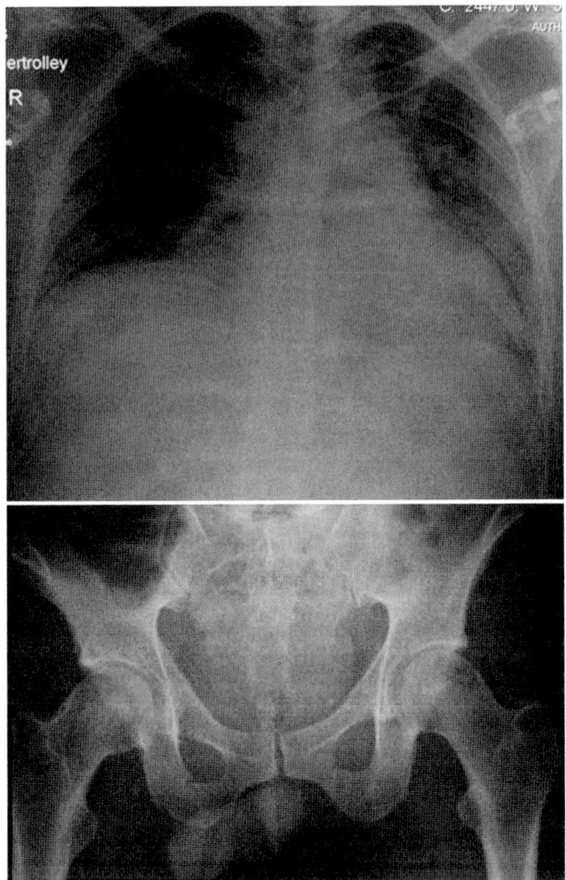

Fig. 8.1

Answers

1. How should the patient be managed in the emergency department?

This man is a typical polytrauma patient who should be managed according to the ATLS protocol. A fatality in the same accident is a strong predictor of major injury. A trauma call should be undertaken with advance warning of his arrival. An anaesthetist should be in attendance to manage the airway. An orthopaedic and general surgeon should assess the patient clinically for injuries that need early management before a CT scan is performed. X-rays of the chest and pelvis should be taken in the resuscitation room to exclude a haemopneumothorax or an unstable pelvic fracture that can be stabilized prior to CT scanning. The lateral cervical spine X-ray may be omitted and the cervical spine kept immobilized if the patient is going to have a CT scan to include this area. A senior emergency medicine clinician should attend the trauma call in a supervisory capacity as the 'team leader'.

2. The chest and pelvis X-rays (Fig. 8.1) are performed during the first 20 minutes. What do they show and how should his management proceed?

The chest X-ray shows diffuse left-sided interstitial shadowing in keeping with a pulmonary contusion. There are some overlying rib fractures (difficult to visualize on this projection). There is no haemo-pneumothorax. The AP pelvis X-ray shows no major disruption of the pelvic ring. However, there is a fracture of the right ischium, which is minimally displaced, and bilateral pubic rami fractures, neither of which require immediate treatment.

Because of concerns over his conscious level he is intubated and ventilated using a rapid-sequence induction. A CT scan is performed, which confirms multiple rib fractures and a sternal fracture with a left pulmonary contusion. There are no visceral injuries or free abdominal fluid, but there is a comminuted pelvic fracture. The spine is appropriately aligned and no fractures are identfied.

Questions

3. Describe the appearances on the CT brain (Fig. 8.2) and their importance.
4. What is his neurosurgical management?
5. What are the central considerations during the next few days?

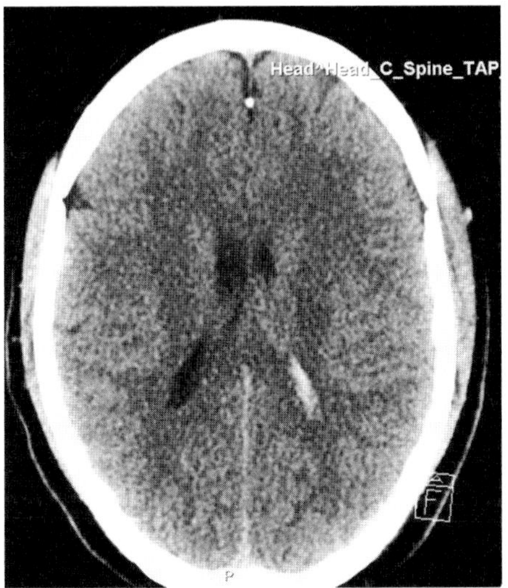

Fig. 8.2

Answers

3. Describe the appearances on the CT brain (Fig. 8.2) and their importance.

There is intraventricular haemorrhage in the left lateral ventricle posteriorly. This is an important finding. Deep haemorrhage within the brain suggests that the shear injury that causes capillary rupture to produce the haemorrhage has been transmitted through the brain from the site of external impact. The shear injury is transmitted through white matter tracts and may be invisible on a CT scan, but it may have major neurological consequences. In the acute phase there may be reactive cerebral oedema with a resultant rise in intracranial pressure. The subsequent neurological sequelae may range from a severe diffuse injury with minimal consciousness to far more subtle problems with higher cognitive and affective function. The most obvious manifestations are related to brainstem dysfunction (reduced level of consciousness, pupillary abnormalities, extension to pain and cardiorespiratory problems). This is the spectrum of injury associated with diffuse axonal injury (DAI).

4. What is his neurosurgical management?

The main concern is how the course of his intracranial injury should be monitored. This man has extensive traumatic injuries and for cardiorespiratory reasons may not be extubated. If he remains sedated and ventilated it is not possible to assess his neurological status clinically, and for this reason an ICP monitor should be placed. This will also enable medical management of intracranial pressure. Another option would be to repeat the CT scan in 12–24 hours to assess radiological progression of the injury, but this does not allow targeted control of intracranial pressure and will not detect events occurring between scans (e.g. an expanding haematoma).

A right frontal ICP monitor is placed with pressures of 10–15mmHg for the next 48 hours. At this point he is extubated, and after a few hours he is speaking in sentences and obeying commands but remains confused. His pelvic fractures are considered stable and are managed non-operatively.

5. What are the central considerations during the next few days?

He should also have regular monitoring of serum sodium levels as he remains at risk of hyponatraemia. Attention to DVT prophylaxis and nutrition is also required. Further assessment of his head injury is required clinically and radiologically. Unless he makes further rapid progress, MRI may be performed to evaluate the extent of DAI. This will also guide the major part of his neurological management which will involve assessment by a multidisciplinary team and a subsequent period of inpatient rehabilitation.

Further reading

Andriessen TM, Jacobs B, Vos PE (2010). Clinical characteristics and pathophysiological mechanisms of focal and diffuse traumatic brain injury. *J Cell Mol Med*; **14**: 2381–92.

Hammoud DA, Wasserman BA (2002). Diffuse axonal injuries: pathophysiology and imaging. *Neuroimaging Clin N Am*; **12**: 205–16.

Kraus MF, Susmaras T, Caughlin BP, Walker CJ, Sweeney JA, Little DM (2007). White matter integrity and cognition in chronic traumatic brain injury: a diffusion tensor imaging study. *Brain*; **130**, 2508–19.

Smith DH, Meaney DF, Shull WH (2003). Diffuse axonal injury in head trauma. *J Head Trauma Rehabil*; **18**: 307–16.

Weiss N, Galanaud D, Carpentier A, Naccache L, Puybasset L (2007). Clinical review. Prognostic value of magnetic resonance imaging in acute brain injury and coma. *Crit Care*; **11**: 230.

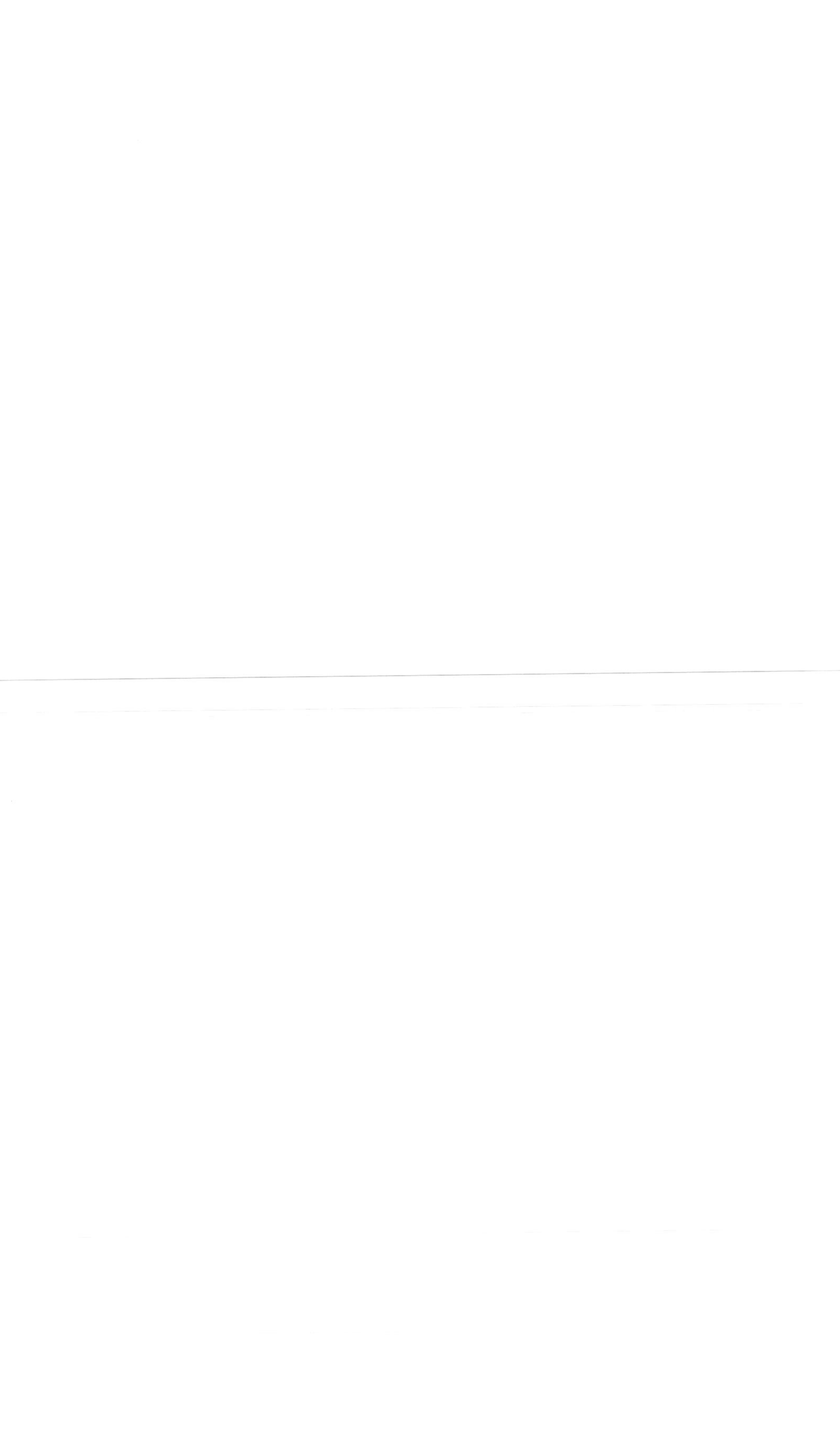

Section 2

Spinal trauma

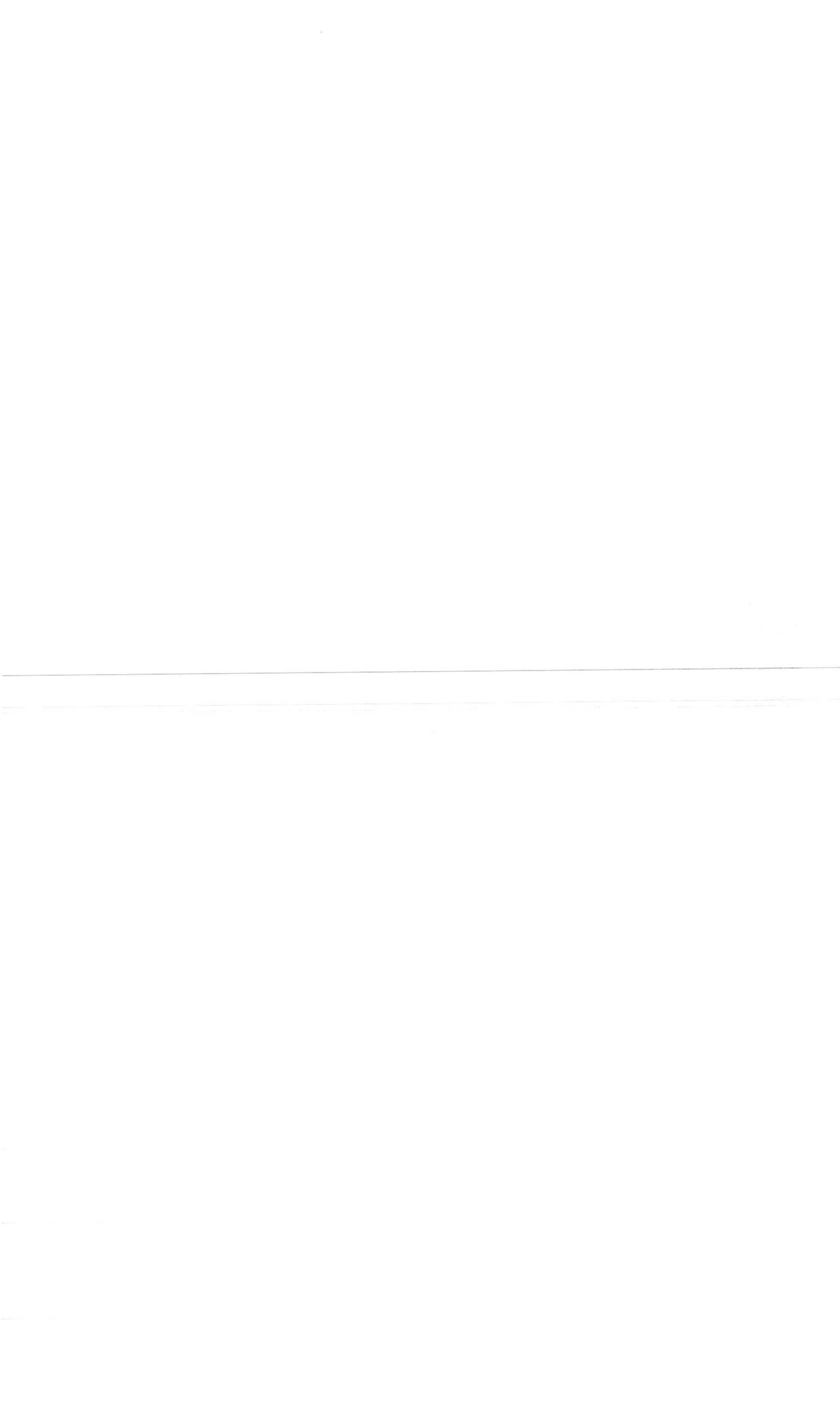

Case 9

A 39-year-old man was brought to the emergency department after falling off a ladder from a height of approximately 5m. He was unsure how he landed but denied loss of consciousness. He had severe neck pain at the scene and the ambulance crew placed him supine on a board with a hard cervical collar and blocks. On examination, he has a laceration on the forehead. His GCS is 15/15 with no focal neurological deficits. The rest of the physical examination is normal.

Questions

1. How can we decide if this patient should have imaging of the cervical spine?
2. The lateral cervical spine and open-mouth odontoid views are shown in Fig. 9.1. Describe any abnormalities. What should be done next?

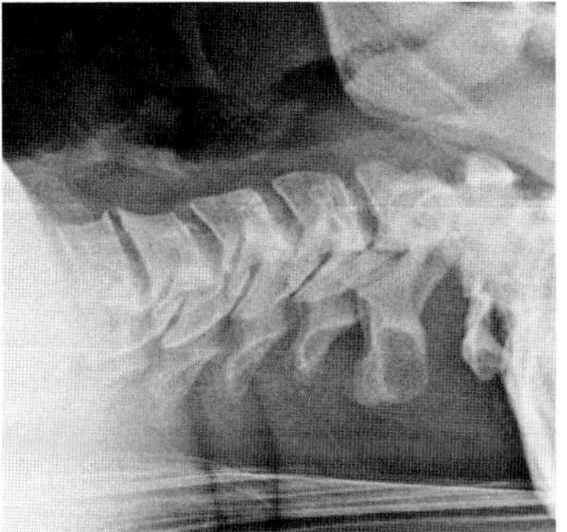
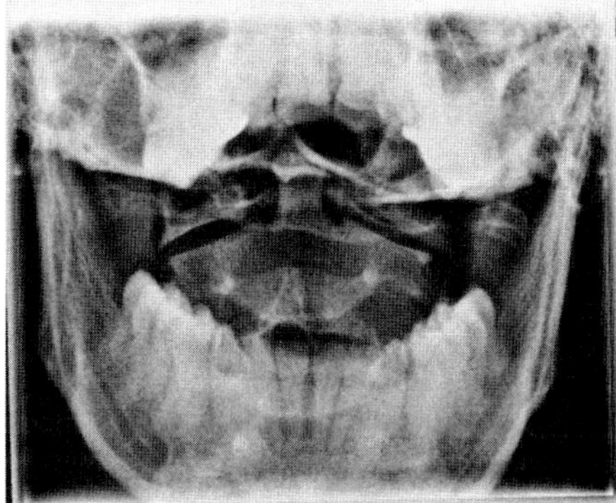

Fig. 9.1

Answers

1. How can we decide if this patient should have imaging of the cervical spine?

The Canadian Cervical Spine Rule is a widely adopted and validated instrument to determine whether a neurologically intact patient who has sustained blunt trauma with a suspected cervical spine injury should have cervical spine imaging. The presence of any of the following major factors mandates a three-view radiograph of the cervical spine:

- age > 65 years
- paraesthesia in extremities
- dangerous mechanism (including fall from >1m or five stairs, RTA >100km/hour or involving roll-over or ejection from a vehicle, bicycle, or recreational vehicle accident).

A patient also qualifies for imaging if they meet one of several minor criteria or if they cannot actively rotate the neck more than 45° to either side. This patient qualifies for imaging on the basis of a dangerous mechanism of injury.

2. The lateral cervical spine and open-mouth odontoid views are shown in Fig. 9.1. Describe any abnormalities. What should be done next?

A lateral cervical spine X-ray should provide adequate views up to the C7/T1 junction. This is an inadequate film as the last visible vertebra is C6 (see 'Interpretation of cervical spine X-rays', p. 73). There is a fracture in the posterior ring of the atlas (A in Fig. 9.2). There is separation of the lateral masses on the PEG view, producing an 'overhang' of C1 on C2 (white arrow in Fig. 9.2: the edge of C1 is not in line with the edge of C2). This is abnormal, and may indicate disruption and instability of the atlanto-axial complex. This patient requires a CT scan of the cervical spine to define these injuries and to enable viewing of the entire cervical spine.

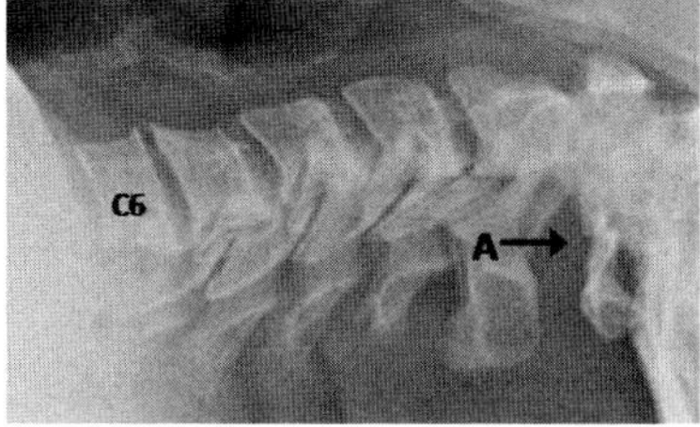

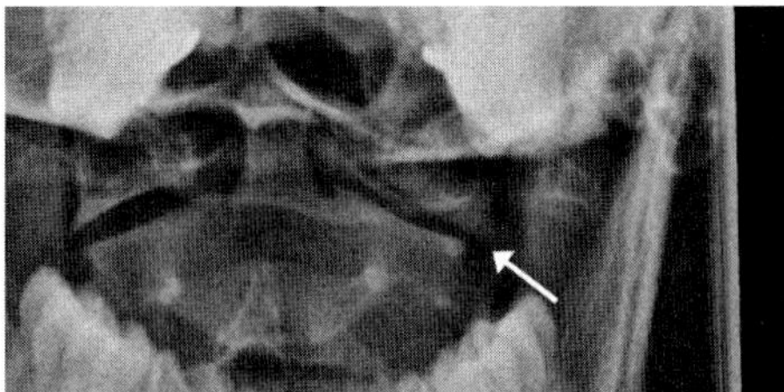

Fig. 9.2

Questions

3. The CT scan at the level of the atlas (C1) is shown in Fig. 9.3.
   a) Describe the abnormalities
   b) How might the patient have landed on the ground?
   c) The patient wants to get up and go for a walk. What would be your advice?
4. No other spinal injuries (apart from the C1 fracture) are found. How should this patient be managed?

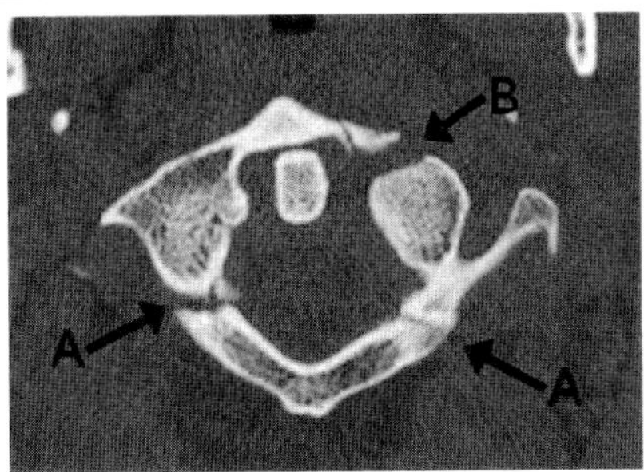

Fig. 9.3

Answers

3. The CT scan at the level of the atlas (C1) is shown in Fig. 9.3.

(a) Describe the abnormalities

There is a burst fracture of the atlas (Jefferson's fracture) involving the posterior laminae bilaterally (A) and the left anterior arch (B).

(b) How might the patient have landed on the ground?

This type of injury is associated with axial loading, suggesting that the patient may have landed on his head.

(c) The patient wants to get up and go for a walk. What would be your advice?

A fracture in the cervical spine is associated with an increased incidence of fractures elsewhere in the spine. Therefore the patient should remain supine and log-rolled until the rest of the spine is imaged and fractures excluded. In most cases plain X-rays of the thoracic and lumbar spine will adequately serve this purpose (see 'Clearing the spine', p. 75).

4. No other spinal injuries (apart from the C1 fracture) are found. How should this patient be managed?

The management of C1 fractures depends on the integrity of the transverse ligament. This can be assessed by MRI, or functional stability can be assessed by flexion–extension views. If the transverse ligament is intact, the treatment is cervical immobilization with a cervical collar or halo vest. If the transverse ligament is disrupted, the treatment is with a halo vest or internal occiput to C2 fixation. In this patient the transverse ligament was intact and a Miami J collar was prescribed for 12 weeks with CT scans scheduled at 6 weeks and 12 weeks to assess healing.

Questions

5. The patient asks what the collar does and whether he can take it off when he showers or goes to bed. How would you advise?
6. The CT scan at 12 weeks after the injury is shown in Fig. 9.4. What does it show, and what is the management?

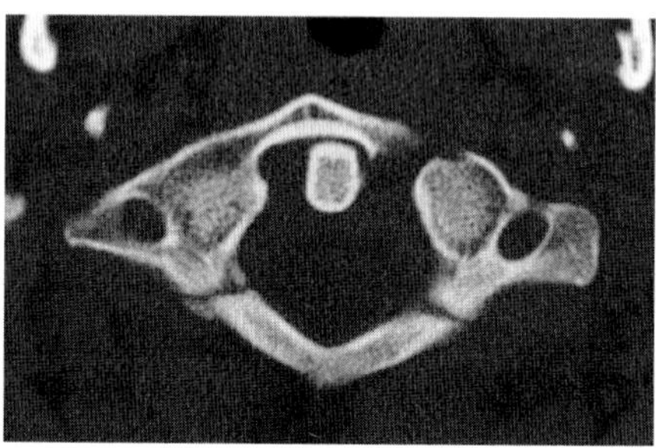

Fig. 9.4

Answers

5. The patient asks what the collar does and whether he can take it off when he showers or goes to bed. How would you advise?

A cervical collar promotes healing by immobilizing the cervical spine in patients with stable fractures. The Miami J collar limits flexion and extension by 55–75%, rotation by 70%, and lateral bending by 60%. In general, the collar needs to be worn at all times, including when bathing and going to sleep, although in certain circumstances the clinician may allow exceptions depending on the type of injury. The collar has removable internal soft pads that can be replaced after bathing.

6. The CT scan at 12 weeks after the injury is shown in Fig. 9.4. What does it show, and what is the management?

The fracture has not united, and the patient will require internal fixation (occipito-cervical fusion).

Further reading

Gibbs MA, Mower WR (2001). Cervical spine injury: a state-of-the-art approach to assessment and management. *Emergency Medicine Practice*; **3**: 1–14.

Stiell IG, Wells GA, Vandemheen KL, *et al.* (2001). The Canadian C-spine rule for radiography in alert and stable trauma patients. *JAMA*; **286**: 1841–8.

Interpretation of cervical spine X-rays

The three-view (lateral, anteroposterior, odontoid) X-ray is the initial mode of imaging the cervical spine in many centres, although it is being replaced with the availability of rapid-access CT scans in emergency departments. Three-view X-rays have been found to have a sensitivity of up to 99% for the identification of cervical spine injuries, depending on the mechanism of injury and clinical suspicion. It is essential to have a systematic method of viewing these X-rays in order to avoid missing abnormalities.

Lateral view

1. Adequacy—an adequate lateral view must include the C7/T1 junction. If this is not the case, the film is inadequate and repeat imaging at a different angle (e.g. swimmer's view or oblique view) or a CT scan is required. This is essential as a large proportion of missed abnormalities are due to inadequate films.
2. Alignment—check the anterior vertebral line, posterior vertebral line, spinolaminar line, and interspinous line (Fig. 9.5). The most important are the posterior spinal and spinolaminar lines which demarcate the spinal canal. If the smooth contour is broken, there is likely to be an abnormality. An exception is the posterior deviation in the spinolaminar line which occurs at C2, which is normal. The anterior spinal line is frequently disrupted by osteophytes, particularly in older patients.
3. Bones—look for fractures of the vertebral bodies, lamina, and spinous processes. The distance between the dens and the anterior arch of C1 (atlantodental interval) should be <4mm in adults and <5mm in children. If not, a fracture may be present.
4. Disc—examine the disc spaces for uniformity of height. Narrowing may indicate a fracture or disc prolapse.
5. Soft tissues—abnormal swelling of the pre-vertebral soft tissue suggests a vertebral fracture.

(continued)

Interpretation of cervical spine X-rays *(continued)*

Anteroposterior view

1. Alignment—observe how the spinous processes line up. Misalignment suggests rotation due to a subluxed or dislocated facet joints.
2. Pedicles—inspect the pedicles for asymmetry (see Case 44).
3. Fractures—look for fractures, although most will also be seen on the lateral view.

Odontoid view

1. Check for the symmetry of space either side of the dens.
2. Check that the C1 and C2 lateral masses are in line. If the sum total of the overhang is >7mm, this may indicate disruption of the transverse ligament.
3. Look for fractures.
4. Beware the central incisors overlying the odontoid process and mimicking a fracture.

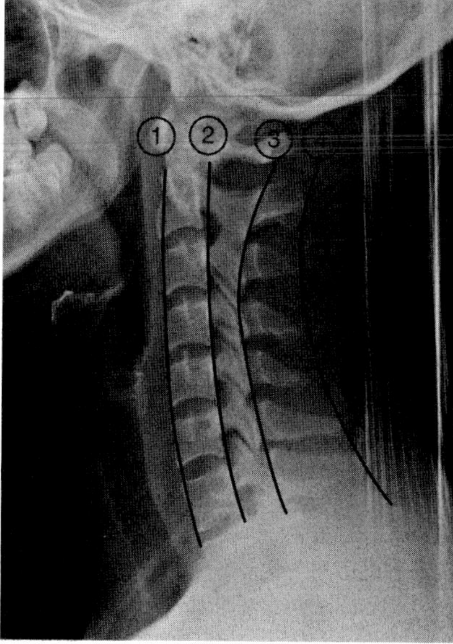

Fig. 9.5 Alignment in the cervical spine: 1, anterior vertebral line (anterior margin of vertebral bodies); 2, posterior vertebral line (posterior margin of vertebral bodies); 3, spinolaminar line (between the bases of the spinous processes); 4, interspinous line (between the tips of the spinous processes).

Clearing the spine

When spinal injury is suspected the potential damage to the spinal cord is a major concern. Therefore the spine is immobilized until injuries are excluded. Immobilization of the cervical spine is achieved by 'three-point immobilization' comprising a hard cervical collar, head blocks, and tape. The thoracolumbar spine is immobilized by bed rest. If turning is required, the patient needs to be 'log-rolled' in bed to maintain the alignment of the spine. The spine can be cleared clinically or radiologically. In general, if there is pain or restricted movement, imaging of the affected part of the spine is required. Imaging of the whole spine should also be performed in trauma scenarios with a high index of suspicion. Radiological clearance of the cervical spine is obtained by three-view X-rays or a CT scan. In most situations the collar can be removed if no fractures are identified. Ligamentous injury is not excluded, and if there is persistent pain flexion–extension views may be performed to check for stability. This is usually performed at least 2 weeks after the injury as muscle spasm in the acute period may limit the range of movement. In comatose patients, a normal CT scan of the cervical spine is generally accepted as adequate to clear the spine and the collar can be removed if there are concerns about raised intracranial pressure. If injury to the thoracolumbar spine is suspected, the patient should undergo imaging. Plain X-rays are usually adequate for this purpose, although in most trauma situations the patient may have had a whole-body CT scan on which the thoracic and lumbar vertebrae can be visualized. Three-point immobilization of the cervical spine should not be attempted if there is a significant pre-existing deformity (e.g. in ankylosing spondylitis). In this scenario putting the patient in a hard cervical collar may exacerbate the injury and produce neurological deficits, and an effort should be made to maintain the spine in its 'normal' position.

Case 10

A 45-year-old woman was admitted, having fallen down the stairs whilst intoxicated. She had severe neck pain at the time but went to bed overnight and only called an ambulance when the pain was still there the next morning, preventing her from getting out of bed. She denies neurological symptoms and examination of her arms and legs is normal. She is immobilized in a hard collar.

Questions

1. How should her possible cervical spine injury be managed? Does she require imaging of any form?
2. What imaging would you request first, and what is its value?

Answers

1. How should her possible cervical spine injury be managed? Does she require imaging of any form?

A high index of suspicion should be maintained for cervical spine injury despite the absence of neurological signs or symptoms. She should be clinically assessed and definitively imaged with CT if there are new neurological signs or symptoms. If not, she may be clinically assessed with a view to 'clearance' if she has minimal or no tenderness to bony palpation and an acceptable pain-free range of active movements after the collar is removed. This can only be considered if she is alert and orientated without a distracting injury such as a long-bone fracture.

Examination reveals midline tenderness to palpation in the upper cervical spine. She has a severely restricted range of active and passive movements of the neck although they do not provoke neurological symptoms.

2. What imaging would you request first, and what is its value?

Initial imaging should be a three-view X-ray of the cervical spine. If this is normal her cervical spine can be considered 'clear' in the context of a low-energy injury with a high sensitivity in this setting. Three-view X-rays are less sensitive when there is higher clinical suspicion and will miss one in seven cervical spine injuries in major trauma patients.

Questions

3. A lateral X-ray is shown (Fig. 10.1). What is the abnormality?
4. Should any further imaging be requested?

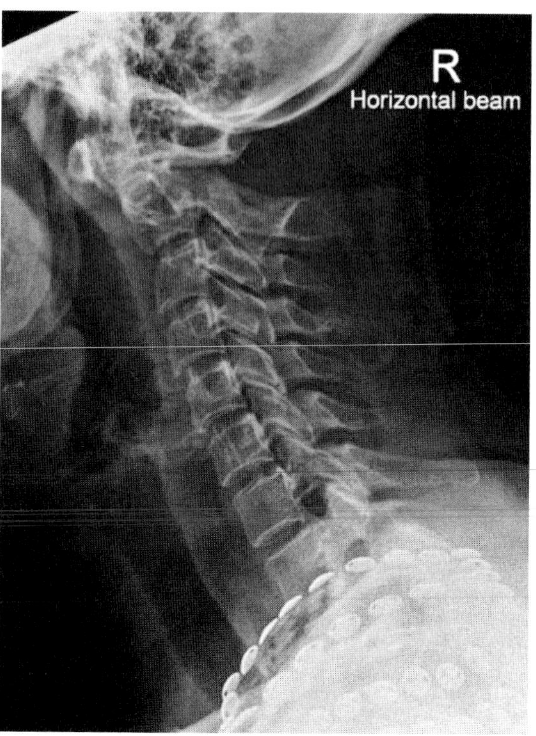

Fig. 10.1

Answers

3. A lateral X-ray is shown (Fig. 10.1). What is the abnormality?

This is a fully adequate lateral X-ray, covering all the cervical spine to T1/2 (unusual after trauma). The imaged structures are normal except for C2 which appears angulated forward.

4. Should any further imaging be requested?

This patient requires a CT scan to clarify the possible anomaly at C2. This is done with sagittal reformats shown and axial source images through the abnormality.

Questions

5. What does Fig. 10.2 show?
6. Is there anything unusual about it?
7. How are these injuries usually classified and managed?

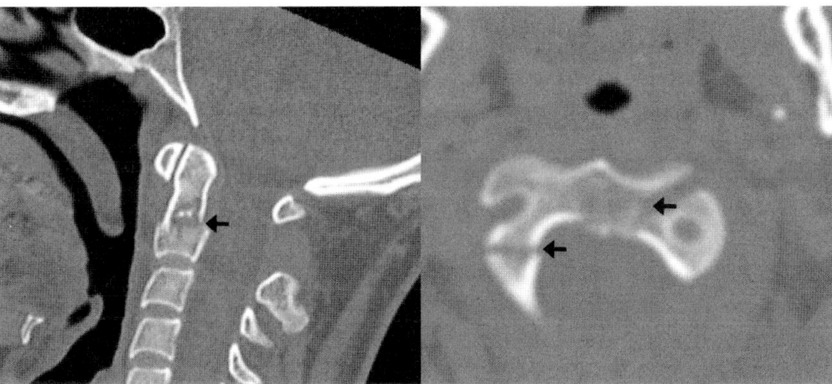

Fig. 10.2

Answers

5. What does Fig. 10.2 show?

The injury is a fracture through C2, confirmed on the axial images (arrows).

6. Is there anything unusual about it?

The unusual aspect is that on the right side the fracture is through the pedicle and on the left side through the body of C2. Bipedicular fractures of C2 are termed 'Hangman's fractures'. Fractures of the body of C2 are usually classified as type 3 odontoid peg fractures. Both may heal with immobilisation only as long as there is not too much diastasis of the fracture fragments which may prevent healing.

7. How are these injuries usually classified and managed?

Odontoid fractures are classified according to Anderson and D'Alonzo as types 1, 2 or 3 (Table 10.1). This case has elements of a type 3 fracture as well as a pedicle fracture. The acceptable anatomical alignment of the fragments and the absence of neurological deficit favours conservative management in a rigid cervical collar.

Table 10.1 Anderson and D'Alonzo (1974) classification

Classification	Description	Treatment
Type 1	Fracture through the tip of the peg, typically an avulsion of the apical ligament of the peg. Usually stable, although uncommon	Usually treated with a rigid collar for associated ligamentous injury but heal with conservative management
Type 2	Very common. There is a transverse or oblique break through the body or base of the odontoid peg. These are usually considered unstable	Often managed conservatively in the first instance with collar or halo immobilization but they have a higher rate of non-union. If instability is demonstrated after an interval of 3 months then operative stabilization is frequently required
Type 3	Involve the body of C2 with comminuted fragments and are also unstable	Usually heal with immobilization in either a collar or a halo vest

Questions

8. The patient's collar is kept on and she is allowed to mobilize and is discharged. In the outpatient clinic 2 weeks later a repeat CT scan is performed as she has worsening neck pain (Fig. 10.3). What does it show and what are the options?
9. What are the options for internal fixation?

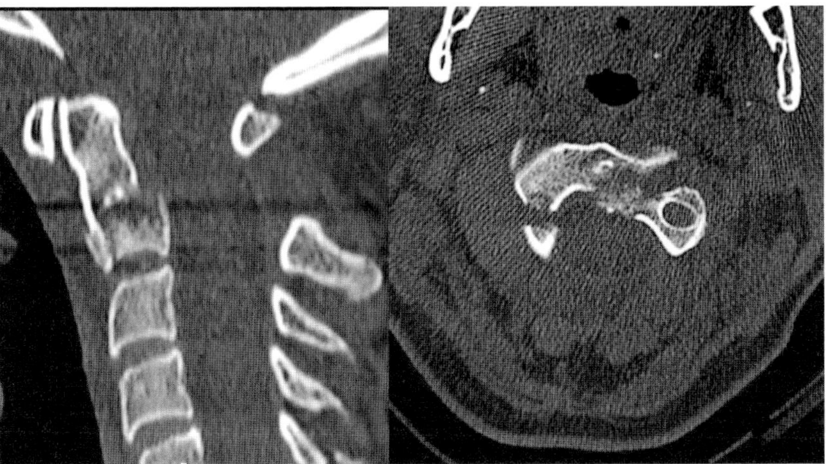

Fig. 10.3

Answers

8. The patient's collar is kept on and she is allowed to mobilize and is discharged. In the outpatient clinic 2 weeks later a repeat CT scan is performed as she has worsening neck pain (Fig. 10.3). What does it show and what are the options?

The fracture has failed to unite. There is worsening diastasis of the fracture compared with the original CT scan. Bony union at this stage is less likely. Therefore continued conservative management is inadvisable and internal fixation is proposed.

9. What are the options for internal fixation?

C2 fractures may often be managed with C1–2 fixation, or fixation of the odontoid peg only with an odontoid screw for type 2 fractures. C1–2 fixation will not be possible for this patient as the anatomy of the C2 fracture makes it unsuitable for holding the screws. At a minimum a C1–3 fixation will be required to bridge C2. In this case an internal fixation from the occiput to C3 and C4 was proposed. This has the advantage of allowing reduction during the fixation, which would not be as easy with C1–3 fixation, and subsequently offering excellent immobilization. The disadvantage is the loss of motion: approximately 50% of cervical spine rotation occurs at C1/2 and 50% of flexion–extension at the occiput–C1 junction. Therefore an occiput to C3/4 fixation in a young person is most disabling, and arrangements should be made to remove the instrumentation (Fig. 10.4) once bony union is confirmed with CT scanning after 3–6 months.

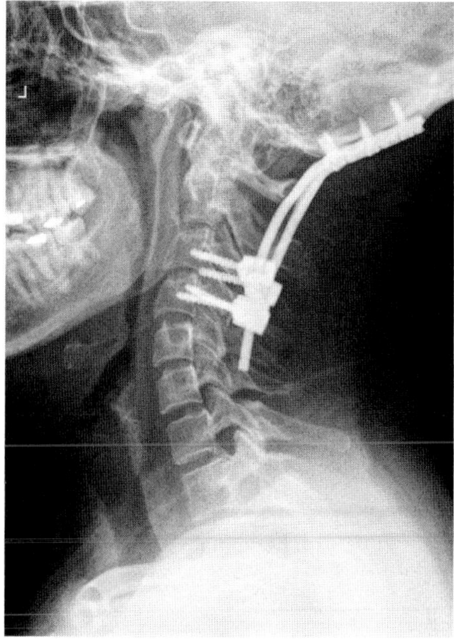

Fig. 10.4

Further reading

Anderson LD, D'Alonzo RT (1974). Fractures of the odontoid process of the axis. *J Bone Joint Surg Am*; **56**: 1663–74.

Elgafy H, Dvorak MF, Vaccaro AR, Ebraheim N (2009). Treatment of displaced type II odontoid fractures in elderly patients. *Am J Orthop*; **38**, 410–16.

Lee C, Rogers LF, Woodring JH, Goldstein SJ, Kim KS (1984). Fractures of the craniovertebral junction associated with other fractures of the spine: overlooked entity? *Am J Neuroradiol*; **5**: 775–81.

Levine AM, Edwards CC (1986). Treatment of injuries in the C1–C2 complex. *Orthop Clin North Am*; **17**: 31–44.

Maak TG, Grauer JN (2006). The contemporary treatment of odontoid injuries. *Spine (Phila Pa 1976)*; **15** (Suppl 11): S53–61.

Case 11

A 32-year-old man is brought into the emergency department as a trauma call. He was a cyclist who had crossed a red traffic light and was hit by a car. He was not wearing a helmet and landed directly on his head. He was immediately unable to move his legs and his spine was immobilized by the attending ambulance crew. He has an open fracture of his left tibia.

In the emergency department he is alert and orientated, but in obvious distress, and has considerable neck pain. He is unable to extend his arms properly although he has preserved elbow flexion and some grip strength. He is able to feel his thumbs on both sides but neither of his little fingers, and his middle fingers feel numb. He has no sensation in his medial upper arms, torso, or legs. He cannot move his legs or feel the leg injury. Rectal examination reveals no anal tone and a urinary catheter is passed without sensation.

Questions

1. What is the clinical diagnosis?
2. What important information is required?

Answers

1. What is the clinical diagnosis?

The clinical diagnosis is of a severe spinal cord injury due to a fracture. The preserved thumb sensation suggests that the cord at the level of C6 is intact, whilst the absent little finger sensation suggests that cord injury is complete at C8. Therefore the level is around C7.

2. What important information is required?

Vital clinical information relates to his heart rate and blood pressure: he may have an important thoracic or abdominal injury with occult blood loss that is masked by the spinal cord injury. He may have other injuries apart from the left tibia that he cannot feel. Therefore he needs a thorough clinical and radiological evaluation.

Questions

3. His heart rate is a little low (55 beats/min) and his blood pressure is 90/55mmHg. He is peripherally warm. An abdominal ultrasound is performed showing no free blood. He goes for a CT scan. The chest and abdomen are normal aside from superficial bruising. The axial images through C6 are shown in Fig. 11.1. What are the findings?
4. Which clinical condition explains his mild bradycardia and hypotension in the setting of no evident blood loss? How should this be managed?
5. How can the severity of spinal cord injury be classified?

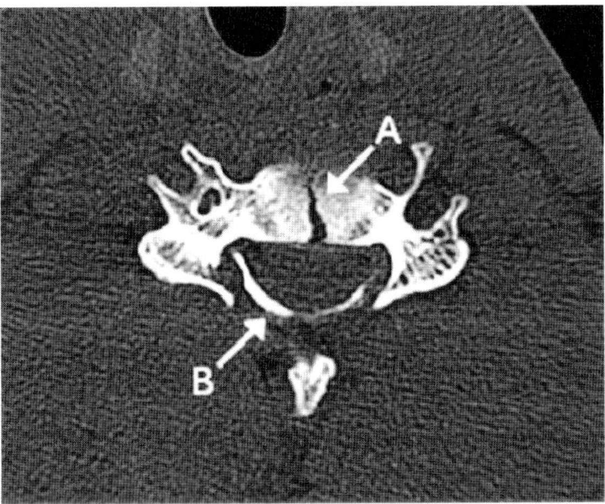

Fig. 11.1

Answers

3. The patient's heart rate is a little low (55bpm) and his blood pressure is 90/55mmHg. He is peripherally warm. An abdominal ultrasound is performed showing no free blood. He goes for a CT scan. The chest and abdomen are normal apart from superficial bruising. The axial images through C6 are shown in Fig. 11.1. What are the findings?

There is a sagittal split fracture through the vertebral body of C6 (A). The lamina below is also seen on this slice and is encroaching on the spinal canal (B), suggesting that the two bones are not aligned normally. This is compatible with a displaced fracture. Clinically the patient has a complete spinal cord injury due to fracture dislocation at C6.

4. Which clinical condition explains his mild bradycardia and hypotension in the setting of no evident blood loss? How should this be managed?

These features are suggestive of spinal shock. This occurs because of interruption of the sympathetic supply which leaves the spinal cord from T1 to around L3 to form the sympathetic chain on either side of the spinal column. The sympathetic chain in turn gives rise to the inferior, middle, and superior cervical ganglia, branches to the peripheral nerves and the splanchnic nerves via which they provide sympathetic supply to the whole body including the head and face. In contrast the majority of parasympathetic supply to the whole body comes from cranial nerves 3, 7, 9, and 10, with the vagus nerve offering all the splanchnic parasympathetic innervation. Therefore a high spinal cord injury has the potential to withdraw all sympathetic nervous system output immediately. The two most clinically obvious manifestations are a mild bradycardia (due to unopposed parasympathetic supply to the heart) and hypotension with warm peripheries due to loss of peripheral vasomotor tone.

The most common cause of hypotension in trauma patients is volume loss, which should be replaced. However, in a patient with spinal shock this will result in hypervolaemia and potentially peripheral and pulmonary oedema. Therefore an urgent assessment of occult blood loss by ultrasound or CT scan should be made. As this is negative, after judicious volume resuscitation the patient will require noradrenaline to augment peripheral vasoconstriction.

5. How can the severity of spinal cord injury be classified?

There are several classification systems but the American Spinal Injury Association (ASIA) impairment scale is one of the most widely used. Individual dermatomes and myotomes are examined and an overall grade is assigned (Table 11.1). The injury in this patient is ASIA grade A.

Table 11.1 ASIA classification system for spinal injuries

ASIA grade	Description
A	Complete injury: no motor or sensory function is preserved in sacral segments S4–S5
B	Incomplete: sensory but not motor function is preserved below the neurological level and includes sacral segments S4–S5
C	Incomplete: motor function is preserved below the neurological level and more than half of the key muscles below the neurological level have a muscle grade <3
D	Incomplete: motor function is preserved below the neurological level and at least half of the key muscles below the neurological level have a muscle grade ≥3
E	Normal: motor and sensory function are normal

Reproduced with permission from American Spinal Injury Association: International Standards for Neurological Classification of Spinal Cord Injury, revised 2011; Atlanta, GA. Reprinted 2011.

Questions

6. The patient undergoes an MRI (Fig. 11.2). What are the findings?
7. What are the nonsurgical aspects of his care?
8. What is the role of surgery?
9. What are the options for stabilization?

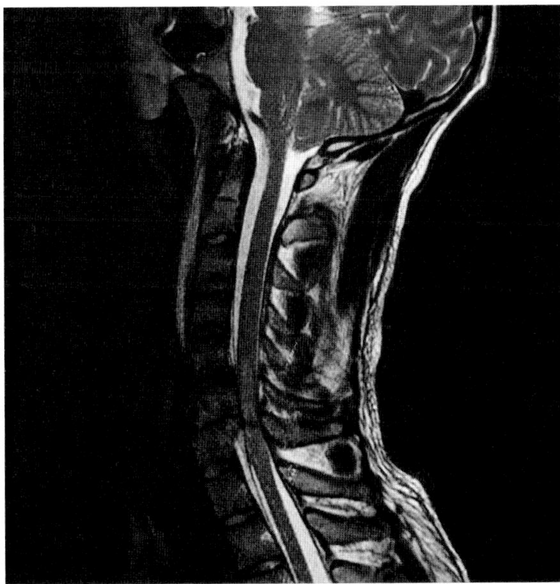

Fig. 11.2

Answers

6. The patient undergoes an MRI (Fig. 11.2). What are the findings?

The vertebral body injury of C6 is demonstrated. The C6/7 disc is disrupted and the posterior longitudinal ligament torn. There is posterior subluxation of C6 on C7. There is mild narrowing of the spinal canal but the spinal cord is also swollen at the level of injury. On this T_2 image the spinal cord at the level of injury returns abnormal high signal with lower signal centrally, suggesting acute oedema and haemorrhage due to a contusional injury.

7. What are the non-surgical aspects of his care?

The medical aspects of his care are those of a patient with an acute spinal cord injury. He needs attention to nutrition, DVT prophylaxis, and bladder and bowel care (a urinary catheter and early administration of stool softeners to prevent severe constipation). He should have early and regular turning to prevent pressure sores. Monitoring of cardiovascular and respiratory function is important in any patient with a spinal cord injury as autonomic reflexes can become exaggerated; for example, bradycardia or blood pressure changes may occur during endotracheal suctioning or bowel evacuation. Ventilatory function should be monitored as he will develop a degree of type 2 respiratory failure which may be masked by the use of supplementary oxygen and oxygen saturation monitoring rather than arterial blood gas and PCO_2.

8. What is the role of surgery?

The role of surgery in patients with complete spinal cord injury is to stabilize the spine to allow nursing and rehabilitation. If the spinal cord injury is complete (complete loss of sensorimotor function within three levels of the radiological injury), he will not recover and rehabilitation will be aimed at education and therapy to allow him to achieve the maximum level of function given his disability. Stabilization should be performed early enough to allow turning and mobilization before he develops complications of spinal cord injury such as pressure sores, DVT, and pneumonia.

9. What are the options for stabilization?

This injury can be managed in various ways. A hard collar alone is not sufficient. The area of the fracture is such that it is likely to unite if treated with halo immobilization. However, reduction of the fracture will be less easily achieved in a halo unless it is applied under anaesthetic with fluoroscopy. Internal fixation of the fracture allows operative assessment of the reduction with X-ray and direct vision and enables the reduced fragments to be maintained in alignment. This was performed using lateral mass screws from C4, C5, and C6 to T1 as shown in Fig. 11.3 (lower segments not shown).

An anterior fusion procedure may additionally be considered so that the fracture can be rendered fully stable in extension and flexion. However, this would require a further surgical operation through a separate incision with potential further morbidity. There is a risk of wound infection if the patient subsequently requires

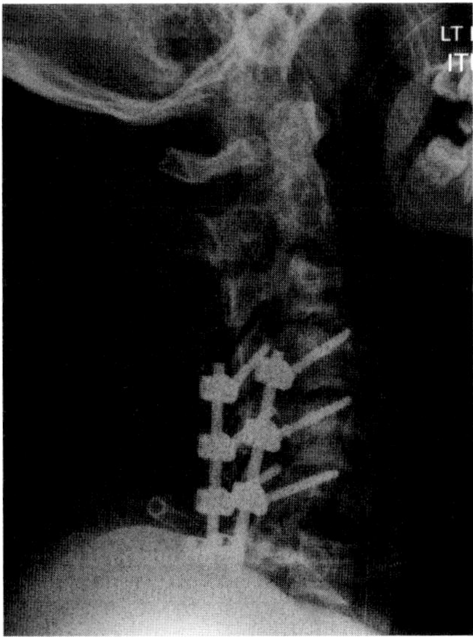

Fig. 11.3

a tracheostomy. The posterior procedure undertaken has been sufficient to stabilize the neck for the purposes of nursing care for the 6 weeks that the fracture will take to heal.

Further reading

American Spinal Injury Association (2003). *Reference Manual for the International Standards for Neurological Classification of Spinal Cord Injury*. Chicago, IL: American Spinal Injury Association.

Baguley IJ (2008). Autonomic complications following central nervous system injury. *Semin Neurol*; **28**: 716–25.

Dvorak MF, Fisher CG, Fehlings MG, Rampersaud YR, Oner FC, Aarabi B (2007). The surgical approach to subaxial cervical spine injuries: an evidence-based algorithm based on the SLIC classification system. *Spine (Phila Pa 1976)*; **32**: 2620–9.

Maynard FM Jr, Bracken MB, Creasey G, *et al.* (1997). International Standards for Neurological and Functional Classification of Spinal Cord Injury. American Spinal Injury Association. *Spinal Cord*; **35**: 266–74.

McMahon D, Tutt M, Cook AMP (2009). Pharmacological management of hemodynamic complications following spinal cord injury. *Orthopedics*; **32**: 331.

Case 12

A 68-year-old man is admitted to the emergency department following a road traffic accident in which he was a front-seat passenger in a stationary car hit from behind by a car travelling at around 20mph. He was wearing a seatbelt and the car had headrests. He had severe neck pain at the scene, and his spine was immobilized by the paramedics with a rigid cervical collar and head blocks. Upon arrival in the emergency department he was complaining of neck pain, heaviness in all limbs, and pins and needles in his hands and feet.

Question

1. The patient undergoes a lateral X-ray of the cervical spine (Fig. 12.1). What does it show?

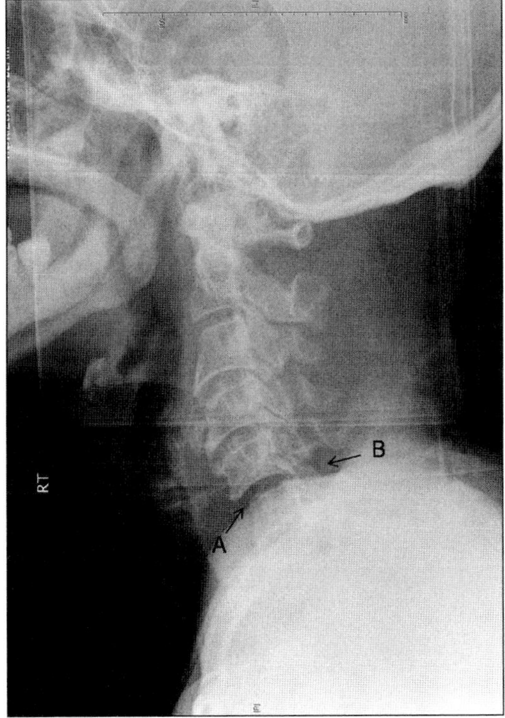

Fig. 12.1

Answer

1. The patient undergoes a lateral X-ray of the cervical spine (Fig. 12.1). What does it show?

First, the X-ray provides an inadequate view as its coverage only extends to the C5/6 level. This is frequently the case in conscious trauma patients with neck pain and a degree of muscle spasm. Obtaining a complete view of the C7–T1 junction by downward shoulder traction is unlikely to be successful. However, a step deformity anteriorly at C5/6 is evident (A). Posteriorly there appears to be widening of the interspinous space (B). This patient should have a cervical spine CT in view of the abnormalities already identified.

Questions

2. The CT is performed. An axial image through C5/6 is shown (Fig. 12.2, left) with C6/7 (Fig. 12.2, right) for comparison. What does it show?
3. The examination findings were as follows: upper limbs: normal tone, power reduced, reflexes absent. Lower limbs: tone increased bilaterally, power reduced, reflexes brisk. Plantars were upgoing. What clinical syndrome does he have?
4. How should the fracture be managed?

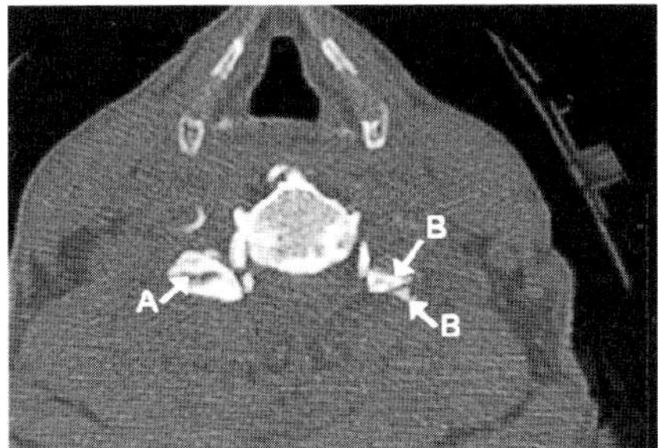

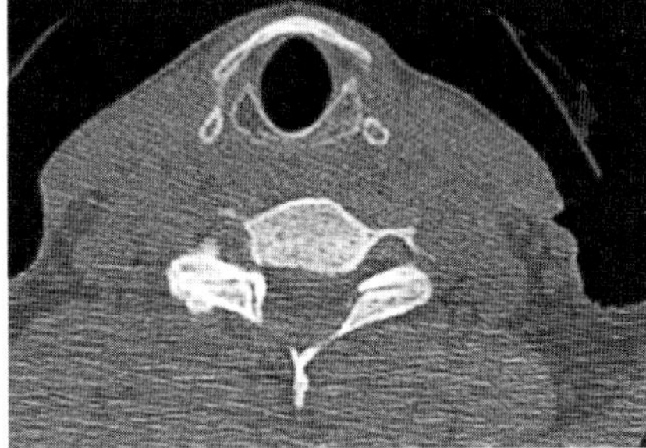

Fig. 12.2

Answers

2. A CT scan is performed. An axial image through C5/6 is shown (Fig. 12.2, left) with C6/7 (Fig. 12.2, right) for comparison. What does it show?

The right C5/6 facet joint has increased joint space (A). The left C5/6 facet is barely seen except for two small adjacent fragments (B). This suggests bilateral facetal misalignment, with the left being almost complete. This is demonstrated more clearly on the sagittal reformatted image (arrows) which shows mild subluxation and joint space widening on the right (Fig. 12.3, left image) whereas on the left the articular facets are 'perched' (Fig. 12.3, right image). There is mild forward displacement of C5 vertebra on C6 and widening of the C5/6 interspinous distance. There is a mild kyphosis at this level.

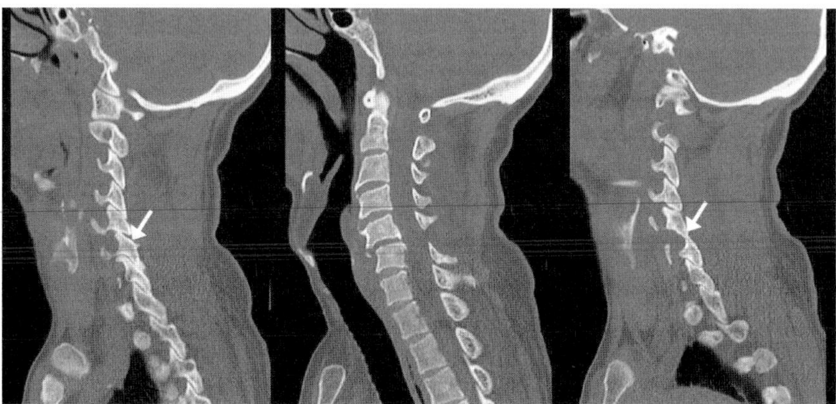

Fig. 12.3

3. The examination findings were as follows: upper limbs: normal tone, power reduced, reflexes absent. Lower limbs: tone increased bilaterally, power reduced, reflexes brisk. Plantars were upgoing. What clinical syndrome does he have?

These findings are consistent with a cervical central cord syndrome, which is a clinical diagnosis, classically affecting the arms more than the legs. The clinical features vary according to the extent of white and grey matter injury to the spinal cord, giving rise to both upper and lower motor neuron signs in the arms, and upper motor neuron signs only in the legs (see 'Types of spinal cord lesions', p. 299).

4. How should the fracture be managed?

Facet joint dislocations are unstable injuries. Treatment is either closed reduction in traction, followed by immobilization, or surgical fixation.

Closed reduction may be attempted using cervical traction with the skull pins positioned a little behind the mid-coronal plane of the skull to encourage a little forward flexion to reduce the perched left C5/6 facet. If this succeeds, the patient will need subsequent immobilization in a hard collar or halo vest to allow healing. The concerns over closed reduction are as follows.

1. It may fail with the facets becoming misaligned again within the 4–6 weeks that the ligaments may take to heal.
2. If it is successful, there is no major fracture to heal and the injury is principally ligamentous. Therefore there may be persistent instability following immobilization.

The alternative is an open reduction and fixation. This will involve a midline posterior approach with enough of the perched facet drilled to enable reduction using a lateral image intensifier for guidance. The fixation can be performed according to individual preference. If enough bone surface has been exposed during the drilling so that bony fusion is expected to take place, simple interspinous wiring may be sufficient, otherwise lateral mass screws will be required.

This patient underwent open operative reduction and interspinous wiring of C5 to C6. He made an uncomplicated recovery from the surgery. His postoperative X-rays are shown in Fig. 12.4. The facets at C5/6 are clearly reduced when compared with the preoperative film.

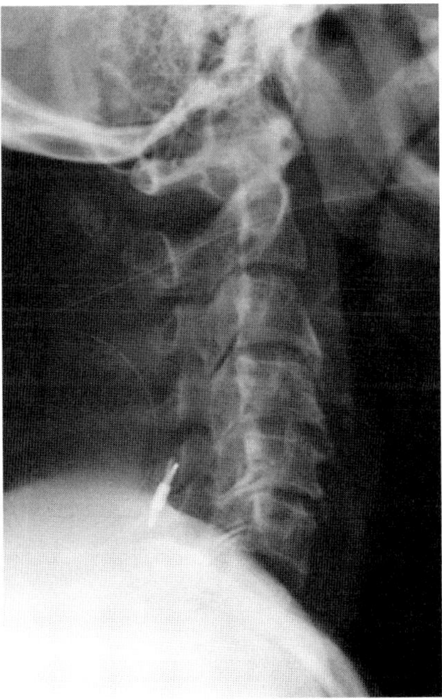

Fig. 12.4

Further reading

Daffner SD, Daffner RH (2002). Computed tomography diagnosis of facet dislocations: the 'hamburger bun' and 'reverse hamburger bun' signs. *J Emerg Med*; **23**: 387–94.

Dvorak MF, Fisher CG, Aarabi B, *et al.* (2007). Clinical outcomes of 90 isolated unilateral facet fractures, subluxations, and dislocations treated surgically and non-operatively. *Spine (Phila Pa 1976)*; **32**: 3007–13.

Hadley MN, Fitzpatrick BC, Sonntag VK, Browner CM (1992). Facet fracture–dislocation injuries of the cervical spine. *Neurosurgery*; **30**: 661–6.

Ivancic PC, Pearson AM, Tominaga Y, Simpson AK, Yue JJ, Panjabi MM (2007). Mechanism of cervical spinal cord injury during bilateral facet dislocation. *Spine (Phila Pa 1976)*; **32**: 2467–73.

Lovely TJ, Carl A (1995). Posterior cervical spine fusion with tension-band wiring. *J Neurosurg*; **83**: 631–5.

Case 13

A 17-year-old man is admitted as a trauma call. He was trying to break into a building and fell from a fence when climbing in. He overbalanced backwards and landed upside down on the top of his head. He had severe neck pain at the time of the injury and did not walk afterwards. Cervical spine X-rays are performed as part of the admitting investigations (Fig. 13.1).

Question

1. What do the X-rays show? Which investigation is required next?

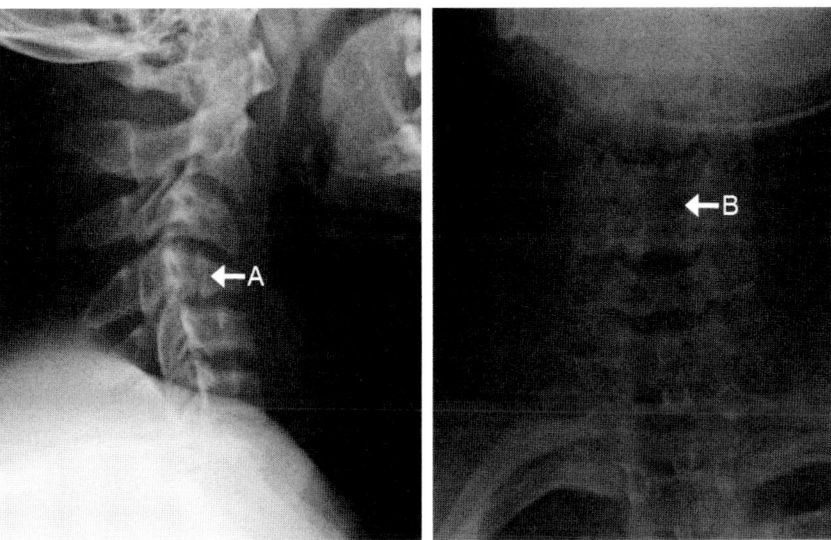

Fig. 13.1

Answer

1. What do the X-rays show? Which investigation is required next?

The X-rays show a wedge fracture of C4 (A) and possibly C3. Therefore the vertebral body is certainly compromised and possibly the posterior elements are as well. Loss of height is apparent on the AP view at the C4/5 level (B). There is a suggestion of a vertical split in the bodies of C3 and C4. These are potentially unstable injuries and CT imaging is required.

Question

2. The coronal view and an axial view at C4 are shown in Fig. 13.2. What do they show?

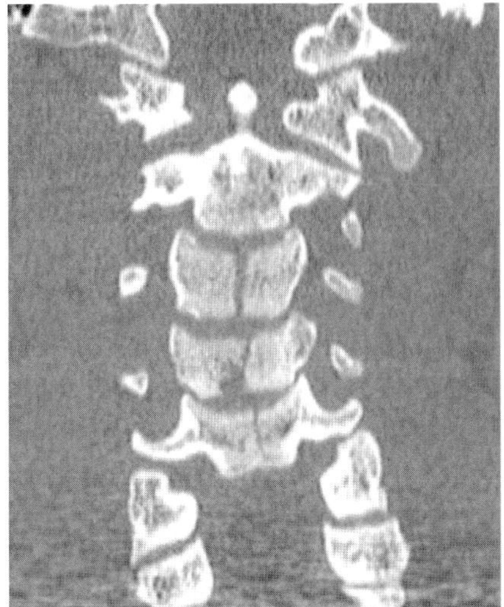

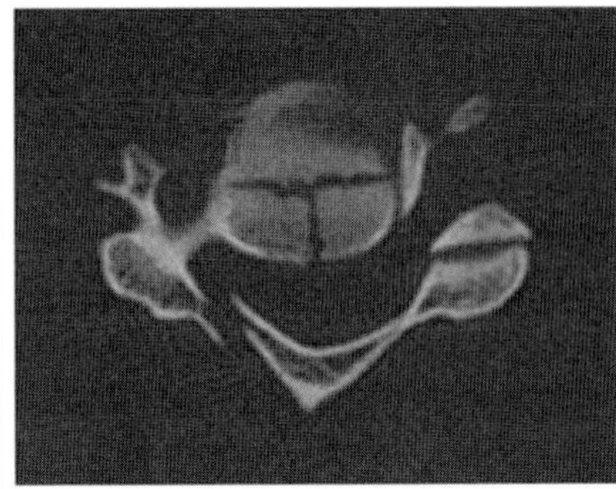

Fig. 13.2

Answer

2. The coronal view and an axial view at C4 are shown in Fig. 13.2. What do they show?

The coronal reformat shows the injury to C4, as well as additional vertical split injuries to C3 and C5. The axial image at C4 (right image) shows a laminar fracture on the right as well as a T-shaped fracture of the vertebral body. This is an unstable injury. Management options are internal fixation, although spanning the fracture with a screw and rod construct would potentially involve fusion from C2 to C6 which is a long immobile segment in any patient, especially a 17-year-old. Anterior fusion would have to be similarly extensive. For these reasons the patient was managed in a halo traction vest, which was removed after 3 months. At this time, flexion-extension X-rays were performed (Fig. 13.3).

The X-rays show appreciable deformity following the trauma. However, there was no abnormal movement of the segment on flexion or extension, and therefore the patient was discharged from clinical follow-up unless he developed further symptoms of pain, worsening deformity, or neurological deficit.

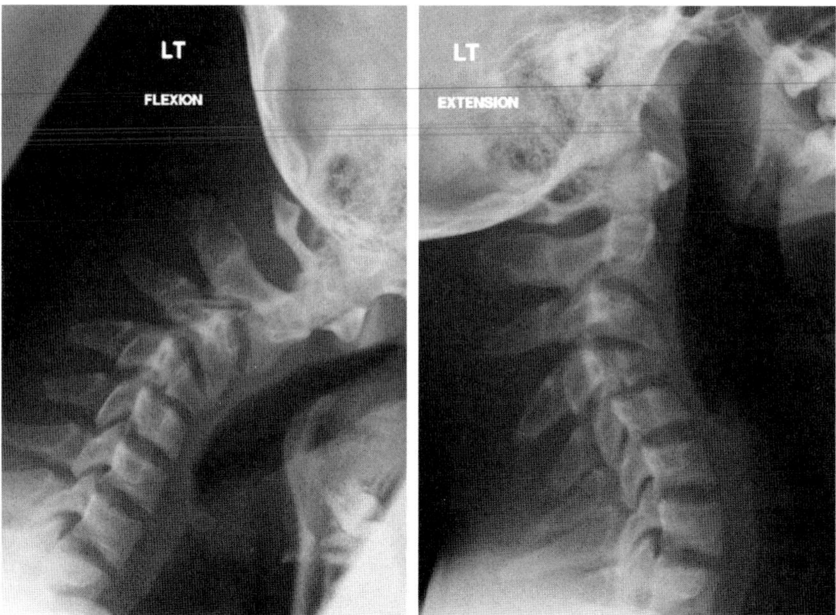

Fig. 13.3

Further reading

Kandziora F, Pflugmacher R, Scholz M, *et al.* (2005). Posterior stabilization of subaxial cervical spine trauma: indications and techniques. *Injury*; **36**: B36–43.

Lemons VR, Wagner FC Jr (1993). Stabilization of subaxial cervical spinal injuries. *Surg Neurol*; **39**: 511–18.

Case 14

A 27-year-old electrician was brought in by ambulance. He had been working at a height of around 3m but fell from a ladder to the ground. He does not know how he landed but had severe back pain and could not get up. The paramedics lifted him and immobilized his neck. On admission he was well with no neurological symptoms in his arms or legs. He has severe low back pain to palpation and to any movement. He has normal perineal sensation and is able to pass urine normally.

Question

1. Plain X-rays of the patient's spine are taken. The abnormal X-ray is shown in Fig. 14.1. Comment on the features and classify the injury. What are the next steps?

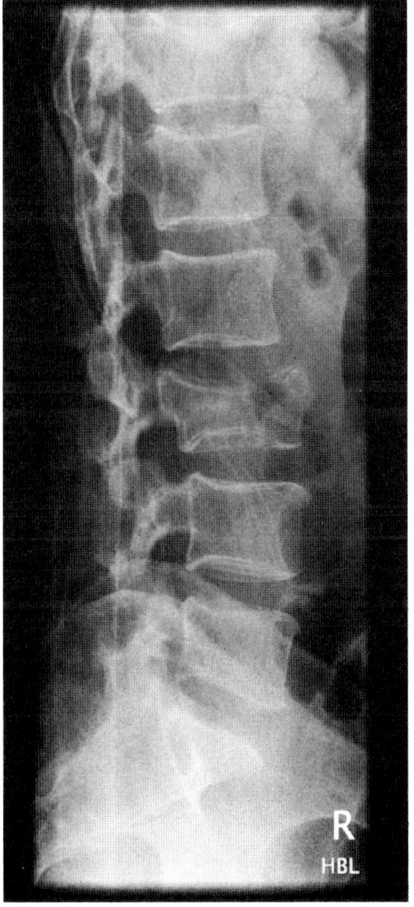

Fig. 14.1

Answer

1. Plain X-rays of the patient's spine are taken. The abnormal X-ray is shown in Fig. 14.1. Comment on the features and classify the injury. What are the next steps?

The X-ray shows an L3 fracture. There is loss of vertebral body height anteriorly and posteriorly. However, the posterior elements (pedicles, pars interarticularis, and facet joints) may be preserved. The spinal canal is narrowed, but is probably not critically compromised as confirmed by the patient's normal neurological status.

Thoracolumbar fractures were classified extensively by Denis (1984). Based on the mechanism of injury and proposed stability the thoracolumbar spine can be divided into three columns: anterior, including the anterior longitudinal ligament and the anterior half of the vertebral body; middle, including the posterior half of the vertebral body, posterior longitudinal ligament and posterior disc elements; posterior, including the facet joints and interspinous and interlaminar ligaments. Compromise of two of these three columns is typically an unstable injury, whilst compromise of one column only is typically a stable injury. This is an anterior and middle column injury—a 'burst' fracture of L3—and as such is probably unstable.

The patient should be kept flat and log-rolled with careful attention to pressure areas and DVT prophylaxis. Older patients are also at risk of pneumonia. A CT scan should be arranged to evaluate the fracture more completely. Whilst this is awaited, a secondary survey should be performed, particularly looking for injuries associated with burst fractures due to falls. These injuries are calcaneal fractures, pilon-type ankle fractures, hip fractures including central acetabular dislocation, and vertical shear injuries of the pelvis.

Question

2. What does the CT scan (Fig. 14.2) show? What are the management options now?

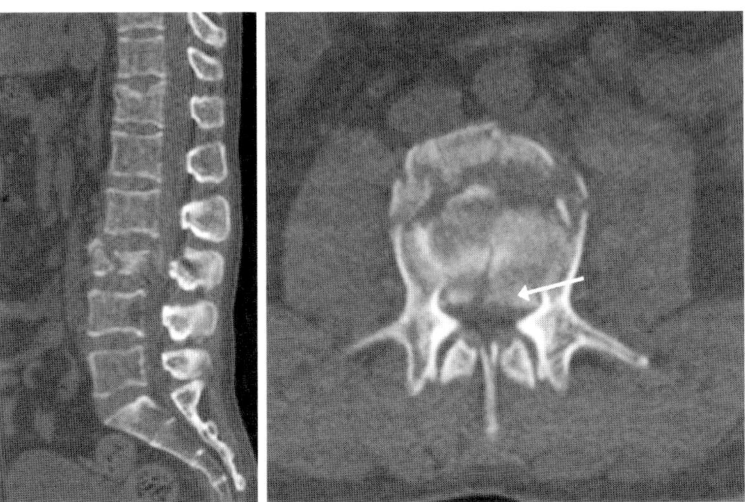

Fig. 14.2

Answer

2. What does the CT scan (Fig. 14.2) show? What are the management options now?

The CT scan confirms anterior, middle, and posterior column injury (the posterior column injury is a fracture through the spinous process of L3). A large bony fragment is retropulsed into the spinal canal (arrow). This is an unstable injury.

The management options are conservative or surgical. Conservative management would involve a period of several weeks' strict bed rest followed by cautious mobilization, perhaps with an external brace. If serial X-rays showed progressive angulation at this time or the patient developed neurological symptoms, he would require surgery. The prospects of conservative management being successful are probably low.

Surgical management would be internal fixation of the fracture with pedicle screws and rods. The vertebral body could reasonably be left to heal with the pedicle screw construct or could also be stabilized with a retroperitoneal approach to replace the fractured body with an expandable metal cage as shown in Fig. 14.3.

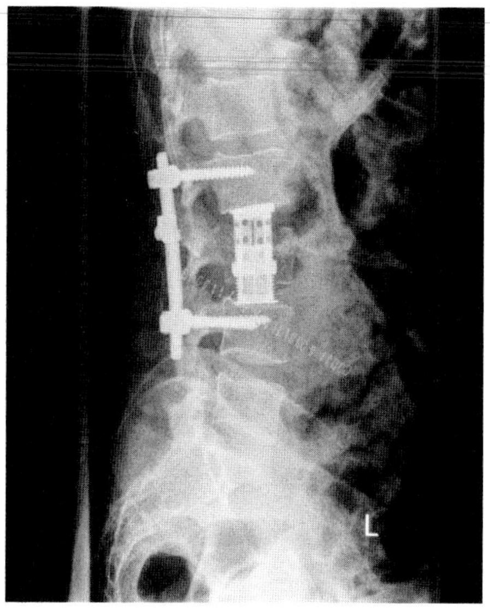

Fig. 14.3

Further reading

Aebi M (2010). Classification of thoracolumbar fractures and dislocations. *Eur Spine J*; **19** (Suppl 1): S2–7.

Ballock RT, Mackersie R, Abitbol JJ, Cervilla V, Resnick D, Garfin SR (1992). Can burst fractures be predicted from plain radiographs? *J Bone Joint Surg Br*; **74**: 147–50.

Denis F (1984). Spinal instability as defined by the three-column spine concept in acute spinal trauma. *Clin Orthop Relat Res*; **189**: 65–76.

Weinstein JN, Collalto P, Lehmann TR (1988). Thoracolumbar 'burst' fractures treated conservatively: a long-term follow-up. *Spine (Phila Pa 1976)*; **13**: 33–8.

Case 15

A 49-year-old builder was admitted to the emergency department. He had been drinking copiously with friends, and when he fell from the wall he was sitting on and did not get up they assumed that he was intoxicated and left him there. A few hours later he was in the same position and an ambulance was called.

On examination he smelled strongly of alcohol. There was facial bruising. He was not eye-opening and only verbalizing. He was not moving any of his limbs spontaneously, and responded weakly to supraorbital but not peripheral painful stimuli. Formal neurological examination was not possible. He was intubated and ventilated in view of the coma.

Questions

1. What is the differential diagnosis of his current condition?
2. A CT scan of head, chest, abdomen, and spine was performed in view of the history of trauma. What are the findings on the image shown in Fig. 15.1?
3. What is the immediate management? Is there a role for steroids?
4. An MRI was performed to establish prognosis, likely ventilator dependence, and potential instability (Fig. 15.2). What does it show and what is the prognosis?

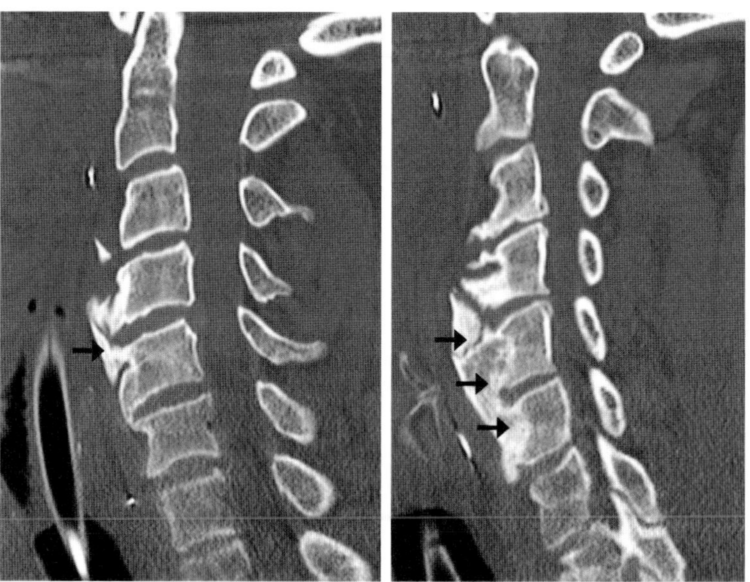

Fig. 15.1

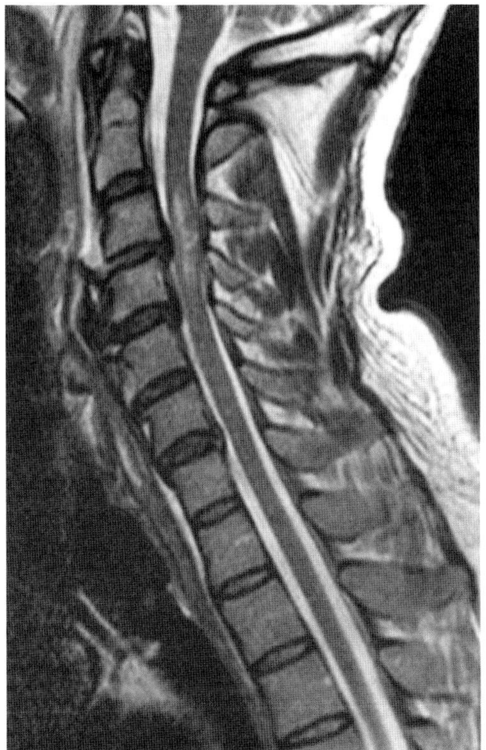

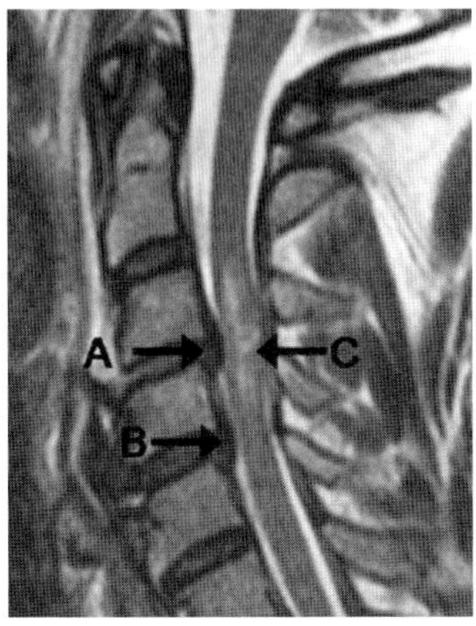

Fig. 15.2

Answers

1. What is the differential diagnosis of his current condition?

The differential diagnosis is wide, but based on the history there are two causative factors: alcohol intoxication and a head or spinal injury. Intracranial trauma is frequently associated with alcohol and therefore it is an error to ascribe coma to alcohol, especially after recent trauma.

2. A CT scan of head, chest, abdomen, and spine was performed in view of the history of trauma. What are the findings on the image shown in Fig. 15.1?

The CT scan shows normal alignment of the cervical vertebrae. The spinal canal is not compromised. However, there is a large osteophyte bridging C3 to C6 anteriorly (arrows) with at least two fracture lines through it. Therefore there has been a significant cervical spine injury, probably of a flexion–extension type, with the potential for cord injury at the time of the event.

3. What is the immediate management? Is there a role for steroids?

The immediate management is supportive. There is no lesion to mandate urgent surgery; the bony injury can be presumed to be unstable, and he should be maintained in a hard cervical collar and log-rolled for the time being. An associated spinal cord injury may be suspected from the findings of response to pain above the clavicles but not below, and an MRI will clarify this. The role of high-dose corticosteroids to reduce spinal cord oedema and improve outcome following acute spinal cord injury has been controversial, but recent meta-analyses suggest no benefit.

4. An MRI was performed to establish prognosis, likely ventilator dependence, and potential instability (Fig. 15.2). What does it show and what is the prognosis?

The MRI shows two modest disc bulges at C3/4 (A) and C4/5 (B). There is signal change in the spinal cord centred on C3/4 (C) with effacement of CSF and swelling of the cord. There is no high signal in the posterior interspinous ligaments, suggesting an absence of ligamentous injury. There is prevertebral soft tissue oedema/haemorrhage extending down from C1, around the anterior osteophytes at C3/4 and C4/5, and into the upper thoracic region. The diagnosis is traumatic spinal cord contusion in an area of pre-existing spinal canal stenosis exacerbated by minor instability due to fracture of bridging osteophytes.

The role of emergency surgery is unproven for acute cord injury such as this. Most surgeons would manage the patient conservatively in the first instance to allow physiological stabilization if there is associated spinal shock. Neurological recovery is often good after this type of injury, presumably because there has not been extensive disruption or compression of the spinal cord. A delayed decompression in a matter of weeks may be performed not to improve neurological recovery but to prevent a further episode.

Further reading

Furlan JC, Noonon V, Cadotte DW, Fehlings MG (2011). Timing of decompressive surgery of spinal cord after traumatic spinal cord injury: an evidence-based examination of pre-clinical and clinical studies. *J Neurotrauma*; **28**: 1371–99.

Hohl JB, Lee JY, Horton JA, Rihn JA (2010). A novel classification system for traumatic central cord syndrome: the Central Cord Injury Scale (CCIS). *Spine (Phila Pa 1976)*; **35**: E238–43.

Nowak DD, Lee JK, Gelb DE, Poelstra KA, Ludwig SC (2009). Central cord syndrome. *J Am Acad Orthop Surg*; **17**: 756–65.

Case 16

A 61-year-old man was referred by the emergency department at 10p.m. He had felt tired after lunch and gone for a walk, but noticed some tingling in his legs so returned home and fell asleep on the sofa. He woke up around 90 minutes later and was unable to feel or move his legs. He was eventually able to call an ambulance and was brought to hospital. His medical history was notable only for hepatitis C infection for which he was under surveillance. On examination he had no discernible power in his legs although his arms were normal. His lower limb reflexes were brisk with upgoing plantars. He had insensate urinary retention with a residual volume of 800mL.

Questions

1. What other features of the history and examination may be important?
2. There is no history of pain. He has a sensory level at the clavicles bilaterally and abdominal breathing. He undergoes an urgent MRI scan (Fig. 16.1). What does it show?
3. What is the underlying aetiology?
4. Is surgery indicated? What should be done?

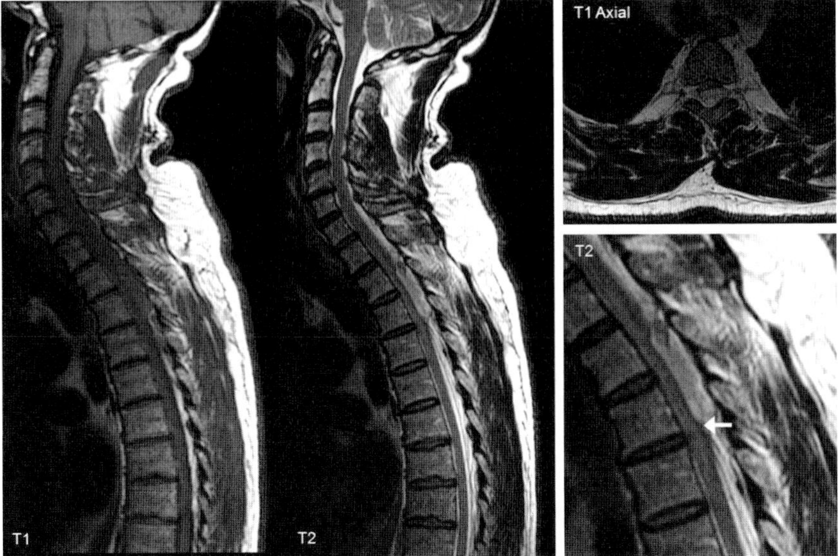

Fig. 16.1

Answers

1. What other features of the history and examination may be important?

There are other clues in the history that may be important. The presence of back pain either previously or during this episode might point to a destructive process such as a tumour or infection. However, the very short history is more in keeping with a vascular event. On examination the level of the sensory deficit may be an important localizing sign; the presence of abdominal breathing (deep inspiration causing an early excursion of the anterior abdominal wall due to intercostal paralysis but retained diaphragmatic function) suggests a high thoracic lesion.

2. There is no history of pain. He has a sensory level at the clavicles bilaterally and abdominal breathing. He undergoes an urgent MRI scan (Fig. 16.1). What does it show?

There is an extensive extra-axial lesion dorsally in the upper spine. It is thickest and most clearly defined at T2/3 where it compresses the spinal cord. Above and below it is ill-defined and effaces the normal high signal of fat on the T_1 sagittal scan from C4/5 to T4. Below the lesion the spinal dura is clearly visible, separating normal extradural fat from CSF in the spinal subarachnoid space. The dura can be traced up to the lesion, where it separates the lesion from the cord, confirming the extradural location of the lesion (arrow).

On T_2 imaging the lesion is slightly darker than CSF but brighter than the spinal cord, and it is slightly brighter than the cord on the T_1 scan. The appearance is typical of an acute spinal extradural haemorrhage. The blood would be very much brighter (similar to fat signal) if the scan were repeated after a few days. A tumour would usually be less extensive, better defined, and arise from bone. A spinal abscess could appear similar on unenhanced imaging, although there may be clinical suspicion and the scan may show associated discitis or paraspinal collection. Collections of pus or haemorrhage do not enhance centrally. An abscess is usually associated with more florid enhancement of surrounding membranes.

3. What is the underlying aetiology?

There is frequently no demonstrable aetiology in such cases. There are reports of spontaneous spinal extradural haematoma from arteriovenous malformations. However, these are usually diagnosed during surgery to remove the clot rather than angiographically before surgery. Surgery almost inevitably finds engorged dural vessels due to preoperative venous stasis, and the pathological importance of these is unclear. Anticoagulation is an important risk factor for spinal epidural haematoma (particularly the use of stronger antiplatelet agents such as clopidogrel). Given the patient's history of hepatitis C infection, a haematologist should be consulted before planning any surgery. Spontaneous or traumatic epidural haematoma can also occur in association with ankylosing spondylitis, often in association with small fractures in the fused spine.

4. Is surgery indicated? What should be done?

Clinically, the patient has a complete spinal cord injury at the affected level. This may not recover and he should be counselled preoperatively that this is a possibility. However, given his current state there is little to be lost with surgery apart from the risks of haemorrhage and infection. His blood results were normal with INR 1.0 and normal liver function tests. The haematologists advised reactive rather than prophylactic use of clotting factors. Therefore he underwent a laminectomy at T2/3 and evacuation of the haematoma. During surgery a little more bleeding was encountered than might normally have been expected, but no abnormal vessels were seen and no transfusion or clotting products were needed.

Further reading

Al-Mutair A, Bednar DA (2010). Spinal epidural hematoma. *J Am Acad Orthop Surg*; **18**: 494–502.

Liao CC, Hsieh PC, Lin TK, Lin CL, Lo YL, Lee SC (2009). Surgical treatment of spontaneous spinal epidural hematoma: a 5-year experience. *J Neurosurg Spine* **11**: 480–6.

Morales Ciancio RA, Drain O, Rillardon L, Guigui P (2008). Acute spontaneous spinal epidural hematoma: an important differential diagnosis in patients under clopidogrel therapy. *Spine J*; **8**: 544–7.

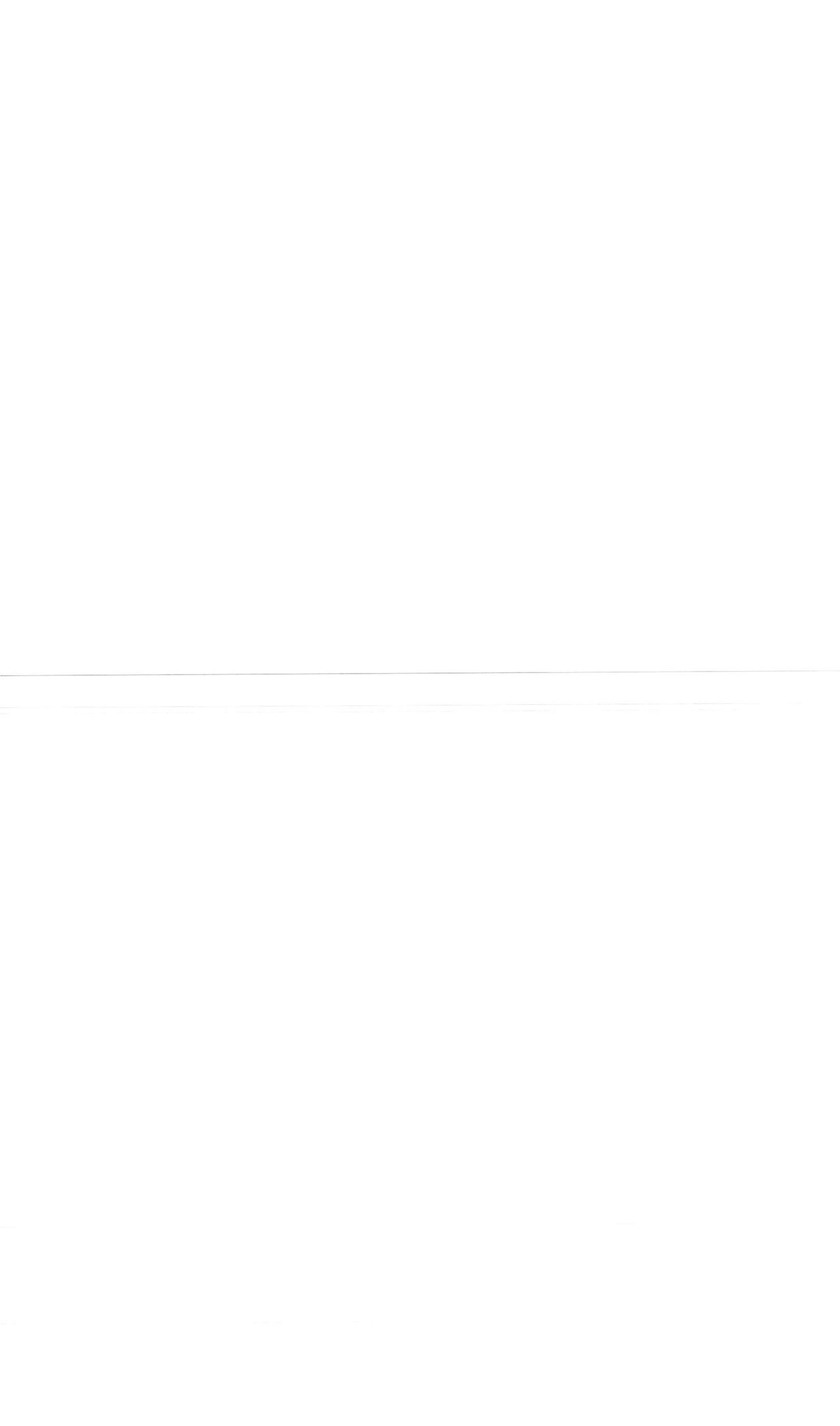

Section 3

Vascular neurosurgery

Question

An MR angiogram of the Circle of Willis is shown here (Fig. 17.1). Identify the labelled structures.

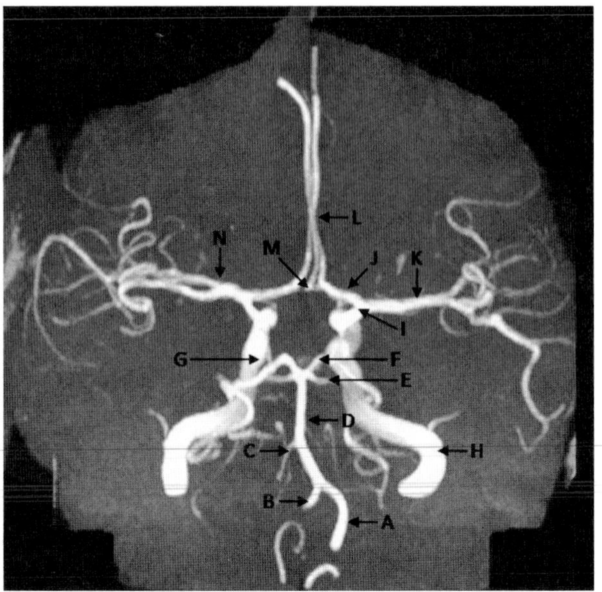

Fig. 17.1

Answer

A = Left vertebral artery; B = Right vertebral artery; C = Right anterior inferior cerebellar artery (AICA); D = Basilar artery; E = Superior cerebellar artery (SCA); F = Left posterior cerebral artery (PCA); G = Arrowhead on the right internal carotid artery (ICA): the right posterior communicating artery (PCom) can be seen branching off the right PCA and advancing anteriorly past the tip of the arrow; H = Left internal carotid artery; I = Left internal carotid artery at the bifurcation into the anterior cerebral and middle cerebral arteries; J = Left anterior cerebral artery (ACA); A1 segment (proximal to anterior communicating artery); K = Left middle cerebral artery (MCA); M1 segment (proximal to bifurcation); L = Anterior cerebral arteries; A2 segment (distal to anterior communicating artery); M = Anterior communicating artery (ACom); N = Bifurcation of right middle cerebral artery. The posterior inferior cerebellar artery (PICA) (not shown in this image) usually branches off the distal part of the vertebral arteries.

Case 17

A 64-year-old man presented to the emergency department after experiencing a severe headache which began suddenly when he was watching TV. He felt nauseous and had vomited several times. At hospital, his GCS was 14/15 (E3, V5, M6), and his pupils were equal and reactive, with no focal neurological deficits. He had a history of hypertension and his blood pressure was 181/122mmHg.

Questions

1. What is the differential diagnosis, and what investigation should be performed?
2. The CT is shown in Fig. 17.2. What is the diagnosis? Identify the arrowed features on the scan.

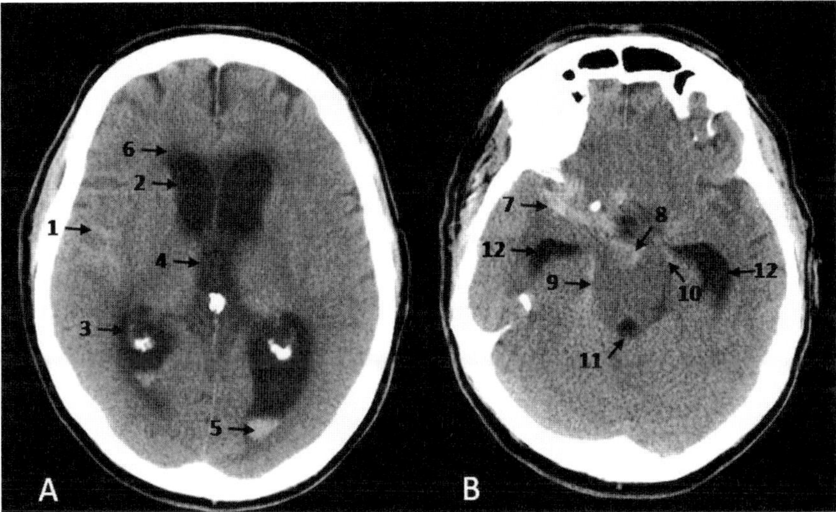

Fig. 17.2

Answers

1. What is the differential diagnosis, and what investigation should be performed?

The differential diagnosis for a severe sudden onset headache includes any variety of intracranial haemorrhage (subarachnoid haemorrhage (SAH), intracerebral haemorrhage, pituitary apoplexy) and migraine. Intracerebral haemorrhage is usually accompanied by lateralizing signs. A CT scan should be performed urgently to exclude intracranial haemorrhage.

2. The CT scan is shown in Fig. 17.2. What is the diagnosis? Identify the arrowed features on the scan.

The diagnosis is subarachnoid haemorrhage.

- Upper slice (A). Blood is seen in the sulci (1), indicating SAH. The frontal (2) and occipital (3) horns of the lateral ventricles are dilated, as is the third ventricle (4). There is intraventricular blood (5). The low-density area around the frontal horns represents transependymal flow (6) due to acute hydrocephalus.
- Lower slice (B). Blood is seen mainly in the right sylvian fissure (7) and also in the interpeduncular cistern (8) and the right (9) and left (10) ambient cisterns. The quadrigeminal cistern (11) appears to be clear of blood. The temporal horns of the lateral ventricles are dilated (12).

Questions

3. What are the causes of subarachnoid haemorrhage? What is the likely cause in this patient?
4. What is the grade of subarachnoid haemorrhage in this patient?
5. What are the general measures that need to be instituted for a patient with aneurysmal subarachnoid haemorrhage, and what are the specific management issues in this case?
6. The following day a catheter angiogram was performed. Fig. 17.3 shows a right internal carotid artery injection. Identify the structures labelled A to E.
7. How would the management of this case have changed had the CT and CTA appearances been as shown in Fig. 17.4?

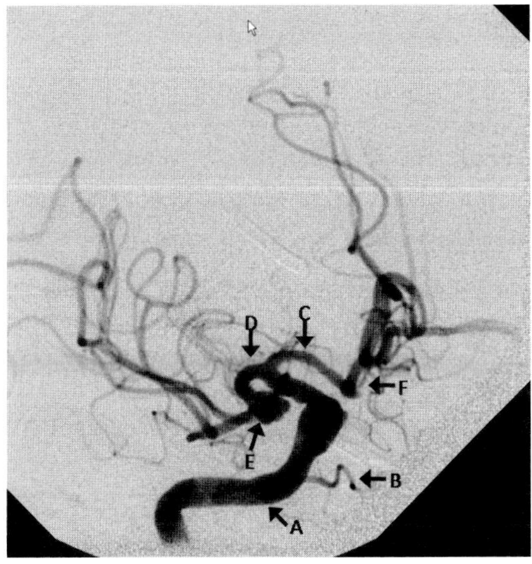

Fig. 17.3

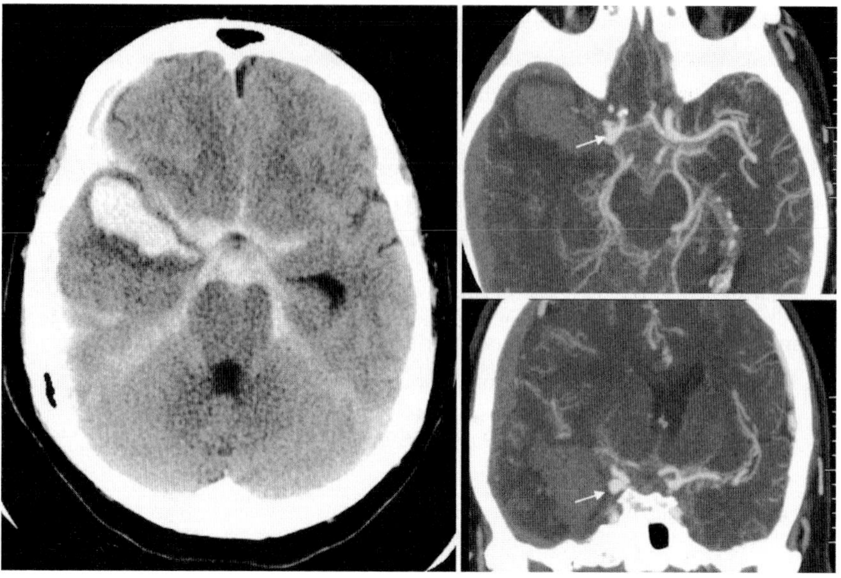

Fig. 17.4

Answers

3. What are the causes of subarachnoid haemorrhage? What is the likely cause in this patient?

Although trauma is a common cause of subarachnoid bleeding, the most common cause of spontaneous SAH is a ruptured cerebral aneurysm, responsible in approximately 70% of cases. Other causes include arteriovenous malformations (5–10%) and rarely vasculitis such as that seen in sickle cell disease or moyamoya disease. In approximately 15–20% of patients all investigations, including catheter angiography, prove negative. In this case the asymmetrical blood distribution is highly suspicious of a ruptured aneurysm on the right middle cerebral, posterior communicating or internal carotid artery (see Fig. 17.5).

4. What is the grade of subarachnoid haemorrhage in this patient?

The patient is currently WFNS grade 2. However, there is hydrocephalus, and the WFNS grade should be applied after the treatment of hydrocephalus if a prognostic value is sought (see 'Grading of subarachnoid haemorrhage', p. 126).

5. What are the general measures that need to be instituted for a patient with aneurysmal subarachnoid haemorrhage, and what are the specific management issues in this case?

The principles of management of patients with SAH are in parallel to support the patient, optimizing cerebral perfusion, and to identify the aneurysm and secure it, by endovascular coiling or craniotomy and clipping, in a timely manner to prevent rebleeding. This should be performed within 48 hours of the ictus.

General measures include:

- management in a high dependency or intensive care setting with frequent neurological observations
- bed rest to minimize fluctuations in blood pressure
- laboratory tests including full blood count, electrolytes, clotting, and grouping
- analgesia, typically paracetamol and codeine
- laxatives to reduce straining
- prophylaxis from DVT with compression stockings or boots (heparin after treatment of the aneurysm if no further surgery is likely)
- adequate hydration (e.g. 3L per day) to reduce risk of volume depletion and cerebral ischaemia
- chest X-ray to exclude neurogenic pulmonary oedema
- ECG to detect myocardial damage
- nimodipine 60mg every 4 hours (po/ng) and a statin for 21 days (see 'Vasospasm and delayed cerebral ischaemia', p. 139)
- specific measures to improve cerebral perfusion may be indicated, such as CSF diversion or haematoma evacuation to reduce intracranial pressure
- cerebral angiography to look for an aneurysm.

The specific issues in this case are as follows.

Management of blood pressure

Patients with SAH often present with an elevated blood pressure. The risk of rupture of aneurysm from maintaining a high blood pressure must be balanced against the risk of ischaemia from lowering the blood pressure. In general, blood pressure should not be aggressively controlled in the acute setting.

Management of hydrocephalus

There is marked hydrocephalus, which could be contributing to the poor neurological state. Therefore immediate CSF diversion is indicated in this patient. The options for drainage are lumbar puncture (LP), lumbar drain, and external ventricular drain (EVD). The first two options are relatively contraindicated in the presence of a mass effect or obstructive hydrocephalus (see 'Lumbar puncture and the risk of coning', p. 167). Otherwise, there is no clear evidence favouring one method over another. LPs carry lower morbidity, but an EVD may be preferable if there is a high blood load to allow controlled drainage of CSF and if there is intraventricular blood which could block CSF flow through the ventricles and hence cause an obstructive hydrocephalus (see 'CSF circulation and hydrocephalus', p. 360). An EVD was placed in this patient.

6. The following day a catheter angiogram was performed. Fig. 17.3 shows a right internal carotid artery injection. Identify the structures labelled A–E.

A = internal carotid artery

B = ophthalmic artery

C = anterior cerebral artery, A1 segment

D = middle cerebral artery, M1 segment

E = aneurysm

F = anterior cerebral artery, A2 segment

At angiography, it was noted that the aneurysm had a broad base and that the superior and inferior divisions of the middle cerebral artery arose from the aneurysm sac. Therefore it was determined that this aneurysm was unsuitable for coiling, and the patient proceeded to craniotomy and clipping of the aneurysm (see 'Coiling versus clipping of cerebral aneurysms', p. 127). The patient made a good recovery but remained intermittently confused. He was discharged to a neurorehabilitation centre.

7. How would the management of this case have changed had the CT and CTA appearances been as shown in Fig. 17.4?

Fig. 17.4 shows, in addition to the subarachnoid blood, a right temporal intracerebral haematoma and an acute subdural haematoma. There is appreciable midline shift. Evacuation of the haematoma is necessary as it is likely to compromise cerebral perfusion. However, the haematoma has arisen directly from the aneurysm, and therefore surgery to evacuate it risks re-rupturing the aneurysm and should be undertaken with this in mind. The CTA confirms a PCom aneurysm at the base of the haematoma (arrow).The options are either to evacuate the haematoma and clip the aneurysm at the same time or to undertake emergency coiling of the aneurysm and proceed to craniotomy and haematoma evacuation under the same anaesthetic, after the aneurysm is secured.

Further reading

Giussani C, Mejdoubi M, Tremoulet M, Roux FE (2008). The role of surgery when endovascular treatment is considered the first choice therapy for ruptured intracranial aneurysms. *J Neurosurg Sci*; **52**: 61–9.

Nowak G, Schwachenwald D, Schwachenwald R, Kehler U, Müller H, Arnold H (1998). Intracerebral hematomas caused by aneurysm rupture. Experience with 67 cases. *Neurosurg Rev*; **21**: 5–9.

Rabinstein AA, Lanzino G, Wijdicks EFM (2010). Multidisciplinary management and emerging therapeutic strategies in aneurysmal subarachnoid haemorrhage. *Lancet Neurol*; **9**: 504–19.

Yoshimoto Y, Wakai S, Satoh A, Hirose Y (1999). Intraparenchymal and intrasylvian haematomas secondary to ruptured middle cerebral artery aneurysms: prognostic factors and therapeutic considerations. *Br J Neurosurg*; **131**: 18–24.

Patterns on bleeding in aneurysmal subarachnoid haemorrhage

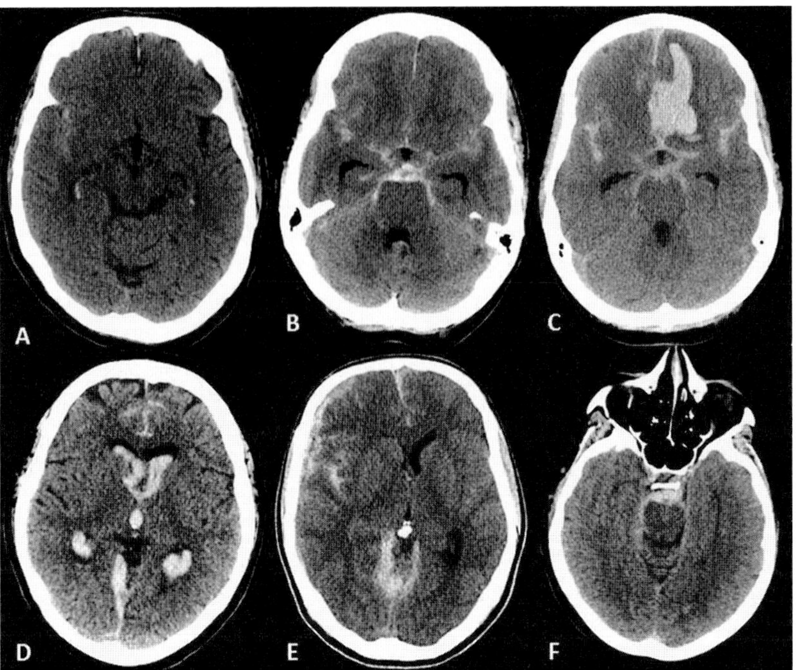

Scan	Location of blood	Likely aneurysm location
A	Sylvian fissure	MCA
B	Basal cisterns	Basilar artery, SCA, PCom
C	Interhemispheric Frontal lobe	ACom, ACA
D	Intraventricular	ACom (through lamina terminalis) Basilar artery (through 3rd ventricle) PICA (through 4th ventricle)
E	Subdural haemorrhage	PCom, ACom (through arachnoid)
F	Perimesencephalic (around brainstem)	Non-aneurysmal (e.g. bleed from pontine vein)

MCA=Middle cerebral artery; SCA=superior cerebellar artery; PCom=posterior communicating artery; ACom=anterior communicating artery; ACA=anterior cerebral artery

Fig. 17.5 Patterns of bleeding in aneurysmal subarachnoid haemorrhage. The location of blood is predictive for the site of the ruptured aneurysm in around 80% of SAH patients. Even in those with apparently 'diffuse' SAH this is often a predictor for a midline or near midline aneurysm such as ACom or PCom. Pattern F is the perimesencephalic distribution of SAH. These patients present as a typical SAH but are usually less distressed and less neurologically disabled. Angiography is usually normal and the bleed is usually considered to be venous, requiring no further treatment.

Grading of subarachnoid haemorrhage

Subarachnoid haemorrhage grading systems are based on clinical or radiological criteria and are useful in determining and communicating the severity of disease among health professionals. Two commonly used scales are described here.

Fisher grading

Fisher *et al.* (1980) used the amount of blood seen on the initial CT scan to predict the subsequent risk of radiological vasospasm (Table 17.1). Patients with thick clots in cisterns or fissures (Fisher grade 3) were most likely to develop vasospasm. The original study was performed using an early CT scanner (EMI 1005) with 16mm axial slices and images printed on film. The blood on the scans was measured using a ruler on the printed films, and Fisher and colleagues acknowledge that their measurements are only applicable to images obtained on their scanner, although they can be translated to other models with appropriate adjustments. One other major shortcoming was that a patient could be classified into more than one grade. A patient with thick subarachnoid blood with an intraventricular clot could be graded as 3 or 4. These and other problems with the original scale have led to modifications being proposed (e.g. Frontera *et al.* 2006 (Table 17.2)).

Table 17.1 Original Fisher scale (Fisher *et al.* 1980)

Fisher grade	Amount of blood on CT scan
1	None
2	Diffuse or thin layer of blood with all vertical layers (vertical fissures or cisterns: inter-hemispheric fissure, insular cistern, and ambient cisterns) <1mm thick
3	>1mm in vertical fissures or cisterns/localized clot
4	Diffuse or no subarachnoid blood, but with intracerebral or intraventricular clots

Table 17.2 Modified Fisher scale (Frontera *et al.* 2006)

Modified Fisher grade	Amount of blood on CT scan
0	None
1	Focal or diffuse thin SAH, no IVH
2	Focal or diffuse thin SAH, with IVH
3	Focal or diffuse thick SAH, no IVH
4	Focal or diffuse thick SAH, with IVH

SAH, subarachnoid haemorrhage; IVH, intraventricular haemorrhage; focal/diffuse/thick/thin, not explicitly defined.

(continued)

Grading of subarachnoid haemorrhage *(continued)*

WFNS (World Federation of Neurological Surgeons) grading

The WFNS grading system (WFNS 1988) (Table 17.3) is based on the Glasgow Coma Scale and shares its benefits and limitations (see 'Glasgow Coma Scale and Coma Score', p. 196). Despite being widely used, it is not uniformly applied, with some clinicians assigning a single score to a patient based on the best pre-treatment (of aneurysm) score on which to base prognosis, whilst others use it to describe the clinical severity of disease at various points in time (e.g. WFNS 3 on admission, WFNS 1 after EVD placement).

Table 17.3 WFNS grading scale (WFNS 1988)

WFNS grade	GCS
1	15
2	13–14, no focal neurological deficit
3	13–14, with focal neurological deficit
4	7–12
5	3–6

NB: A patient who is alert and orientated (GCS 15/15) but has a focal neurological deficit (e.g. a hemiparesis) is classified as grade 3. Reproduced with permission from World Federation of Neurological Societies.

Coiling versus clipping of cerebral aneurysms

Craniotomy and clipping of the aneurysm has been the traditional method of securing an aneurysm. Coil embolization was introduced in the 1990s as an alternative method to secure aneurysms. In the UK, coiling is performed by radiologists, but in many other parts of the world both clipping and coiling are performed by neurosurgeons. The controversial International Subarachnoid Haemorrhage Trial (ISAT) (Molyneux *et al.* 2002) demonstrated that for a selected population (good grade, anterior circulation aneurysms suitable for both coiling and clipping and for which there was uncertainty about the best mode of treatment) coiling was associated with a lower risk of dependency or death at 1 year (relative/absolute risk reduction in dependency (modified Rankin score of 3–6) or death at 1 year of 22.6%/6.9%, respectively). This difference was not seen at 5 years (Molyneux *et al.* 2009; Bakker *et al.* 2010; Raper and Allan 2010). There are many factors that make a particular aneurysm more suitable for coiling or clipping, and treatment decisions should be made on an individual basis by a multidisciplinary team (neurologist, radiologist, and neurosurgeon) depending on the location and configuration of the aneurysm and patient characteristics (Table 17.4).

(continued)

Coiling versus clipping of cerebral aneurysms *(continued)*

Table 17.4 Factors that influence whether an aneurysm is best managed with clipping or with coiling

Favours coiling	Favours clipping
◆ Posterior circulation aneurysms (relatively difficult to access surgically) ◆ Poor-grade patients ◆ Elderly ◆ Presence of medical comorbidities ◆ Raised intracranial pressure	◆ Wide necked aneurysms ◆ Aneurysms incorporating branching arteries ◆ Coexisting haematoma requiring evacuation ◆ Acute brainstem compression

References

Bakker NA, Metzemaekers JDM, Groen RJM, *et al.* (2010) International Subarachnoid Aneurysm Trial 2009: endovascular coiling of ruptured intracranial aneurysms has no significant advantage over neurosurgical clipping. *Neurosurgery*; **66**: 961–2.

Fisher CM, Kistler JP, Davis JM (1980). Relation of cerebral vasospasm to subarachnoid hemorrhage visualized by CT scanning. *Neurosurgery*; **6**: 1–9.

Frontera JA, Claassen J, Schmidt JM, *et al.* (2006). Prediction of symptomatic vasospasm after subarachnoid hemorrhage: the modified Fisher scale. *Neurosurgery*; **59**: 21–7.

Molyneux A, Kerr R, Stratton I, *et al.* (2002). International Subarachnoid Aneurysm Trial (ISAT) Collaborative Group: International Subarachnoid Aneurysm Trial (ISAT) of neurosurgical clipping versus endovascular coiling in 2143 patients with ruptured intracranial aneurysms: a randomised trial. *Lancet*; **360**:1267–74.

Molyneux AJ, Kerr RSC, Birks J, *et al.* (2009). Risk of recurrent subarachnoid haemorrhage, death, or dependence and standardised mortality ratios after clipping or coiling of an intracranial aneurysm in the International Subarachnoid Aneurysm Trial (ISAT): long-term follow-up. *Lancet Neurol*; **8**: 427–33.

Raper DMS, Allan R (2010). International Subarachnoid Trial in the long run: critical evaluation of the long-term follow-up data from the ISAT Trial of clipping vs coiling for ruptured intracranial aneurysms. *Neurosurgery*; **66**: 1166–9.

WFNS (World Federation of Neurological Surgeons) (1988). Report of World Federation of Neurological Surgeons Committee on a universal subarachnoid hemorrhage grading scale. *J Neurosurg*; **68**: 6.

Case 18

A 49-year-old woman presented to hospital having suffered a sudden-onset severe headache 6 days previously. She felt nauseous at the time of the headache, although she did not vomit. The headache reached maximum intensity 24 hours after onset and then eased, but has persisted. Three days prior to admission she noticed that her left eyelid was drooping. She attended her general practitioner who arranged for her to be seen in the emergency department. On examination, she was alert and orientated (GCS 15/15). Her left eyelid was closed and she could not open it. When the eyelid was lifted, the left pupil was dilated and the eye was found to be looking down and out. No other neurological deficits were found.

Questions

1. Explain the clinical signs.
2. What is the differential diagnosis, and which investigations should be performed?
3. A CT scan is performed (Fig. 18.1). What does it show, and what should be done?

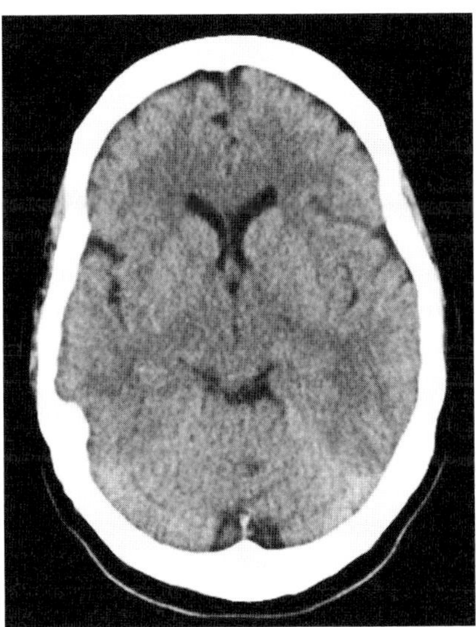

Fig. 18.1

Answers

1. Explain the clinical signs.

The patient has a left oculomotor (third) nerve palsy. The motor portion of the third nerve supplies the levator palpebrae superioris and the extraocular muscles except the lateral rectus and superior oblique. The parasympathetic part of the third nerve supplies the sphincter pupillae muscle in the iris. Therefore denervation of this nerve leads to ptosis, mydriasis (dilation of pupil), and an eye that looks down (due to unopposed superior oblique) and out (due to unopposed lateral rectus) (see 'Assessment of eye movements', p. 140).

2. What is the differential diagnosis, and which investigations should be performed?

The differential diagnosis includes any lesion affecting the third nerve. However, with the history of a sudden-onset severe headache, the priority is to exclude a SAH from an aneurysm compressing the third nerve. Another less common cause of sudden-onset headache with a third nerve palsy is pituitary apoplexy. In this case the intracavernous segment of the third nerve is compressed by the expanding pituitary mass.

The sensitivity of CT for blood in the first 24 hours after SAH is about 95%. This decreases to about 70% after 3 days. At 6 days post ictus, a CT scan is not sensitive enough to detect SAH. However, in most hospitals CT is the most readily available investigation and it should still be performed first to exclude other potential intracranial pathology responsible for the headache.

3. A CT scan is performed (Fig. 18.1). What does it show, and what should be done?

The scan is normal. The pituitary fossa is not seen on this slice, but this was also normal. A lumbar puncture (LP) may be performed to exclude SAH, although it would be reasonable to proceed directly to cerebral angiography as an aneurysm, if found, will require urgent treatment in this context (with headache and a third nerve palsy) whether or not it has bled.

Questions

4. When should the LP be performed, and for what reason?
5. How should this patient be managed until the result of the LP is available?
6. The LP confirms subarachnoid haemorrhage and a catheter angiogram is performed (Fig. 18.2). Identify the structures labelled A to F. Where is the aneurysm?
7. Explain how a posterior communicating artery aneurysm can cause a third nerve palsy. Which other aneurysms can cause a third nerve palsy?

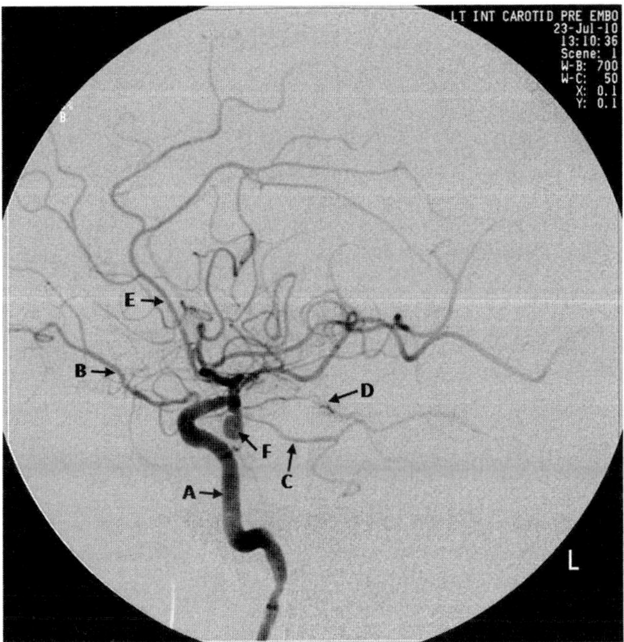

Fig. 18.2

Answers

4. When should the LP be performed, and for what reason?

The timing of the LP depends on which diagnostic test for SAH is being used. Spectrophotometry is commonly used in the UK, in which a positive result (i.e. diagnosis of SAH) rests on the detection of bilirubin in the CSF. In this case, the LP should be performed after 12 hours of headache onset, as it takes up to 12 hours for bilirubin to be reliably detected in the CSF after the time of haemorrhage (see 'The use of lumbar puncture in the diagnosis of subarachnoid haemorrhage', p. 141).

5. How should this patient be managed until the result of the LP is available?

The standard medical treatment for SAH should be applied pending the results of the LP (see Case 17).

6. The LP confirms subarachnoid haemorrhage and a catheter angiogram is performed (Fig. 18.2). Identify the structures labelled A–F. Where is the aneurysm?

A = internal carotid artery

B = ophthalmic artery

C = posterior cerebral artery

D = anterior choroidal artery

E = anterior cerebral artery

F = aneurysm, which arises from the posterior communicating artery.

7. Explain how a posterior communicating artery aneurysm can cause a third nerve palsy. Which other aneurysms can cause a third nerve palsy?

The paired oculomotor nerves exit the midbrain anteriorly. They lie between the posterior cerebral artery above and the superior cerebellar artery below, either side of the basilar artery. They then pass forward, via the lateral wall of the cavernous sinus, to enter the orbit via the superior orbital fissure. The third nerve passes by the point where the posterior communicating artery branches off the internal carotid, the site of origin of most posterior communicating artery aneurysms (Fig. 18.3). Superior cerebellar artery and basilar tip aneurysms can also present with a third nerve palsy, as can aneurysms of the internal carotid artery within the cavernous sinus.

The patient underwent coil embolization of the aneurysm. The post-procedure angiogram (Fig. 18.4) shows obliteration of the aneurysm, just visible as a subtraction artefact.

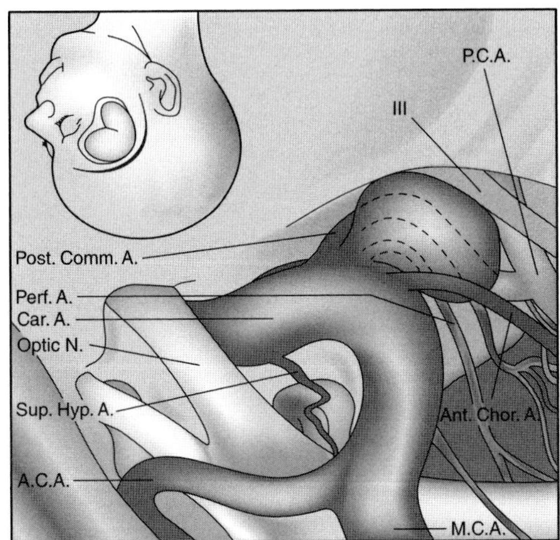

Fig. 18.3 Relationship of the oculomotor nerve to posterior communicating artery aneurysms. Adapted with permission from *Neurosurgery* 2002 Oct; **51**(4 Suppl): S121–58. © Lippencott, Williams & Wilkins, 2002.

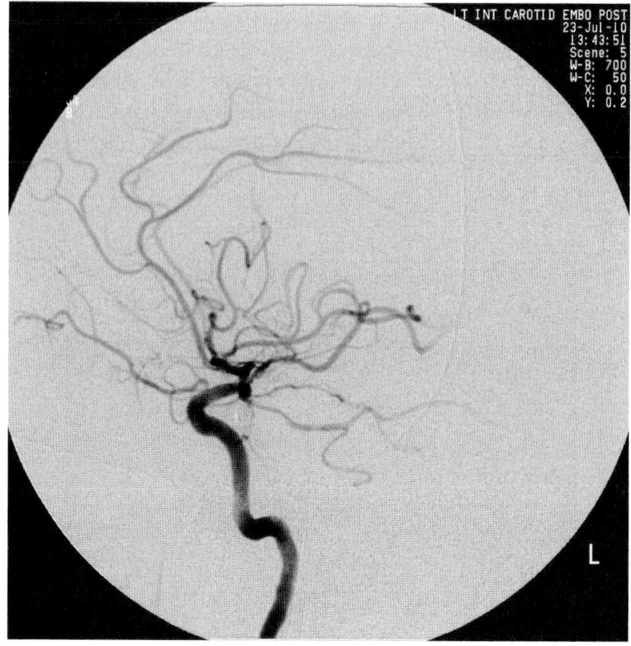
LT INT CAROTID EMBO POST
23-Jul-10
13:43:51
Scene: 5
W-B: 700
W-C: 50
X: 0.0
Y: 0.2
L

Fig. 18.4

Questions

8. The patient makes a good recovery and returns to the ward with no neurological deficits. Twelve hours later, you are informed that the patient has deteriorated. On examination, the patient is drowsy, and her GCS is 11/15 (E3, V3, M5).
   (a) What are the common causes of deterioration in this scenario?
   (b) How should the patient be managed?
9. A CT is performed (Fig. 18.5). Describe the findings on the scan and features A–F.
10. Explain what has happened. What should be done now?

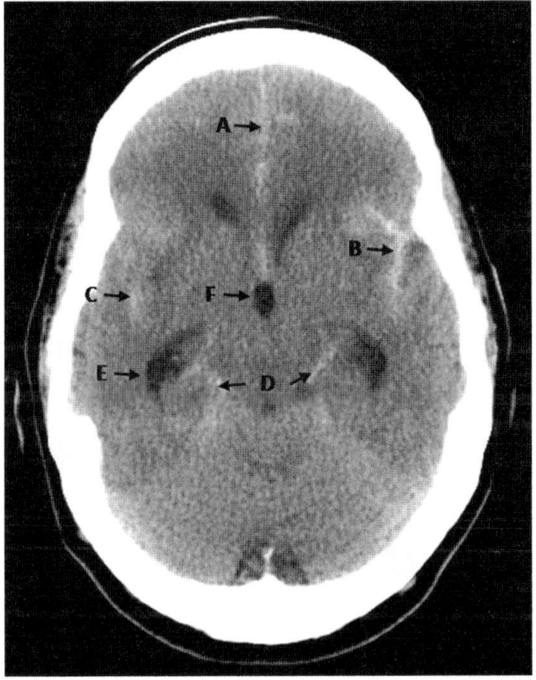

Fig. 18.5

Answers

8. The patient makes a good recovery and returns to the ward with no neurological deficits. Twelve hours later, you are informed the patient has deteriorated. On examination, the patient is drowsy and her GCS is 11/15 (E3, V3, M5).

(a) What are the common causes of deterioration in this scenario?

The common causes for neurological deterioration after SAH are:

- re-bleed from aneurysm (unlikely in this scenario as the aneurysm has been secured)
- vasospasm
- hyponatraemia
- hydrocephalus
- seizures
- hospital-acquired infections.

(b) How should the patient be managed?

After ensuring that the patient's airway is safe and that blood pressure and oxygenation are stable, the patient requires an urgent CT scan and a blood test to include electrolytes and inflammatory markers. Adequate hydration should be ensured as dehydration increases the risk of vasospasm.

9. A CT is performed (Fig. 18.5). Describe the findings on the scan and features A–F.

Blood is seen in the inter-hemispheric fissure (A), both sylvian fissures, left (B) more than right (C), and both ambient cisterns (D). There is hydrocephalus, indicated by enlargement of the temporal horns of the lateral ventricles (E) and dilation of the third ventricle (F).

10. Explain what has happened. What should be done now?

The presence of subarachnoid blood on this scan confirms that the patient has re-bled (as the CT scan on admission was normal). This may have occurred from the aneurysm that was treated, or from a separate aneurysm that was not identified on initial imaging. The patient should have urgent repeat angiography to determine whether the treated aneurysm is secure and also to look for additional aneurysms. The repeat angiogram in this patient showed that the treated aneurysm was apparently secure and no additional vascular abnormalities were demonstrated. The patient proceeded to a craniotomy and a small remnant of the aneurysm neck, which was not seen on angiography, was found. This was clipped.

Questions

11. The day after surgery, you are alerted as the patient has developed left sided weakness. On examination, the patient is drowsy with a GCS of 11/15 (E3, V3, M5). There is partial ptosis of the left eyelid. The pupils are both reactive; the left is size 4 and the right is size 3. There is grade 4/5 weakness in the left arm and leg. What are the potential causes of deterioration?
12. The patient has a CT scan, which shows no new changes.
    (a) What is the diagnosis?
    (b) How should the patient be managed?

Answers

11. The day after surgery, you are alerted as the patient has developed left-sided weakness. On examination, the patient is drowsy with a GCS of 11/15 (E3, V3, M5). There is partial ptosis of the left eyelid. The pupils are both reactive; the left is size 4 and the right is size 3. There is grade 4/5 weakness in the left arm and leg. What are the potential causes of deterioration?

The causes of neurological deterioration listed in Answer 6 apply to any deteriorating patient with SAH. However, the presence of lateralizing signs in this scenario make hyponatraemia, hydrocephalus, and hospital-acquired infections relatively less likely. Additionally, a postoperative haematoma requires consideration in this scenario as the patient has just had a craniotomy, and an urgent CT scan should be performed to exclude this.

12. The patient has a CT scan which shows no new changes.

(a) What is the diagnosis?

The CT scan excludes postoperative haematoma and a re-bleed. Therefore the likely diagnosis is delayed cerebral ischaemia (DCI) due to vasospasm.

(b) How should the patient be managed?

Treatment strategies for DCI are controversial and vary considerably, but have traditionally been based on volume resuscitation and induced hypertension (see 'Vasospasm and delayed cerebral ischaemia', p. 139).

Further reading

Bederson JB, Connolly ES, Batjer HH, *et al.* (2009). Guidelines for the management of aneurysmal subarachnoid hemorrhage. *Stroke*; **40**: 994–1025.

Bhatia R, Hughes D, Crocker M, Strong AJ (2006). Aneurysmal subarachnoid haemorrhage in a patient with thyrotoxicosis. *Br J Neurosurg*; **20**: 165–8.

Dankbaar JW, de Rooij NK, Velthuis BK, Frijns CJ, Rinkel GJ, van der Schaaf IC (2009). Diagnosing delayed cerebral ischemia with different CT modalities in patients with subarachnoid hemorrhage with clinical deterioration. *Stroke*; **40**: 3493–8.

Dorhout Mees SM, Rinkel GJ, Feigin VL, *et al.* (2007). Calcium antagonists for aneurysmal subarachnoid haemorrhage. *Cochrane Database Syst Rev*; **18**: CD000277.

Edlow JA, Caplan LR (2000). Avoiding pitfalls in the diagnosis of subarachnoid haemorrhage. *N Engl J Med*; **342**: 29–36.

Kassell NF, Sasaki T, Colohan AR, Nazar G (1985). Cerebral vasospasm following aneurysmal subarachnoid hemorrhage. *Stroke*; **16**: 562–72.

Lazaridis C, Naval N (2010). Risk factors and medical management of vasospasm after subarachnoid hemorrhage. *Neurosurg Clin N Am*; **21**: 353–64.

van Gijn J, Rinkel GJE (2005). How To Do It. Investigate the CSF in a patient with sudden headache and a normal CT brain scan. *Pract Neurol*; **5**: 362–5.

Vasospasm and delayed cerebral ischaemia

Vasospasm refers to the spasm or narrowing of the cerebral vasculature that may follow SAH. It is often seen in aneurysmal SAH but is rare in non-aneurysmal SAH (including traumatic SAH, perimesencephalic SAH, and SAH from vascular malformations). The cause of vasospasm is not clearly established, although various endothelial mediators are thought to play a role. Radiological vasospasm (vasospasm seen on angiography (Fig. 18.6) is reported to occur in up to 70% of patients with aneurysmal SAH and may or may not lead to a clinically detectable neurological deficit. The terms **delayed cerebral ischaemia (DCI)**, **delayed ischaemic neurological deficit (DIND)**, or **symptomatic vasospasm** are used when vasospasm leads to a clinical neurological deficit. This occurs in approximately 30% of patients with aneurysmal SAH, typically 7–14 days after ictus but may occur at any time up to 21 days after the haemorrhage. The deficit may be reversible with treatment, or may be permanent if cerebral infarction occurs.

The only intervention that has been shown in a large randomized trial to improve outcome associated with DCI is the use of nimodipine. Pickard *et al.* (1989) found that the administration of 60mg oral nimodipine every 4 hours for 21 days reduced the risk of cerebral infarction by 34% and poor outcomes by 40%. When DCI

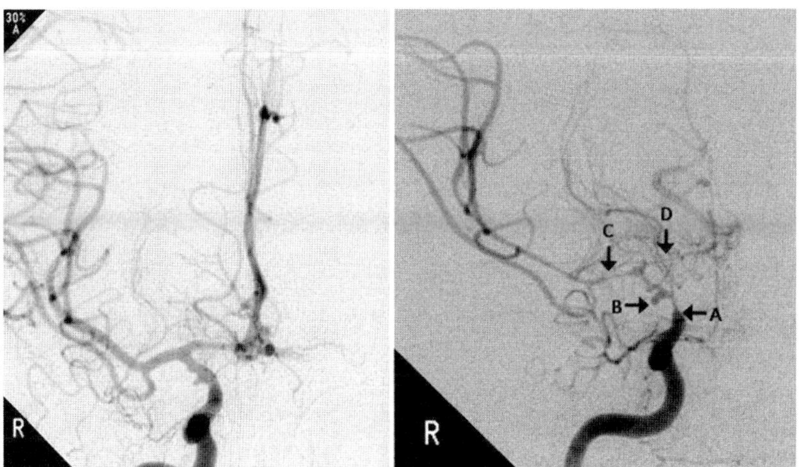

Fig. 18.6 AP right internal carotid angiogram on admission (left) and after 4 days with evolving left hemiparesis (right) of a 41-year-old man with a subarachnoid haemorrhage. By day 4 there is severely reduced calibre of the terminal internal carotid artery which begins just proximal to the aneurysm (A, transition point; B, aneurysm). The proximal MCA (C) and ACA (D) are both very severely attenuated compared with the earlier angiogram. This is diagnostic of severe vasospasm. Reproduced with permission from *Br J Neurosurg* 2006 Jun; **20**(3):165–8, © Informa Healthcare, 2011.

(continued)

Vasospasm and delayed cerebral ischaemia *(continued)*

occurs, the overall goal of treatment is to augment cerebral blood flow to the affected area. 'Triple-H' therapy (haemodilution, hypertension, hypervolaemia), first described by Kosnik *et al.* (1976) was developed for this purpose and has been widely used. The relative contribution of each component of the triple-H is not known. Adequate hydration must be ensured (this may be guided by CVP monitoring) and inotropes may be used to augment the mean arterial pressure. Endovascular therapies for DCI such as transluminal angioplasty and intra-arterial release of vasodilators have not been proven in randomized studies but may be used in refractory cases, with good results having been reported in individual cases (Rabinstein *et al.* 2010).

Assessment of eye movements

Eye movements are tested by asking the patient to follow your finger as it moves in the patient's field of view. The extra-ocular muscles exert their maximum action in specific directions, as shown in Fig. 18.7. The muscles that mediate horizontal

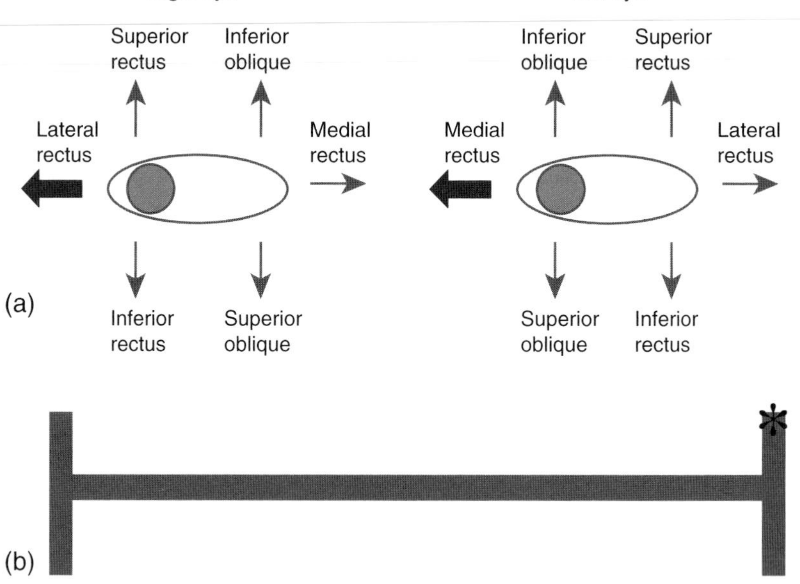

Fig. 18.7 Assessment of eye movements. (a) The directions in which the maximal actions of the extra-ocular muscles can be tested. Note that looking in one direction involves opposite pairs of muscles in each eye. For example, looking right (as in the figure) involves the lateral rectus of the right eye and the medial rectus of the left eye (thick arrows). (b) Using an H-shape can expose the movements of each muscle. For example, the location marked with an asterisk will testt the superior rectus of the left eye and the inferior oblique of the right eye.

(continued)

Assessment of eye movements *(continued)*

movements are easy to remember. For vertical movements, note that the oblique muscles principally act when the eyeball is turned medially whereas the superior and inferior rectus muscles principally act when the eyeball is turned laterally. Using the H-shape to examine eye movements can test the actions of individual muscles (Fig. 18.7). Remember that although each muscle has a particular direction in which it acts maximally, the movement of the eye in a particular direction depends on the coordinated movement of all muscles as the non-dominant ones relax or exert tone. Diplopia results when the two eyes fail to coordinate their movements, which commonly occurs due to cranial nerve deficits (e.g. from a compressive tumour or aneurysm) resulting in paralysis of the extra-ocular muscles. The patient must always be asked whether they 'see double' during assessment of their eye movements, as subtle cranial nerve deficits will not be apparent to the person testing eye movements but will manifest as diplopia. See Table 18.1 for a list of features of ocular cranial nerve palsies.

Table 18.1 Features of ocular cranial nerve palsies

Oculomotor (III)	The affected eye looks 'down and out' in the resting position due to the unopposed action of the lateral rectus and superior oblique. There would also be ptosis and the pupil will be fixed and dilated.
Trochlear (IV)	Isolated fourth nerve palsies are rare. The affected eye looks up and slightly medially in the resting position. Diplopia is maximal when the patient looks 'down and in'. Tilting the head to the unaffected side attenuates the diplopia and some patients may adopt this posture.
Abducens (VI)	The resting position may be normal although the affected eye may be looking slightly medially. The patient is unable to abduct the affected eye. Diplopia is maximal on horizontal gaze in the direction of the affected eye, and the patient may compensate by turning the head in the direction of maximal diplopia.

The use of lumbar puncture in the diagnosis of subarachnoid haemorrhage

Historically the interpretation of LP results for suspected SAH has been controversial. The issues are the reliability of the various methods to analyse CSF and the ability to distinguish SAH from a traumatic LP in which the spinal needle punctures a blood vessel.

Visual inspection at the time of LP

CSF that appears blood-stained at the time of LP is consistent with both SAH and a traumatic tap. If frank blood is aspirated, a traumatic tap is more likely (and more so if the blood then clears), although the patient may also have had an SAH and the diagnosis cannot be excluded.

(continued)

The use of lumbar puncture in the diagnosis of subarachnoid haemorrhage *(continued)*

Comparing the number of red blood cells in serial samples

In SAH the number of red blood cells in the CSF will be uniformly raised in all bottles. A decreasing number of red blood cells in sequential bottles is more consistent with a traumatic tap, although again the patient may also have had an SAH and the diagnosis cannot be excluded.

Absolute number of red blood cells

If the red cell count in the CSF is only mildly elevated (i.e. several hundred) SAH is less likely as the red blood cell count in SAH usually has a magnitude of thousands. However, a very high red cell count is also consistent with a traumatic tap.

Visual inspection for 'xanthochromia'

Most North American centres use this method. The CSF is inspected after it has been centrifuged. The result is positive if it has an orange tinge (the sample is held against a white background). A traumatic tap may also produce a positive result. However, a recent retrospective study has found that this method yields a sensitivity of 93%, a specificity of 95%, a positive predictive value of 72%, and a negative predictive value of 99% (Dupont *et al.* 2008). Some advocates of this method argue that waiting 12 hours before performing an LP (see below) is an unacceptable risk to the patient as the risk of re-bleeding is highest in the first 24 hours.

Spectrophotometry

This method differentiates between SAH and a traumatic tap by detecting oxyhaemoglobin and bilirubin in the CSF (UK NEQAS 2008). Any blood that enters the CSF (from SAH or a traumatic tap) will be converted to oxyhaemoglobin, as this process occurs both *in vivo* (in the subarachnoid space in the case of SAH) and *in vitro* (in the collecting container, either from SAH or traumatic tap). In contrast, the breakdown of red blood cells into bilirubin only occurs *in vivo* (and takes at least 12 hours) and thus cannot result from a traumatic tap. Therefore a CSF sample taken 12 hours after headache onset which is positive for bilirubin is consistent with SAH. High CSF protein or serum bilirubin may also result in raised CSF bilirubin.

Ultimately the decision to investigate for SAH depends on the clinical history. If there is any doubt about the LP result, cerebral angiography should be performed to look for an aneurysm. Vasospasm, which suggests recent haemorrhage, can also be detected on angiography. Alternatively an MRI scan with gradient echo and MRA sequences can demonstrate the presence of blood and aneurysm.

References

Dupont SA, Wijdicks EFM, Manno EM, Rabinstein AA (2008). Thunderclap headache and normal computed tomographic results: value of cerebrospinal fluid analysis. *Mayo Clin Proc*; **83**: 1326–31.

Kosnik EJ, Hunt WE (1976). Postoperative hypertension in the management of patients with intracranial arterial aneurysms. *J Neurosurg*; **45**: 148–54.

Pickard JD, Murray GD, Illingworth R, *et al*. (1989). Effect of oral nimodipine on cerebral infarction and outcome after subarachnoid haemorrhage: British Aneurysm Nimodipine Trial. *BMJ*; **298**: 636–42.

Rabinstein AA, Lanzino G, Wijdicks EFM (2010). Multidisciplinary management and emerging therapeutic strategies in subarachnoid haemorrhage. *Lancet Neurol*; **9**: 504–19.

UK NEQAS Specialist Advisory Group for EQA of CSF Proteins and Biochemistry (2008). Revised national guidelines for analysis of cerebrospinal fluid for bilirubin in suspected subarachnoid haemorrhage. *Ann Clin Biochem*; **45**: 238–44.

Case 19

A 48-year-old man was found collapsed at work. He cried out briefly and then fell to the floor. He was seen to shake and stop breathing for a short period, and he was taken to hospital immediately. On arrival in the emergency department he was comatose, flexing with the left arm, and localizing with the right. He was snoring and not making any sounds. His pupils were sluggishly reactive to light and his blood pressure was 200/110mmHg.

Question

1. What is the likely diagnosis? How should his immediate management proceed?

Answer

1. What is the likely diagnosis? How should his immediate management proceed?

The differential diagnosis of sudden collapse and coma includes cardiac events and hypoxic brain injury. The suggestion of seizure activity makes an intracerebral event more likely. He may have had a seizure and currently be recovering in a post-ictal phase, although an intracerebral haemorrhage must be ruled out.

His immediate management should consist of a primary survey, intravenous access, laboratory blood tests, and an ECG. Unless there is certainty that he is improving neurologically after a seizure he is likely to require intubation for safe ongoing management including transfer to CT. Patients with intracerebral (especially subarachnoid) haemorrhage frequently have a troponin rise and ECG abnormalities. This very rarely reflects a primary coronary event but rather the sudden myocardial stress caused by an extreme surge in sympathetic activity in association with the ictus of subarachnoid haemorrhage.

His blood pressure may be raised due to chronic hypertension or acutely as part of an autoregulation response. It should not be aggressively controlled in the acute setting. Giving an anaesthetic in order to intubate him for safe management will likely lower systolic pressure, and this is acceptable, but efforts to control blood pressure using conventional antihypertensives should be deferred unless the blood pressure settles at an unacceptable level, usually >200mmHg.

Question

2. He is intubated and taken for a CT scan (Fig. 19.1). What is shown and what is the likely aetiology and prognosis? How should his management proceed?

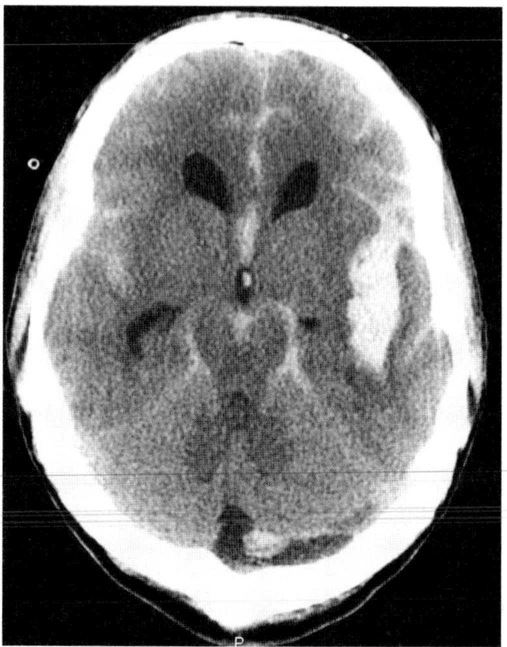

Fig. 19.1

Answer

2. He is intubated and taken for a CT scan (Fig. 19.1). What is shown and what is the likely aetiology and prognosis? How should his management proceed?

There are three key findings. First, there is diffuse subarachnoid blood in keeping with an aneurysmal haemorrhage. Secondly, there is a large intracerebral haematoma arising in the left sylvian fissure and extending into the temporal lobe. However, there is no midline shift from the haematoma and the ventricles are symmetrical. Thirdly, there is hydrocephalus.

The left sylvian fissure haemorrhage is highly suggestive of a ruptured left middle cerebral artery aneurysm, usually arising at the junction between the proximal MCA (M1) and the first branches (M2). The M1 usually splits into two branches (a bifurcation), one of which then splits into two itself. Occasionally all three M2 branches arise from the M1 (a trifurcation).

This man is by all criteria a poor-grade SAH. His WFNS grade is 4, his Fisher grade is 4, and his Hunt and Hess grade is also 4. Each of these grading systems has consistently been shown to correlate with worse outcome in terms of death and major disability. The risk of vasospasm and ischaemia leading to irreversible stroke is higher in poor-grade SAH patients. Their complication rate in terms of ventilator-acquired pneumonia, DVT, and infection is also higher. Treatment to secure the aneurysm may also be more challenging as endovascular access may be limited by vasospasm; surgery to clip the aneurysm often finds a swollen brain, making access without resection of brain impossible (resection of the brain is not normally necessary in aneurysm surgery, as access to the aneurysm is obtained via cerebral fissures).

The priority is management of the hydrocephalus. This should be undertaken as soon as possible with an external ventricular drain (EVD). His neurological state may then be reassessed by weaning the sedation. If he improves after ventricular drainage, he might have a slightly better prognosis: the WFNS and Hunt and Hess grading systems do not distinguish between coma due to high blood load and coma due to hydrocephalus, although they are undoubtedly of different prognostic value. Angiography (typically CT angiography) should then be performed to confirm the location and character of the aneurysm and the options for its treatment. The CTA (Fig. 19.2) reveals two aneurysms: the left MCA aneurysm underlying the haematoma as expected and a smaller unruptured ACom aneurysm (arrows). The CTA also shows diffuse vasospasm, causing attenuation of the visualized anterior circulation vessels bilaterally.

Question

3. When should the aneurysm(s) be treated, and how?

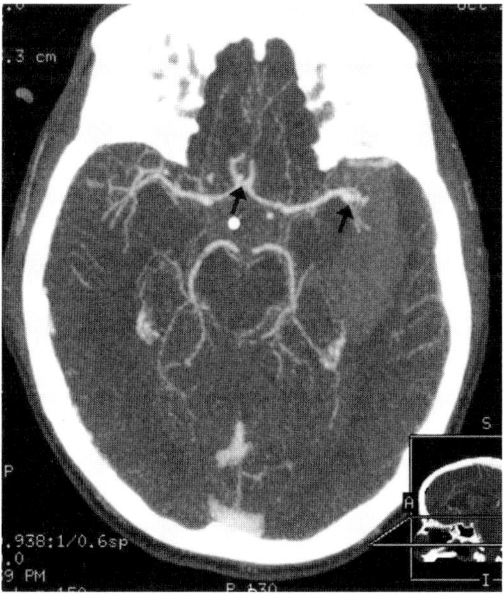

Fig. 19.2

Answer

3. When should the aneurysm(s) be treated, and how?

The left MCA aneurysm should be secured as soon as possible to reduce the risk of a re-bleed which is likely to be fatal. However, as above, surgery will be challenging and may itself pose an unacceptably high risk. Coiling is likely to be a lower-risk procedure, although there is a much higher chance of recurrence of MCA aneurysms with coiling as the neck of the aneurysm often cannot be completely secured with coiling.

This man underwent a combined approach to the MCA aneurysm: he was coiled on day 3 post bleed with the expected suboptimal angiographic result leaving a large neck remnant. However, the aneurysm was considered protected and he then underwent conventional management of his vasospasm and hydrocephalus, both of which settled by day 12 post bleed. By day 22 he was alert and orientated with a very mild residual right hemiparesis, and he underwent a scheduled craniotomy and clipping of the ACom and residual MCA aneurysms from which he made a good recovery.

Further reading

Kaku Y, Yamashita K, Kokuzawa J, Hatsuda N, Andoh T (2010). Treatment of ruptured cerebral aneurysms: clip and coil, not clip versus coil. *Acta Neurochir Suppl*; **107**: 9–13.

Kassel NF, Torner JC, Haley EC Jr, Jane JA, Adams HP, Kongable GL (1990). The international cooperative study on the timing of aneurysm surgery. Part 1: overall management results. *J Neurosurg*; **73**: 18–36.

Kassel NF, Torner JC, Jane JA, Haley EC Jr, Adams HP (1990). The international cooperative study on the timing of aneurysm surgery. Part 2: surgical results. *J Neurosurg*; **73**: 37–47.

Nishimura S, Fujita T, Sakata H, *et al.* (2009). Choice of intentional partial coiling for a ruptured intracranial aneurysm in the acute stage followed by clipping in the chronic stage. *No Shinkei Geka*; **37**: 757–63.

Case 20

A 49-year-old woman presented to the emergency department with a one-week history of severe headache. The onset was sudden. It did not cause her to lose consciousness although she vomited once. Since then her headaches had continued, and they were so severe that she had been unable to leave the house for 3 days. She had been taking paracetamol and codeine analgesia to little effect. Her medical history was unremarkable but she had smoked 20 cigarettes daily since her teens. On examination she was alert and orientated and the neurological examination was unremarkable. She had no papilloedema. The physicians arranged a head CT scan following which she was referred to neurosurgery.

Question

1. What are the arrowed abnormalities (Fig. 20.1) and suggested management?

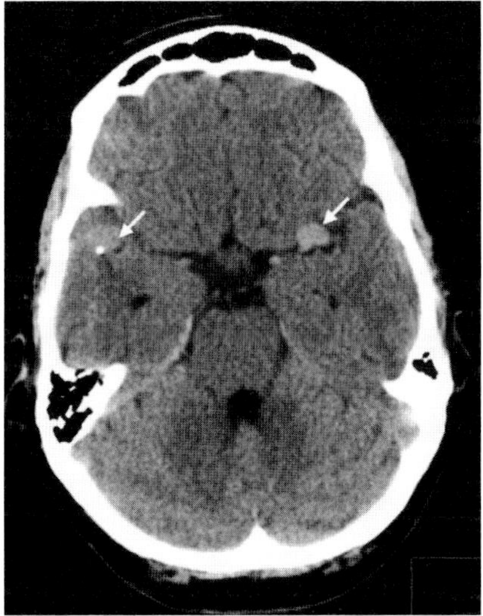

Fig. 20.1

Answer

1. What are the arrowed abnormalities (Fig. 20.1) and suggested management?

Two areas of hyperdensity are seen in the sylvian fissures bilaterally. Given the history of a sudden-onset headache, SAH is possible and these lesions would be suspicious for MCA aneurysms. It is also possible that the aneurysms have not bled and that there is another cause for her headache. It is reasonable for her to undergo an LP, not to diagnose an aneurysm (which will only be found on angiography) but to establish whether or not she has suffered a SAH. This information is required to decide on how this patient should be managed if an aneurysm is subsequently confirmed.

Her LP confirmed SAH. A CT angiogram was arranged and representative images from the maximum intensity projection (MIP) images are shown.

Question

2. What is seen in Fig. 20.2, and what therapeutic challenges now arise?

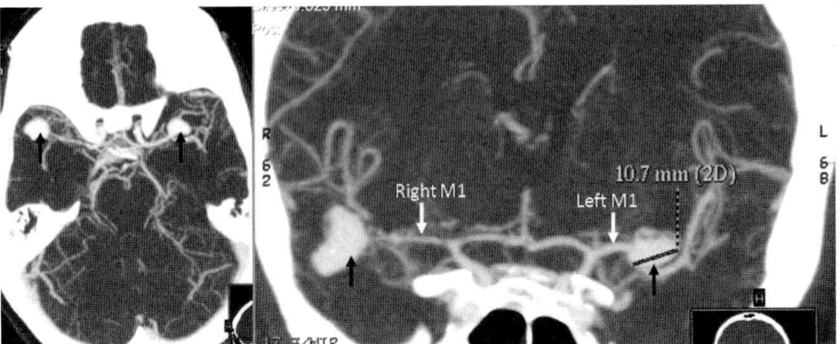

Fig. 20.2

Answer

2. What is seen in Fig. 20.2, and what therapeutic challenges now arise?

There are bilateral MCA aneurysms (black arrows) which are approximately the same size. 'Mirror' aneurysms in this configuration are seen occasionally. There is vasospasm of the right middle cerebral artery M1 segment, which is narrowed and irregular.

As with any patient presenting with SAH and more than one aneurysm, it is necessary to determine which aneurysm has bled (and therefore requires treatment). Sometimes more than one aneurysm may be treated in the same session. For example, a PCom and an ACom aneurysm in a favourable anatomical configuration could be coiled in the same session or clipped in the same operation from the same side. This is not the case with these aneurysms which will require either coiling via an approach from the right ICA and then a separate approach via the left ICA, or if neither can be coiled, as is often the case with MCA aneurysms, clipping via separate bilateral craniotomies. A single surgical procedure to peform sequential bilateral MCA aneurysm clippings is possible but will more than double the risk to the patient of a single procedure because of bilateral brain retraction. Therefore there should be a concerted effort to establish which aneurysm has bled.

Question

3. How can one identify which aneurysm has bled?

Answer

3. How can one identify which aneurysm has bled?

The most common way of identifying which aneurysm has bled is to review the pattern of the subarachnoid blood on the presenting CT scan. The location of the blood at presentation corresponds to the aneurysm in around 80% of SAHs (see 'Patterns of bleeding in aneurysmal subarachnoid haemorrhage', p. 125). Unfortunately, this patient has presented a week after a clinically modest SAH. There is no blood on the presenting CT and this cannot be used to point to one aneurysm or the other.

An MRI can be used to look for asymmetric subarachnoid blood with greater sensitivity than CT. There may also be signs of recent rupture on angiography. Specifically, aneurysm morphology associated with a secondary bleb or 'Murphy's teat' points to higher rupture risk; this is more often seen at surgery but may be defined angiographically. The angiogram may show localized vasospasm around one aneurysm more than around another, suggesting recent subarachnoid blood. The CTA images show vasospasm of the right M1 segment with none on the corresponding left M1 artery (note that the M1 is thinner on the right than the left, indicating vasospasm (Fig. 20.2, white arrows)). An MRI was performed (Fig. 20.3); the most sensitive sequence for recent subrachnoid haemorrhage is FLAIR

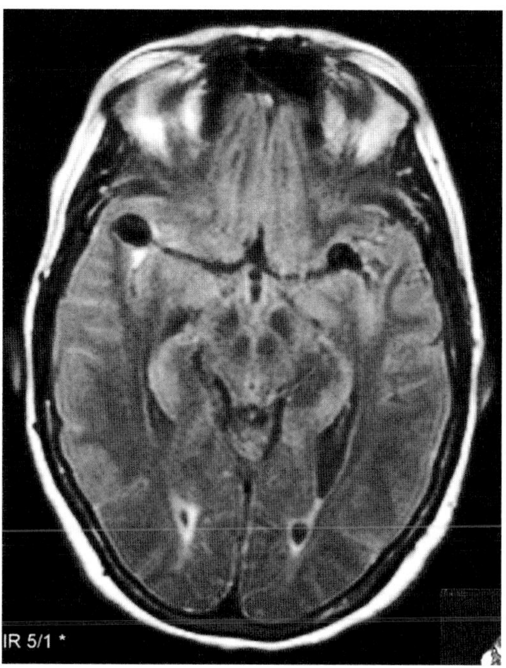

Fig. 20.3

(fluid attenuated inversion recovery). This shows bilateral MCA aneurysms as oval low-signal flow voids. On the right there is a small amount of high signal around the aneurysm, confirming this to be the side of rupture.

Accordingly, the right MCA aneurysm was considered to have ruptured and, as it was deemed favourable for endovascular treatment because of its small neck, was managed with coiling with a good angiographic result. The patient went home 10 days later and returned for an elective craniotomy and clipping of the left MCA aneurysm 3 months later (the left MCA aneurysm was not considered suitable for coiling).

Further reading

Hino A, Fujimoto M, Iwamoto Y, Yamaki T, Katsumori T (2000). False localization of rupture site in patients with multiple cerebral aneurysms and subarachnoid hemorrhage. *Neurosurgery*; **46**: 825–30.

Karttunen AI, Jartti PH, UkkolaVA, Sajanti J, Haapea M (2003). Value of the quantity and distribution of subarachnoid haemorrhage on CT in the localization of a ruptured cerebral aneurysm. *Acta Neurochir (Wien)*; **145**: 655–61.

Marshall SA, Kathuria S, Nyquist P, Gandhi D (2010). Noninvasive imaging techniques in the diagnosis and management of aneurysmal subarachnoid hemorrhage. *Neurosurg Clin N Am*; **21**: 305–23.

Rajesh A, Praveen A, Purohit AK, Sahu BP (2010). Unilateral craniotomy for bilateral cerebral aneurysms. *J Clin Neurosci*; **17**: 1294–7.

Case 21

A 59-year-old man experienced a sudden-onset right-sided headache whilst walking in the street. He vomited and was unable to move his left side. He was brought by ambulance to the emergency department where his GCS was 8/15 (E1, V1, M6) and his pupils were equal and reactive. His blood pressure was 210/105mmHg. A CT scan was performed, and is shown in Fig. 21.1.

Questions

1. Describe the appearances on the CT scan and features A–D.
2. Why is the patient hemiplegic?
3. What is the diagnosis and what could be the cause?

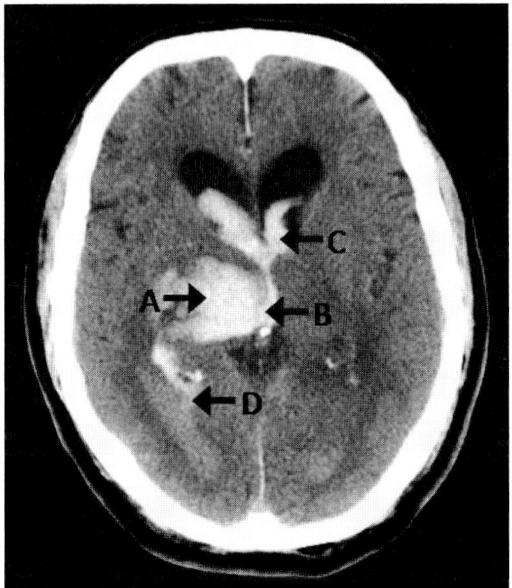

Fig. 21.1

Answers

1. Describe the appearances on the CT scan and features A–D.

There is a large high-density lesion in the region of the right thalamus representing acute haemorrhage (A). The blood extends into the third ventricle (B), the frontal horns of the lateral ventricles (C), and the occipital horns of the lateral ventricles (D). The frontal horns are dilated, indicating hydrocephalus.

2. Why is the patient hemiplegic?

The hemiplegia is due to involvement of the internal capsule, which lies adjacent to the thalamus and basal ganglia.

3. What is the diagnosis and what could be the cause?

The patient has suffered a spontaneous intracerebral haemorrhage. The differential diagnosis includes hypertensive haemorrhage, bleeding from an underlying lesion such as an AVM or tumour, and coagulopathy. Hypertensive haemorrhage is most frequently seen in this location in a patient of this age.

Questions

4. In which areas of the brain do hypertensive haemorrhages occur most often, and why?
5. What is the management of this patient?
6. What are the options for the treatment of hydrocephalus, and how should this patient be treated?

Answers

4. In which areas of the brain do hypertensive haemorrhages occur most often, and why?

The most common location for spontaneous intracerebral haemorrhage is the basal ganglia, followed by cerebrum (lobar haemorrhage) followed by the cerebellum. These areas are susceptible because they are supplied by small arteries that directly branch off major arteries (e.g. the lenticulostriate arteries supplying the basal ganglia and the thalamoperforating arteries supplying the thalamus). The walls of these susceptible arteries have been found to contain fat cells and fibrin-like material, a process termed lipohyalinosis, and these small arteries develop microaneurysms (Charcot–Bouchard aneurysms).

5. What is the management of this patient?

Patients with spontaneous subcortical haemorrhage should be admitted to a stroke unit and receive intravenous fluids, DVT prophylaxis, and a nasogastric tube for feeding if required. The role of surgery in evacuation of spontaneous intracerebral haematomas is controversial (see 'Surgery for spontaneous intracerebral haematomas', p. 167), but is generally not recommended when the haemorrhage is subcortical as the deficit from the haematoma is unlikely to improve with surgery. However, treatment of the hydrocephalus may lead to neurological improvement.

6. What are the options for the treatment of hydrocephalus, and how should this patient be treated?

Options for the treatment of hydrocephalus include LP, a lumbar drain, and external ventricular drain. This patient has haemorrhage extending into the third (and most probably the fourth) ventricle, and performing a LP/lumbar drain in this situation carries the risk of coning (see 'Lumbar puncture and the risk of coning', p. 167). He underwent placement of an EVD.

Questions

7. Five days after placement of the drain you are contacted by a nurse who is worried that the drain may be blocked. The patient has improved clinically since admission and his GCS is 14/15 (E4, V4, M6). What should be done now?
8. The drain is flushed with saline but remains blocked and it is removed. Does it need to be replaced?

Answers

7. Five days after placement of the drain you are contacted by a nurse who is worried that the drain may be blocked. The patient has improved clinically since admission and his GCS is 14/15 (E4, V4, M6). What should be done now?

A blocked EVD can lead to acutely raised intracranial pressure and is a potential emergency. An urgent assessment of the patient and the EVD apparatus is required. If the CSF 'swings' in the drain when it is lowered, obstruction is unlikely and the non-drainage is probably due to the EVD being set higher than the CSF pressure. If the CSF does not swing, obstruction is suspected (see 'External ventricular drains: indications and management of common problems', p. 167).

8. The drain is flushed with saline but remains blocked and is removed. Does it need to be replaced?

This depends on whether ventricular drainage is still required. This will be informed by a CT scan to assess the size of the ventricles (Fig. 21.2).

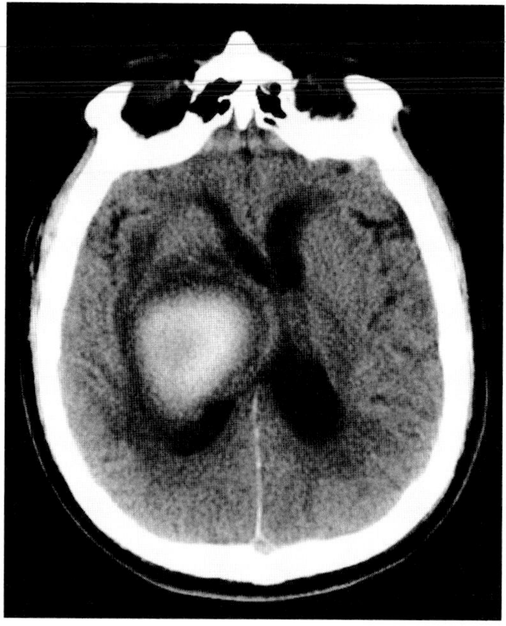

Fig. 21.2

Questions

9. Does the patient need another EVD? What other neurosurgical input is required?
10. The CT scan of a similarly aged patient with an acute onset left hemiparesis is shown in Fig. 21.3. Would your management be different, and why?
11. Another common location for spontaneous intracerebral haematoma is the cerebellum. How would you manage a 69-year-old man with a cerebellar haematoma as shown here in Fig. 21.4?

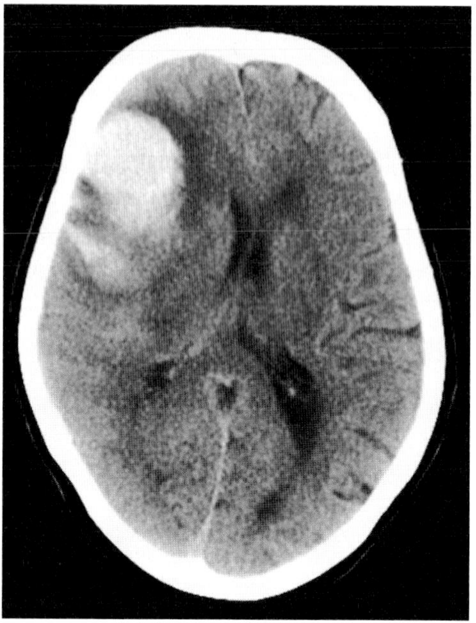

Fig. 21.3

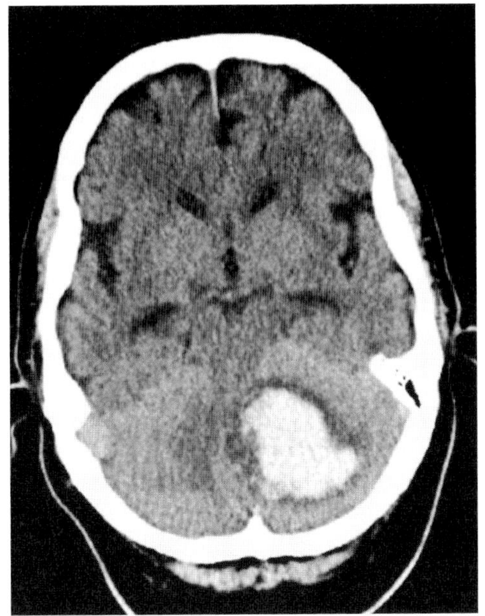

Fig. 21.4

Answers

9. Does the patient need another EVD? What other neurosurgical input is required?

The ventricles have decompressed and the patient has clinically improved. Another EVD is not necessary. The patient requires ongoing stroke rehabilitation and an interval CT scan to check for recurrence of hydrocephalus and evolution of the haemorrhage.

10. The CT scan of a similarly aged patient with an acute onset left hemiparesis is shown in Fig. 21.3. Would your management be different, and why?

This is a superficial lobar haemorrhage. There is no associated intraventricular blood or hydrocephalus. There may be an unproven benefit for surgery in these cases to relieve local mass effect and improve the associated deficit. If the patient is otherwise medically well, direct evacuation of the haematoma would often be appropriate. Evacuation of the haematoma partly depends on whether the clot is thought to have caused the deficit by direct damage to eloquent brain or by local mass effect. In the latter situation surgery is more likely to have benefit.

11. Another common location for spontaneous intracerebral haematoma is the cerebellum. How would you manage a 69-year-old man with a cerebellar haematoma as shown in Fig. 21.4?

Cerebellar haematomas are more often treated surgically than supratentorial haematomas because the local mass effect can cause distortion of the fourth ventricle and obstructive hydrocephalus, the prevention of which results in a far better outcome. Many people will rehabilitate better from the bleed itself in the cerebellum rather than one in more eloquent brain. This patient has early hydrocephalus and the surgical options are to treat the hydrocephalus only with an EVD, to evacuate the clot (and anticipate that the hydrocephalus will settle), or to evacuate the clot and place an EVD at the same time with a view to weaning it over the next few days. Evacuation of the clot would be preferred in this case as there is radiological evidence of brainstem compression, which would not be relieved by EVD placement.

Further reading

Cohen ZR, Ram Z, Knoller N, Peles E, Hadani M (2002). Management and outcome of non-traumatic cerebellar haemorrhage. *Cerebrovasc Dis*; **14**: 207–13.

Mayer SA, Rincon F (2002). Treatment of intracerebral haemorrhage. *Lancet Neurol*; **4**: 662–72.

Mendelow AD, Gregson BA, Fernandes HM, *et al.* (2005). Early surgery versus initial conservative treatment in patients with spontaneous supratentorial intracerebral haematomas in the International Surgical Trial in Intracerebral Haemorrhage (STICH): a randomised trial. *Lancet*; **365**: 387–97.

Morioka J, Fujii M, Kato S, *et al.* (2006). Japan Standard Stroke Registry Group (JSSR). Surgery for spontaneous intracerebral hemorrhage has greater remedial value than conservative therapy. *Surg Neurol*; **65**: 67–72.

Surgery for spontaneous intracerebral haematomas

Surgically removing spontaneous intracerebral haematomas removes the mass effect and reduces the toxic effect of the blood clot, reduces brain oedema, and preserves brain tissue. The decision to operate depends on a balance of factors including the patient's age and fitness, location of the clot, neurological status, and expected improvement with surgery.

Superficial lobar haematomas are relatively easier to access, whereas deep subcortical haematomas are more difficult to access and are surrounded by delicate structures. A recent randomized study (STICH) showed that there was no significant difference in outcome between surgery and early conservative management for patients with spontaneous intracerebral haematomas in which the clinician was uncertain whether surgery or conservative management would be beneficial. This study covered a variety of cases including superficial and deep haematomas. Randomized trials are currently underway to examine if there is a difference in outcome according to the location of haemorrhage (Mendelow and Unterberg 2007).

Lumbar puncture and the risk of coning

An LP can induce a pressure gradient in the subarachnoid space and in some circumstances cause downward displacement of the brain, brainstem compression, and death ('coning'). The risk is precipitated in the presence of mass lesions or obstructive hydrocephalus. Supratentorial mass lesions and obstructive hydrocephalus (both of which lead to mass effect in the supratentorial compartment) may precipitate transtentorial herniation, followed by tonsillar herniation. Infratentorial mass lesions may precipitate tonsillar herniation. The space around the foramen magnum can be inspected for abundance of CSF on a CT scan to assess the risk of brainstem compression from tonsillar herniation. If a patient's conscious level deteriorates during an LP, CSF (or saline) should be introduced back into the subarachnoid space.

External ventricular drains: indications and management of common problems

The EVD is one of the most frequently performed procedures in neurosurgery. It involves placing a catheter within a ventricular cavity (most often the frontal horn of the lateral ventricle and on the right side to minimize risk to the language areas) which is externalized through the skin and connected to a drainage device (Fig. 21.5). The zero level on the manometer is placed at the level of the foramen of Monro (approximately at the level of the external auditory meatus). The level of

(continued)

External ventricular drains: indications and management of common problems *(continued)*

CSF in the manometer reflects the intracranial pressure. The height of the manometer is adjusted to set the level for drainage, and CSF will drain when the intracranial pressure exceeds that level. At intracranial pressures less than this, the CSF will 'swing' in the tubing (without draining) at the ICP. A port is provided for sampling and antibiotic administration.

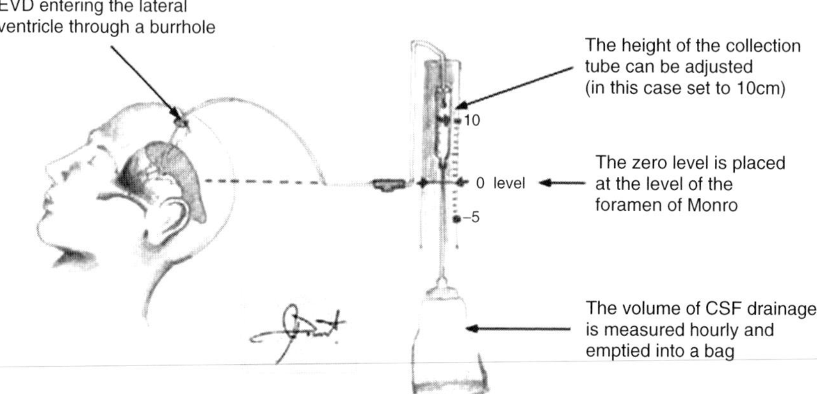

Fig. 21.5 External ventricular drainage system.

Indications for EVDs

- Treatment of hydrocephalus: provides controlled, continuous drainage of CSF
- Treatment of ventriculitis: antibiotics can be administered 'intrathecally' through the EVD
- Continuous measurement of intracranial pressure.

(continued)

External ventricular drains: indications and management of common problems *(continued)*

Complications of EVDs

- Intraoperatively: bleeding, malposition of drain, rarely stroke (from malpositioned drain)
- Postoperatively: infection (skin infection, ventriculitis), CSF leak, blockage of drain, seizures.

Common problems with EVDs

Infection

- The most frequent complication: leads to ventriculitis.
- The catheter should be replaced and intrathecal and intravenous antibiotics should be commenced.

Blockage

- Check patency by lowering the drain: If CSF swings, drain is patent
- Check apparatus for disconnection/leaks
- Check inside tubing for debris
- Consider CT scan to check position of drain
- Consider aspirating from drain
- Consider flushing drain with saline
- If you can flush but not aspirate from a drain which is not draining, the drain may be left *in situ* if it is used for administration of antibiotics; otherwise it should be removed
- If you cannot flush or aspirate from the drain which is not draining, it should be removed
- Any manipulation of the EVD apparatus involving access to CSF must be performed under sterile conditions.

CSF leak

- Occurs where the drain exits the scalp
- Check length of drain to see whether it has been displaced (or has come out)
- Place a suture to tighten the space between drain and scalp, or lower drain level to drain more CSF through the drain
- A CSF leak must not be left to continue as it will result in ventriculitis.

Reference

Mendelow AD, Unterberg A (2007). Surgical treatment of intracerebral haemorrhage. *Curr Opin Crit Care*; **13**: 169–74.

Case 22

A 54-year-old man is referred from a local hospital. He has been admitted there following a sudden collapse. He has been persistently confused since the event with a severe headache. On examination he has a marked (2/5) weakness of his left arm; the leg is also weak but slightly less so. His GCS is 12/15 (E3, V3, M6) and his pupils are equal and reactive. His blood pressure is 130/80mmHg.

Questions

1. The patient undergoes a CT scan (Fig. 22.1). What are the findings, what are the possible underlying diagnoses, and how should he be managed?
2. What vascular imaging should be offered, and why?

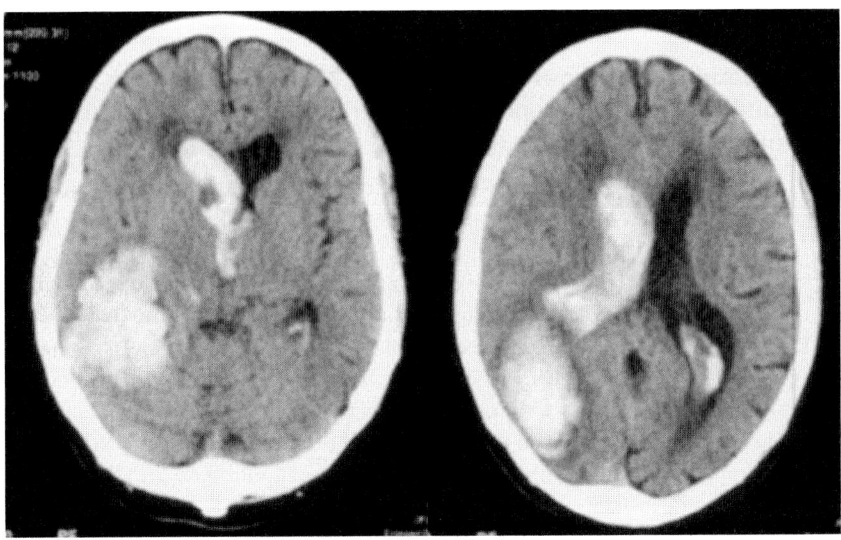

Fig. 22.1

Answers

1. The patient undergoes a CT scan (Fig. 22.1). What are the findings, what are the possible underlying diagnoses, and how should he be managed?

There is a large right temporo-occipital intracerebral haematoma which has ruptured into the ventricles. There is moderate hydrocephalus.

This is not a typical location for hypertensive haemorrhage. He is relatively young and his blood pressure is not elevated. Therefore an underlying vascular malformation is possible, most commonly an arteriovenous malformation (AVM). Haemorrhage from a tumour or cavernoma is possible but unlikely, as these are typically more confined. The haemorrhage is parenchymal without any blood in the sylvian fissure making a ruptured aneurysm unlikely.

The early management is supportive. Given the degree of intraventricular blood, hydrocephalus, and neurological impairment, he should have an EVD placed. Surgery for the haematoma can be considered, but the underlying cause should be considered first so that intraoperative problems can be anticipated (e.g. haemorrhage from an AVM).

2. What vascular imaging should be offered, and why?

Many centres employ CT angiography as first-line assessment of patients with SAH to look for intracranial aneurysms. If this patient has a vascular pathology it is much more likely to be an AVM. Catheter angiography is preferred for AVMs as it offers dynamic information during the contrast injection and allows better visualization of the feeding arteries supplying the AVM nidus, as well as showing which veins drain the AVM. However, it is invasive and more complex and time consuming to perform if the patient requires emergency surgery. In this case a CT angiogram should show abnormal vasculature prior to emergency surgery, although it might not be sufficient for definitive elective treatment.

Questions

3. He undergoes a CTA immediately and catheter angiogram 2 days later, which are shown in Fig. 22.2.
   (a) What images are shown?
   (b) Identify the features labelled 1 to 6.
   (c) What is the abnormality and what are its salient features?
4. This patient is managed with an EVD and supportive care and gradually improves during the next five days. What are the treatment options in this case? How may his surgical risk be assessed?

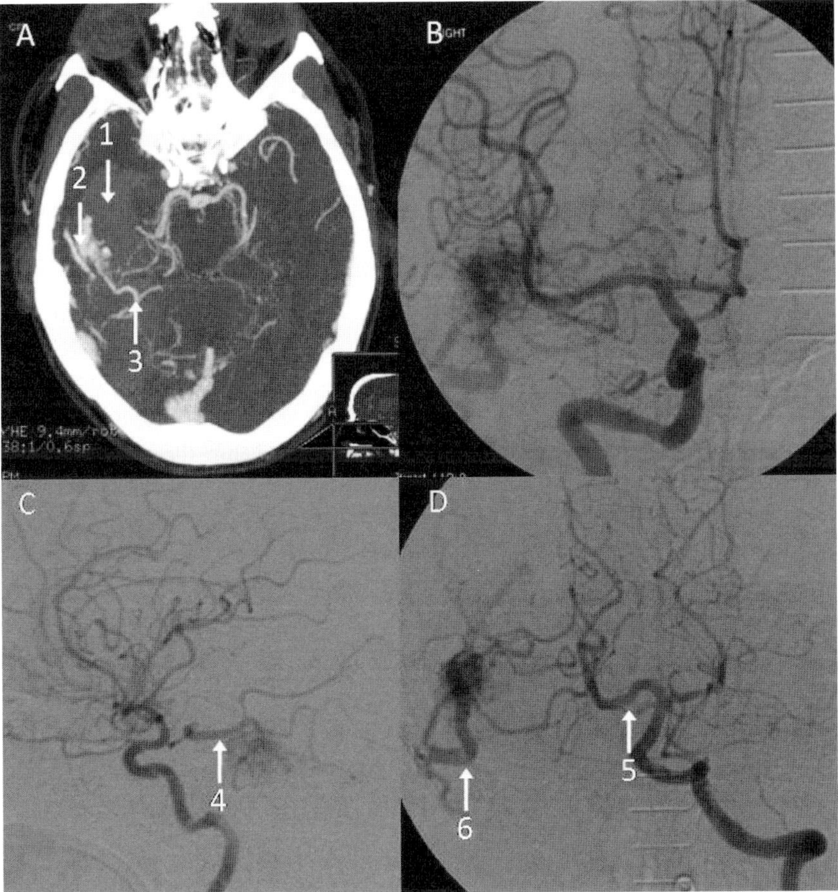

Fig. 22.2

3. He undergoes a CTA immediately and catheter angiogram 2 days later, which are shown in Fig. 22.2.

(a) What images are shown?

The images are an axial maximum intensity projection (MIP) of the CTA (A), an AP and a lateral projection of the right internal carotid artery angiogram (B and C), and an AP view of the left vertebral artery angiogram (D).

(b) Identify the features labelled 1–6.

The CTA shows the haematoma (1), with some abnormal blood vessels posterolaterally in the haematoma bed (2). There appears to be some supply to them from the right posterior cerebral artery (3). The carotid angiogram shows the abnormal tangle of blood vessels with supply coming through a fetal posterior communicating artery (4) which partly feeds the posterior cerebral artery (5). The vertebral angiogram also shows supply from the posterior cerebral artery and in addition, during the arterial phase as shown, there is filling of the veins draining the AVM (6), before the normal cerebral venous phase. Early venous filling is the hallmark of arteriovenous shunting. Overall the nidus is around 2.5cm in diameter.

(c) What is the abnormality and what are its salient features?

The arterial supply and venous drainage of the AVM are the most important features, along with the overall size of the nidus. If endovascular therapy is to be attempted, either prior to surgical resection or radiosurgery, the vessels supplying the AVM must be wide enough to allow catheter access. Similarly, if these vessels also supply eloquent brain areas close to the AVM nidus, achieving a safe catheter position for embolization will be more difficult and the risk of embolization causing a stroke would be higher. Surgical planning requires knowledge of the arterial supply so that appropriate vessels can be ligated in turn before the nidus is excised. The venous drainage must be established and ligated last before excision of the nidus, otherwise intranidal pressure will rise and this may cause severe intraoperative haemorrhage. Finally, the overall size of the AVM must be established as smaller lesions (<3cm in diameter) may be treated with stereotactic radiosurgery. Although there is a lag of usually 2 years but up to 5 years before radiosurgery results in AVM obliteration, it is a treatment with low morbidity and therefore is preferred for smaller AVMs in eloquent brain areas.

4. This patient is managed with an EVD and supportive care and gradually improves during the next five days. What are the treatment options in this case? How may his surgical risk be assessed?

The treatment options in any AVM are conservative, embolization alone with curative intent, surgery alone, radiosurgery alone, or embolization followed by surgery or radiosurgery. The most important aspect is multispecialty discussion. Embolization alone is not usually curative and should be performed for larger AVMs prior to surgery. It may be tried with curative intent in surgically inaccessible

AVMs following failed radiosurgery or with palliative intent for large AVMs presenting with unusual features (e.g. steal phenomena or hydrocephalus due to raised venous pressure).

Surgical risk for AVMs has been classified according to the Spetzler–Martin scale. The AVM is scored in three areas: eloquence of surrounding brain (non-eloquent = 0, eloquent = 1), presence of deep draining veins (present = 1, absent = 0), and size of the nidus (<3cm = 1, 3–6cm = 2, >6cm = 3). The total score ranges from 1 to 5. In the original series of operated AVMs the morbidity and mortality increased with increasing grade. For grade 1 AVMs (small non-eloquent brain, superficial venous drainage) the surgical morbidity and mortality should be very low and surgery is the treatment of choice. For larger AVMs in non-eloquent brain embolization should be performed prior to surgery. Smaller eloquent AVMs should be managed by radiosurgery, possibly in combination with prior embolization. High-grade (4 and 5) AVMs are considered inoperable and should be treated with embolization to reduce the size of the nidus and then re-evaluated.

This patient's AVM is small (<3cm), with superficial venous drainage as demonstrated on the AP vertebral angiogram. The adjacent brain is not completely non-eloquent; however, there has been a recent haemorrhage and therefore the AVM may already be partly dissected from the adjacent brain. In this case surgery may not exacerbate the deficit and should be strongly considered in the early phase. The risks of a second haemorrhage are far lower for ruptured AVMs than for aneurysms (5–17% per year for AVMs compared with 2% per day for aneurysms) and therefore there is not the same mandate for urgent AVM excision as there is for protection of a ruptured aneurysm. However, if the patient is sufficiently well there is a strong argument in this case for early surgery for the AVM.

This patient underwent a right temporal craniotomy for the AVM which was systematically isolated from its arterial supply and excised. A postoperative angiogram confirmed no abnormal blood vessels or early venous filling. The EVD was removed after 2 weeks but he developed ongoing hydrocephalus and required a VP shunt. He was discharged to rehabilitation and was still making progress after 6 months.

Further reading

Fukuoka S, Takanashi M, Seo Y, Suematsu K, Nakamura J (1998). Radiosurgery for arteriovenous malformations with gamma-knife: a multivariate analysis of factors influencing the complete obliteration rate. *J Clin Neurosci*; **5** (Suppl): 68–71.

Katsaridis V, Papagiannaki C, Aimar E (2008). Curative embolization of cerebral arteriovenous malformations (AVMs) with Onyx in 101 patients. *Neuroradiology*; **50**: 589–97.

Spetzler RF, Martin NA (1986). A proposed grading system for arteriovenous malformations. *J Neurosurg*; **65**: 476–83.

Zhao J, Wang S, Li J, Qi W, Sui D, Zhao Y (2005). Clinical characteristics and surgical results of patients with cerebral arteriovenous malformation. *Surg Neurol*; **63**: 156–61.

Case 23

A 60-year-old man presented with a 2-month history of progressive unsteadiness. He reported having a painful sensation over the previous 18 months which began in the feet and gradually ascended in the legs. Intermittently, he also found it difficult to pass urine. His medical history was unremarkable and he was not on regular medication. On examination, he was alert and orientated. In the lower limbs, the tone was increased, power was normal, and reflexes were brisk. Proprioception was impaired bilaterally in the toes and plantars were upgoing bilaterally. Romberg's test was negative and there were no cerebellar signs. A sensory level was identified at the level of T3. The upper limbs were normal.

Questions

1. Where is the lesion likely to be?
2. Explain how a spinal cord lesion leads to problems with micturition.
3. How should this patient be managed?

Answers

1. Where is the lesion likely to be?

The signs point to a lesion in the upper thoracic spinal cord. The relevant findings are the upper motor neuron signs in the lower limbs, the T3 sensory level, and extensor plantars. Impaired proprioception in this context suggests dorsal column involvement (see 'Types of spinal cord lesions', p. 299).

2. Explain how a spinal cord lesion leads to problems with micturition.

A lesion in the spinal cord can interfere with the central micturition pathway which runs in the spinal cord (see 'Disorders of micturition in neurosurgery', p. 342).

3. How should this patient be managed?

The patient requires an urgent MRI scan of the spine. He also requires a bladder scan before and after voiding. If he is found to have a residual volume, a urology opinion is indicated.

Questions

4. The MRI scan is shown in Fig. 23.1.
   a) Describe the findings and features A–C.
   b) What is the diagnosis?
   c) What further investigations are required?
5. Describe the vascular supply to the spinal cord.

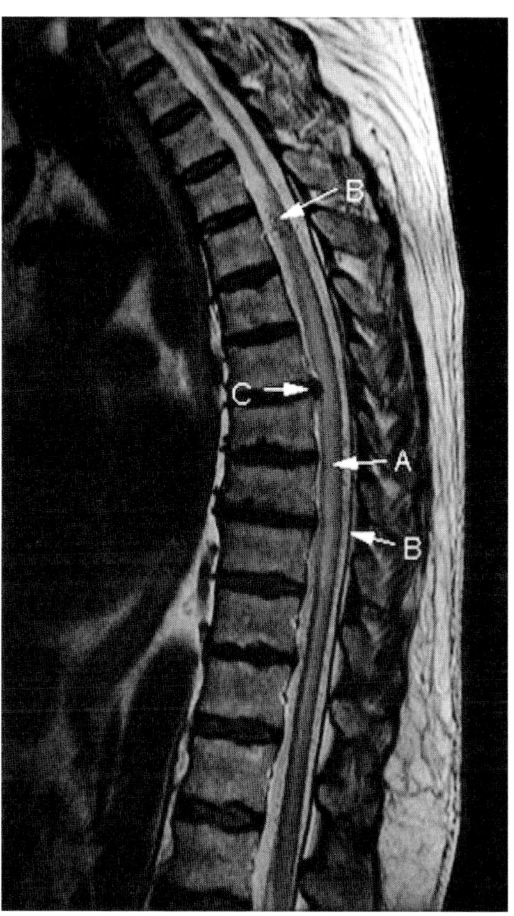

Fig. 23.1

Answers

4. The MRI scan is shown in Fig. 23.1. a) Describe the findings and structures A–C. b) What is the diagnosis? c) What further investigations are required?

There is an area of diffuse high signal in the spinal cord extending from the T3/4 level to around T12 (A). Prominent vessels are present around the cord between these levels, indicated by small areas of hypointensity or flow voids on the cord surface (B). The appearances are highly suggestive of a spinal vascular malformation. The high signal in the cord represents oedema. A mild disc bulge is also present (C) which is not compressing the spinal cord and is therefore unrelated to the presenting symptoms. Further investigations to define the vascular abnormality are required.

5. Describe the vascular supply to the spinal cord

The spinal cord is supplied by an arterial anastomotic network consisting of the anterior spinal artery, paired posterior spinal arteries, and anterior and posterior segmental arteries arising from the vertebral, posterior intercostal, lumbar, or sacral arteries (depending on the level of the spinal cord) which enter the spinal canal through the intervertebral foramina. Segmental arteries supply the spinal nerve roots and may extend intradurally to anastomose with the anterior or posterior spinal arteries. The spinal veins have a similar configuration to the arteries. There are usually three anterior and three posterior spinal veins that lie on the surface of the spinal cord and drain into the epidural venous plexus. This plexus

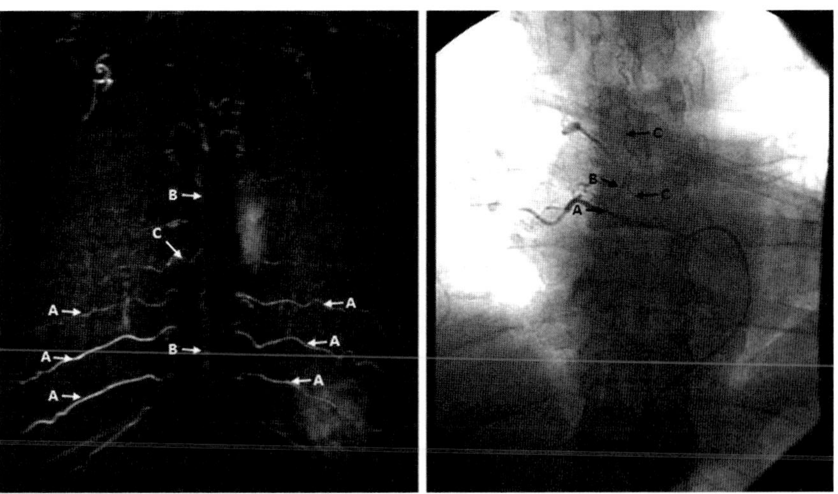

Fig. 23.2

drains into the segmental veins, but also communicates with the intracranial venous sinuses through the foramen magnum.

An MR angiogram is performed (Fig. 23.2(left)). This shows the intercostal arteries (A) and reveals a prominent tortuous early filling midline draining vein (B), which has a connection to a right intercostal artery (C). The appearances are consistent with a spinal dural arteriovenous fistula. This was confirmed by catheter angiography (Fig. 23.2(right)), which shows an intercostal artery (A), the fistula at the level of T7 (B), and the filling central vein (C).

Questions

6. How are spinal vascular malformations classified?
7. Explain how spinal dural fistulas can cause myelopathy. Why did the patient's symptoms begin in the feet?
8. What is the management of this case?

Answers

6. How are spinal vascular malformations classified?

The classification of spinal vascular malformations has evolved with radiological and surgical advances which have allowed more accurate descriptions of the pathological processes involved. A commonly used classification system based on the work of American, English, and French investigators is as follows: Type 1 lesions are dural arteriovenous fistulas in which a segmental artery forms a fistula with a draining vein at the dural sleeve of a nerve root. Type 2 (glomus) lesions consist of a compact intramedullary nidus. Type 3 (juvenile) lesions are large intramedullary lesions which may extend extradurally or extraspinally. Type 4 lesions are intradural, extramedullay arteriovenous fistulas with a direct connection between the vascular supply of the spinal cord (usually the anterior spinal artery) and a vein. This patient has a Type 1 arteriovenous malformation (dural AV fistula). This type accounts for the majority of spinal vascular malformations.

7. Explain how spinal dural fistulas can cause myelopathy. Why did the patient's symptoms begin in the feet?

In type 1 spinal AVMs, arteriovenous shunting leads to chronic venous hypertension in the intradural venous system. This leads to slower flow in the arterial system, impaired oxygenation, and ischaemic myelopathy. Spinal cord oedema begins in the most dependent part of the cord; hence symptoms are usually of an ascending nature. In extradural AVMs, myelopathy may result from compression of the cord due to engorged extradural veins.

8. What is the management of this case?

The patient has progressive symptoms and therefore should be offered treatment to obliterate the fistula. The options are surgical division of the fistula or endovascular embolization. Surgical division offers the highest rate of success, although the risks are of an open operation. The endovascular option is less invasive but is associated with an appreciable recurrence rate (approximately 50%). This patient underwent surgical division of the fistula. His postoperative MRI scan (Fig. 23.3) shows a marked reduction in the amount of cord swelling (note the reduction in hyperintensity in the cord). The fistula and the central vein are no longer evident on the MR angiogram. His symptoms progressively improved over a period of 6 months.

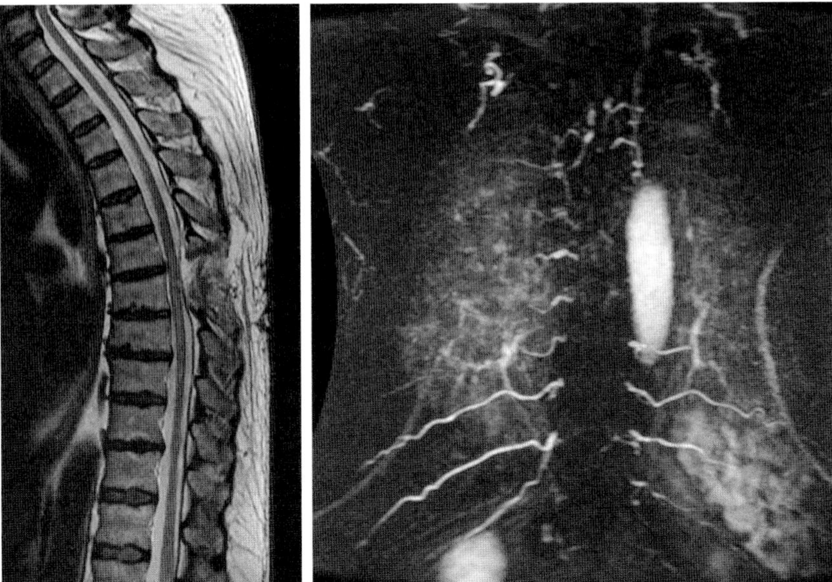

Fig. 23.3

Further reading

Black P (2006). Spinal vascular malformations: an historical perspective. *Neurosurg Focus*; **21**: E11.

Kim LJ, Spetzler RF (2006). Classification and surgical management of spinal arteriovenous lesions: arteriovenous fistulae and arteriovenous malformations. *Neurosurgery*; **59** (Suppl 3): 195–201.

Case 24

A 35-year-old man presents with a sudden onset of severe headache that occurred whilst gardening. He is a previously healthy non-smoker. Of note, when aged 26 he suffered a single generalized seizure that was not investigated. In the emergency department he is alert and orientated with no photophobia or neck stiffness, and his headache is settling by the time he is reviewed after 4 hours. He has no discernible neurological deficit.

Questions

1. What is the differential diagnosis?
2. A CT scan is done (Fig. 24.1). Comment on the findings and the management options. How would you advise the patient?

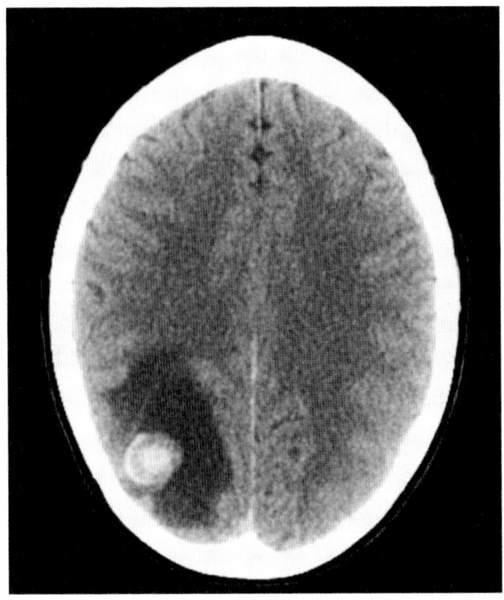

Fig. 24.1

Answers

1. What is the differential diagnosis?

The differential diagnosis includes vascular events such as subarachnoid haemorrhage, although typically patients with SAH are more unwell. Other types of intracranial haemorrhage should be considered, although frequently they are associated with focal neurological deficits. Non-haemorrhagic causes such as migraine and cluster headache should also be considered, although typically such patients have a prior history of these events.

2. A CT scan is done (Fig. 24.1). Comment on the findings and the management options. How would you advise the patient?

There is a well-circumscribed subcortical hyperdensity in the right parietal region with an appreciable amount of surrounding oedema. This is an acute haemorrhage. The location of the haemorrhage and the age of the patient mandate a search for an underlying abnormality that may have bled, such as a tumour or vascular malformation. If no structural lesion is found, the patient should be investigated for medical causes such as vasculitis or amyloid angiopathy.

The management should initially be conservative given the good neurological condition of the patient. If he deteriorates repeat imaging should be performed to look for further haemorrhage. In planning further investigations, the underlying cause should be considered. The bleed has none of the features of an aneurysmal haemorrhage and urgent investigation is probably not necessary. MRI scanning should be delayed for 6 weeks to allow the haematoma to involute and to increase the diagnostic certainty. Angiography may be required depending on the MRI findings.

During this interval (assuming he is to be discharged) he should be given general advice about recurrence of symptoms and, if so, the need to return to hospital. He must be advised that he should not drive because of the presence of a supratentorial haemorrhage of unknown aetiology and the associated risk of seizures. For the same reasons he should be counselled about swimming alone and working in dangerous situations (e.g. at heights).

Question

3. His headache settles and he goes home. An MRI scan is performed at 6 weeks as planned (Fig. 24.2). What does it show and what is the diagnosis? Should he have an angiogram?

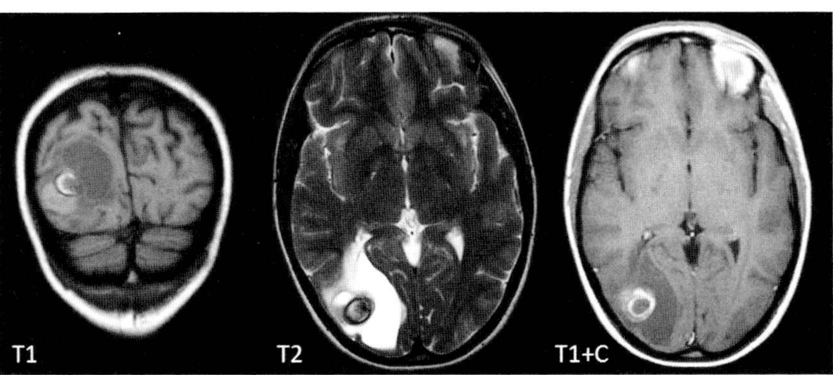

Fig. 24.2

Answer

3. His headache settles and he goes home. An MRI scan is performed at 6 weeks as planned (Fig. 24.2). What does it show and what is the diagnosis? Should he have an angiogram?

The coronal T_1, axial T_2, and axial T_1 post contrast scans are shown. The abnormality and an associated fluid-filled cavity within it (bright on T_2) are seen. The mass has high signal elements on T_1 and low signal, even a black rim, on T_2. It does not enhance appreciably. These are the characteristic findings of a cavernoma; however, a metastasis is still possible. The black rim on T_2 reflects haemosiderin deposition from haemorrhage. An angiogram is not required. If an angiogram is performed it will probably be normal, although occasionally a late venous 'blush' may be seen reflecting the venous nature of the vascular channels in the cavernoma. The near-normal angiographic appearances of cavernomas has led to them being described previously as 'angiographically occult vascular malformations'.

Questions

4. What is the natural history of cavernomas and how would you counsel him?
5. What is the role of radiosurgery for cavernomas?
6. How would you advise a patient who presented with dipolopia and was found to have a single haemorrhage from a cavernoma located in the brainstem as shown in Fig. 24.3?

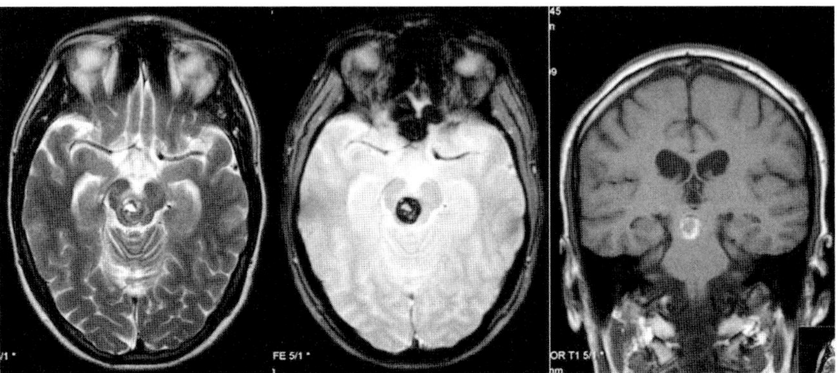

Fig. 24.3

Answers

4. What is the natural history of cavernomas and how would you counsel him?

Cavernomas are characterized by recurrent haemorrhages that are typically small as they are under venous pressure. As such, a cavernoma in this location is unlikely to be life-threatening. Surgery is typically curative and depending on the location may carry low morbidity. This patient's cavernoma is fairly superficially located at the boundary between the parietal and occipital lobes. As such, surgery using image guidance to locate it should carry low risk. The principle risks of surgery are epilepsy and focal neurological deficits. In this case this may be a non-dominant parietal lobe syndrome, which might include problems of spatial perception (classically getting lost in an otherwise familiar location) or dressing apraxia. Conversely, the risks of not treating him are also low. The overall risk of haemorrhage from a cavernoma is 0.5–2% per year, and a haemorrhage from a cavernoma in this location is likely to be well tolerated. Therefore he should probably not be offered immediate surgery unless he has difficulty with the uncertainty of conservative management.

5. What is the role of radiosurgery for cavernomas?

Radiosurgery has been used extensively with safety and good long-term results for intracranial arteriovenous malformations. It has also been used for cavernomas with equivocal results. Therefore the role is currently unproven; however, it appears to be safe and thus may be given if there is no alternative and conservative management is not acceptable. It is more appropriate for surgically inaccessible lesions such as those in the thalamus, or brainstem. This patient's lesion is superficial and surgically accessible, and if he wishes for active treatment he should undergo open surgery. This was performed because of concern over the diagnosis; happily it proved to be a cavernoma rather than a metastasis.

6. How would you advise a patient who presented with dipolopia and was found to have a single haemorrhage from a cavernoma located in the brainstem as shown in Fig. 24.3?

The patient should be told of the diagnosis but reassured that the risks of recurrent haemorrhage are statistically low (of the order of 0.5–2.0% per year) but this may be more clinically apparent in eloquent areas of the brain, particularly the brainstem. A gradual recovery is to be expected from this bleeding episode, and therefore he should be offered rehabilitation as necessary and ophthalmological follow-up in case the diplopia does not resolve. He may be disqualified from driving because of his diplopia, although driving may be permitted if he can satisfy the authorities that his diplopia is mild or is managed well with prisms, or that he can drive safely with one eye covered. Counselling of the patient with an element of reassurance is most important at this stage as he may become extremely anxious at the prospect of a further haemorrhage. This is particularly important for a brainstem cavernoma as the treatment options are very limited. Most experienced surgeons would reserve surgery for brainstem cavernomas for patients with recurrent bleeds and progressive deficits with a lesion that is surgically accessible, i.e. rising to the surface of the structure it involves.

As with the previous case, there is an unproven role of radiosurgery for cavernomas. However, it may be the only option available, and this should be explored for such cases.

Further reading

Duckworth EA (2010). Modern management of brainstem cavernous malformations. *Neurol Clin*; **28**: 887–98.

Kondziolka D, Lunsford LD, Kestle JR (1995). The natural history of cerebral cavernous malformations. *J Neurosurg*; **83**: 820–4.

Monaco EA, Khan AA, Niranjan A, *et al.* (2010). Stereotactic radiosurgery for the treatment of symptomatic brainstem cavernous malformations. *Neurosurg Focus*; **29**: E11.

Pollock BE (2008). Radiosurgery for cavernous malformations: theory and practice. *Clin Neurosurg*; **55**: 97–100.

Porter PJ, Willinsky RA, Harper W, Wallace MC (1997). Cerebral cavernous malformations: natural history and prognosis after clinical deterioration with or without hemorrhage. *J Neurosurg*; **87**: 190–7.

Case 25

A 55-year-old man arrived in the emergency department having been found collapsed in his kitchen 6 hours previously. He was last seen well by his wife an hour before he was found. On arrival in the emergency department, he was alert and eye-opening spontaneously, and obeying commands with his left hand (he was unable to move his right side). He was attempting to speak but was unable to do so. His pulse rate was 126bpm and the rhythm was atrial fibrillation. His blood pressure was 203/110mmHg.

Questions

1. What is this patient's GCS?
2. What type of dysphasia does this patient have?
3. A CT scan is performed (Fig. 25.1). Describe the appearances on the scan.
4. What is the medical management of this case?
5. Is this patient a candidate for a decompressive craniectomy? How should the decision be reached?

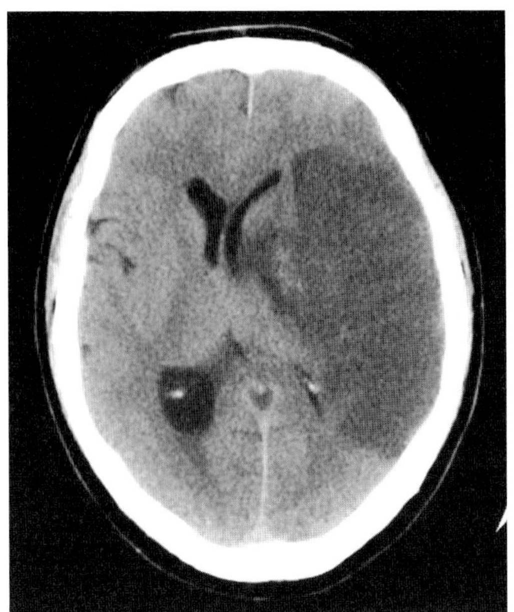

Fig. 25.1

Answers

1. What is this patient's GCS?

His GCS is (E4, VD, M6 = 10D). He is unable to speak, presumably due to damage to the language areas in the left hemisphere. His verbal score is therefore recorded as D (dysphasic). There are various other situations in which components of the GCS are not possible to assess; for example the verbal score when a patient is intubated. In this situation the verbal score is recorded as T (intubated) and not 1 (none). Recording a response as 1 when in fact assessment is not possible may lead to a falsely unfavourable prognosis (see 'Glasgow Coma Scale and Coma Score', p. 196).

2. What type of dysphasia does this patient have?

This patient has an expressive dysphasia as he is obeying commands, indicating that his comprehension is intact.

3. A CT scan is performed (Fig. 25.1). Describe the appearances on the scan.

There is a large area of low attenuation in the left frontal, temporal, and parietal regions and in the posterior parts of the basal ganglia. This is an acute infarct and it involves the entire left middle cerebral artery territory. There is some early haemorrhagic transformation indicated by patchy high density in the left putamen. The caudate head is spared as it is supplied by anterior cerebral artery perforators. There is effacement of the frontal horn of the left lateral ventricle with midline shift. There is also contralateral compartmental hydrocephalus of the trigone of the right lateral ventricle.

4. What is the medical management of this case?

Thrombolysis should be considered for acute cerebral infarction, but this is not appropriate in this case as the presentation is too late. The patient should receive aspirin, intravenous fluids, thromboprophylaxis with compression stockings, a swallowing assessment, and if necessary a nasogastric tube for feeding and medication. Further considerations are as follows.

(a) Management of blood pressure: the blood pressure is elevated, but in this setting probably represents a compensatory response to cerebral infarction to maintain cerebral perfusion pressure (see 'Cerebral blood flow and autoregulation', p. 50). Lowering the blood pressure risks precipitating further ischaemia. On the other hand, a grossly elevated blood pressure may increase the risk of haemorrhage into the infarct. In general, hypertension in the immediate period after a stroke is best left alone. If antihypertensive agents are to be used, an intravenous infusion that can be stopped rapidly (e.g. labetalol) should be used.

(b) Management of atrial fibrillation (AF): the ventricular rate should be controlled with an appropriate agent. Cardioversion should not be performed if the duration of AF is unknown, as it may precipitate embolization of a cardiac thrombus. If the patient remains in AF, anticoagulation should be considered at a later stage (typically 2 weeks) to reduce the risk of systemic embolization. Anticoagulation should not be introduced in the immediate period after a stroke because it may precipitate haemorrhage into the infracted brain.

(c) After the patient recovers from the acute episode, investigations should be performed to search for the underlying cause of the stroke, including carotid doppler ultrasound to look for atherosclerotic plaques, cardiac echocardiography to look for thrombi, valve disease, and septal defects, and routine blood tests including full blood count, urea and electrolytes, cholesterol level, and glucose.

5. Is this patient a candidate for a decompressive craniectomy? How should the decision be reached?

There are three randomized trials (DESTINY, DECIMAL, and HAMLET) to date comparing decompressive hemicraniectomy with medical management for malignant middle cerebral artery infarction. None of the studies individually showed a difference in the primary outcome, although a meta-analysis of the three studies appears to show that surgery reduces mortality in patients under the age of 60 who undergo surgery within 48 hours. Many, although not all, patients who are salvaged with surgery are left with a significant disability (modified Rankin score ≥4). The decision to operate should be made on an individual basis, taking into account the patient's neurological status, previous level of functioning, and comorbidities and discussions with the family. This patient underwent surgery, and his postoperative scan is shown in Fig. 25.2 (left). Note the brain herniating through the craniectomy defect and the resolution of midline shift. The outcome without surgery would have been transtentorial herniation. After surgery this patient remained aphasic and hemiplegic, and he was transferred to a neurorehabilitation centre for

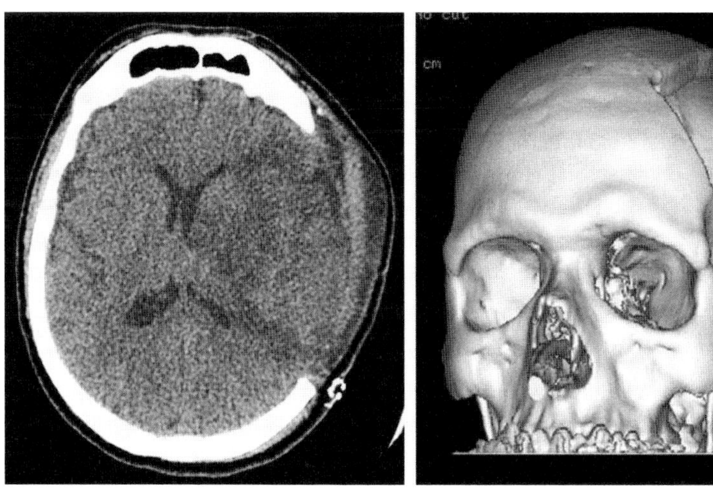

Fig. 25.2

further care. If he regains independence a cranioplasty will be required at a future date, and a CT scan was performed to plan the shape of the prosthesis (Fig. 25.2 (right), showing the craniectomy defect).

Further reading

Hofmeijer J, Kappelle LJ, Algra A, *et al.* (2009). Surgical decompression for space-occupying cerebral infarction (the Hemicraniectomy after middle cerebral artery infarction with Life-threatening Edema Trial (HAMLET)): a multicentre, open, randomised trial. *Lancet Neurol*; **8**: 326–33.

Mitchell P, Gregson BA, Crossman J, *et al.* (2009). Reassessment of the HAMLET study. *Lancet Neurol*; **8**: 602–3.

Glasgow Coma Scale and Coma Score

The Glasgow Coma Scale was developed to allow accurate and reproducible assessment of the level of consciousness in individual patients and to facilitate effective communication of this between health professionals (Teasdale and Jennett 1974). The original scale consisted of the three domains of eye-opening, verbal response, and motor response, each of which were numerically rated according to the patient's best response from a minimum of 1 (no response) to a maximum of 4 for eye opening, 5 for verbal response, and 5 for motor response. The motor domain was later expanded to include two types of flexion response (thereby increasing the maximum score in the motor domain to 6), but it was found that most health professionals could not reliably differentiate between the two flexion responses. Therefore it has been recommended that the distinction between normal and abnormal flexion is not attempted for routine clinical purposes (Teasdale and Murray 2000).

The difficulty arises because the 15-point GCS (incorporating the distinction between normal and abnormal flexion) has been adopted in most hospitals worldwide—a GCS of 14 implies that the patient is not neurologically intact. However, the GCS was not designed to be used as a total score for clinical purposes (rather, the total score was used for collating data in research). The practice of adding up and reporting only the total score can be very misleading because of its numerous possible permutations. For example, a patient with a total GCS of 11 can simply be intoxicated with alcohol (E2, V3, M6) or severely impaired neurologically (E3, V3, M5). Furthermore, in some situations it is not possible to assess a particular component of the scale, such as the verbal score in an intubated patient or the eye response in a patient whose eyes are shut due to periorbital oedema. In these situations the response should be recorded as such (e.g. intubated or otherwise not possible to assess) rather than ascribing a score of 1, as in some cases this erroneous practice has led to the conclusion that some patients with a GCS of 3 did better than those with a GCS of 4. Therefore in clinical practice the GCS should always be reported in terms of the individual responses in the three domains and not solely as the total score.

References

Teasdale G, Jennett B (1974). Assessment of coma and impaired consciousness: a practical scale. *Lancet*; **2**: 81–4.

Teasdale G, Murray L (2000). Revisiting the Glasgow Coma Scale and Coma Score. *Intensive Care Med*; **26**:153–4.

Case 26

A 68-year-old woman presented with a sudden onset of left arm weakness whilst eating breakfast such that she dropped her fork and was unable to pick it up. This lasted for around 30 minutes, after which there was a gradual recovery to normal. She attended the emergency department where a CT scan was performed. The contrast enhanced scan is shown in Fig. 26.1. Her medical history includes coronary heart disease, diabetes, hypertension, and multiple strokes.

Questions

1. What does the scan show and does it explain her symptoms?
2. What is the initial step in the management of this case? Does the patient require admission to hospital?

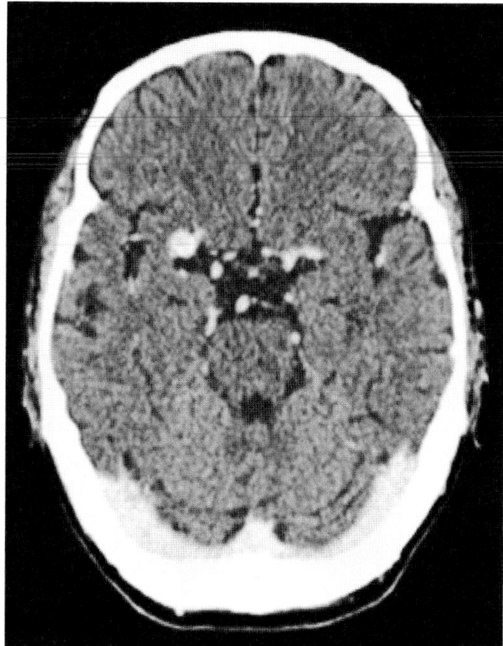

Fig. 26.1

Answers

1. What does the scan show and does it explain her symptoms?

The scan shows a circular hyperdense area adjacent to the right middle cerebral artery, which is likely to be an aneurysm. Note that the density is the same as the adjacent blood vessels. There is no subarachnoid blood, suggesting that this is an incidental finding. There are small low-density areas in the left side of the pons which may be due to small-vessel disease. The patient's symptoms were thought more likely to be due to a transient ischaemic attack (TIA).

2. What is the initial step in the management of this case? Does the patient require admission to hospital?

The initial management is to investigate the TIA in the conventional manner with echocardiography, carotid ultrasound, and risk factor control. Subsequently, the risks of aneurysm rupture should be weighed against the risks of the procedure to secure the aneurysm and to decide whether it would be in the patient's best interests to treat it. The rupture risk of an unruptured MCA aneurysm of this size (the report on Fig. 26.1 indicated this to be an 8mm aneurysm) is about 0.5–1% per year. The risk of aneurysm rupture should be weighed against long-term morbidity from other causes, which are appreciable in this patient by virtue of age and the presence of cerebrovascular disease. If the relative risk to life from aneurysm rupture is small, treatment of the aneurysm may not be justified. The patient does not have to be admitted to hospital—this discussion should take place in the outpatient setting (see 'Unruptured aneurysms', p. 199).

Unruptured aneurysms

Unruptured intracranial aneurysms are increasing in incidence for a number of reasons. First, more people are undergoing high-resolution brain imaging for symptoms that in the past would not have warranted imaging of sufficient quality to show a small aneurysm. Minor headaches, migraines, and vertigo are routinely investigated using MRI and therefore asymptomatic aneurysms may be discovered. Secondly, increased education of the relatives of patients with subarachnoid haemorrhage is resulting in more screening investigations for first-degree relatives of these patients.

Occasionally unruptured aneurysms present symptomatically. The most common is visual disturbance, typically a third nerve palsy due to a PCom or SCA aneurysm, or reduced acuity in one eye due to optic nerve compression by an ophthalmic artery or a terminal carotid aneurysm. Giant aneurysms(>25mm diameter) can occasionally present with cortical deficits due to mass effect. Large aneurysms are usually lined with thrombus, and if there is turbulent flow within the aneurysm itself this thrombus may act as a source of emboli. In this case aneurysms may present with transient ischaemic attacks (TIAs) in the downstream territory.

(continued)

Unruptured aneurysms *(continued)*

The majority of unruptured aneurysms are treated specifically to prevent rupture. Large aneurysms are difficult to clip or coil and may require complex vascular surgical procedures including bypass. Only rarely are aneurysms treated for reasons other than to prevent rupture, and these are managed on an individual basis. Various factors must be considered to inform decision-making around treatment of an unruptured aneurysm:

- What is the life expectancy of the patient?
- What is the annual risk of rupture of the aneurysm?
- What are the consequences of aneurysmal rupture likely to be (cavernous carotid aneurysms may cause a carotid-cavernous fistula which is a more benign problem than a full subarachnoid haemorrhage)?
- How can the aneurysm be treated? Is it suitable for coiling and will coiling provide an angiographically good and durable result? If it is suitable for clipping, what are the risks associated with the surgery?

The risk of rupture of unruptured aneurysms was considered in the International Study of Unruptured Intracranial Aneurysms (ISUIA) (Wiebers *et al.* 2003) (Table 26.1). Aneurysms were classified as anterior (ICA, ACA/ACom, MCA) or posterior (PCom, Basilar, PCA).

Therefore individualized counselling is vital for patients with unruptured aneurysms. Surveillance is warranted in case the aneurysm increases in size; this may increase the associated rupture risk. Whether conservative management or intervention is proposed, other issues must be considered; the most important of these are control of hypertension and cessation of smoking. Patients who undergo aneurysm repair should be advised that their risk of recurrence is increased fourfold if they continue to smoke (Ortiz *et al.* 2008).

Table 26.1 Five-year risk of aneurysm rupture: ISUIA study

Aneurysm size (mm)	Five-year rupture risk (%)		Five-year rupture risk (cavernous carotid) (%)
	Anterior	Posterior	
<7	0	2.5	0
7–12	2.6	14.5	0
13–24	14.5	18.4	3.0
>24	40	50	6.4

References

Ortiz R, Stefanski M, Rosenwasser R, Veznedaroglu E (2008). Cigarette smoking as a risk factor for recurrence of aneurysms treated by endosaccular occlusion. *J Neurosurg*; **108**: 672–5.

Wiebers DO, Whisnant JP, Huston J 3rd, *et al.* (2003). International Study of Unruptured Intracranial Aneurysms Investigators. Unruptured intracranial aneurysms: natural history, clinical outcome, and risks of surgical and endovascular treatment. *Lancet*; **362**: 103–10.

Case 27

A 43-year-old woman is admitted with a sudden severe headache in good neurological condition. She has marked photophobia and is vomiting. Her CT scan shows subarachnoid blood and angiograms confirm a right PCom aneurysm. The patient undergoes coiling of the aneurysm as in view of the neck it is considered likely to provide a good angiographic result. The angiograms before and after coiling are shown in Fig. 27.1. She makes a good recovery which continues when she is seen in outpatients 6 weeks later.

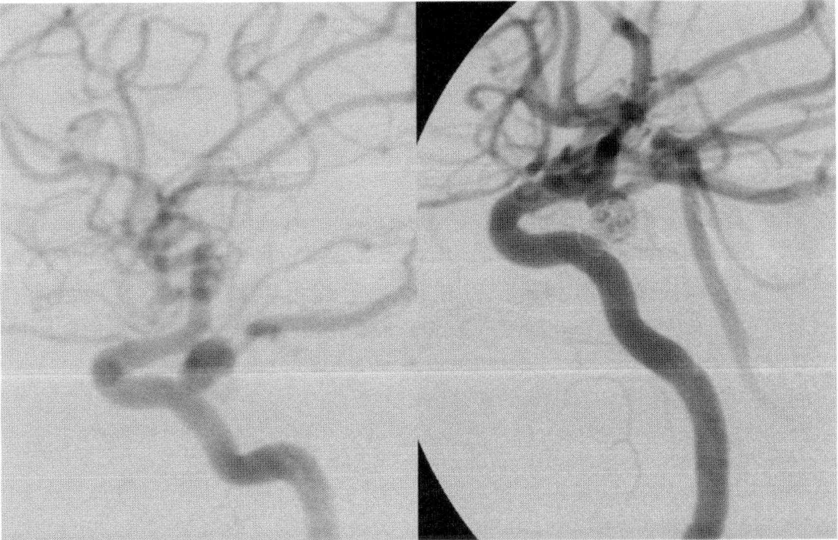

Fig. 27.1

Questions

1. How would you follow her up and when?
2. The patient's sister has come with her and wants to know if she should be screened for unruptured aneurysms. How would you counsel her?

Answers

1. How would you follow her up and when?

The options for follow-up are strongly dictated by local preference for the modality of choice. Follow-up is not to detect imminent rupture but rather to detect recurrence of the aneurysm neck which might over time and result in an unstable aneurysm with a risk of re-rupture. CTA is the modality of choice for diagnosis of the ruptured aneurysm initially, but there will be too much artefact from the coils to make it of any value in surveillance of the coiled aneurysm. MR angiography or catheter angiography can be used instead. The latter carries additional risks, however small, of arterial puncture and stroke, and therefore should be reserved for cases where the MRA is unclear.

The timing of the follow-up imaging is also debated. An early post-procedure MRA may be done to offer baseline comparison for the next scan which can be done at 6 months, assuming that the coiling is deemed satisfactory. If scans at 6 months and 1 year show stable coiling, the follow-up interval is increased.

2. The patient's sister has come with her and wants to know if she should be screened for unruptured aneurysms. How would you counsel her?

Screening for unruptured aneurysms should be offered to any individual with two first-degree relatives with aneurysmal subarachnoid haemorrhage. Patients with associated disease (e.g. adult polycystic kidney disease) may be offered a screening CTA or high-quality MRA. There are emerging groups of patients with lesser indications for screening angiography—for example, those with relatives with unruptured aneurysms. They may be offered screening, but should be counselled that small aneurysms in difficult locations to access surgically may be left or monitored and the act of screening them may provoke more anxiety than it assures.

Questions

3. The patient undergoes an MR angiogram which suggests a neck recurrence. This is evaluated with a catheter angiogram which is shown in Fig. 27.2. How does it compare to the previous angiogram at the end of the coiling?
4. Given the patient's age (45) and good recovery from the haemorrhage the recurrence merits re-treatment. What are the options and which would you prefer?

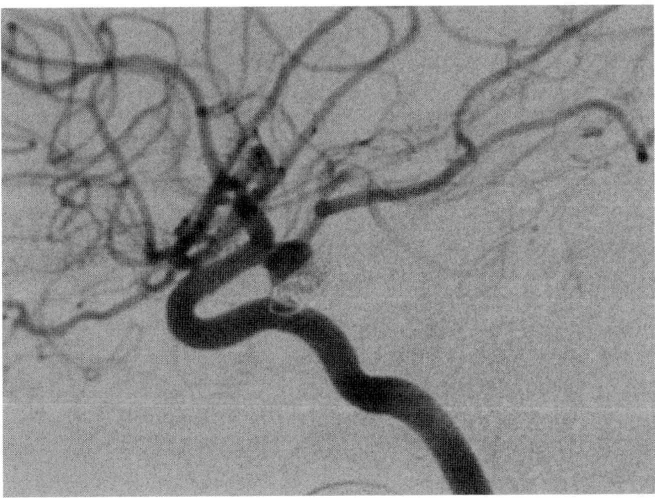

Fig. 27.2

Answers

3. The patient undergoes an MR angiogram which suggests a neck recurrence. This is evaluated with a catheter angiogram which is shown in Fig. 27.2. How does it compare to the previous angiogram at the end of the coiling?

There is appreciable recurrence of the neck of the aneurysm due to compaction of the coils into the dome.

4. Given the patient's age (45) and good recovery from the haemorrhage, the recurrence merits re-treatment. What are the options and which would you prefer?

The options are again endovascular or surgical management. Endovascular treatment can be offered if the patient has a strong preference. However, the aim of treatment now is very different to the aim of the original coiling. The aim now is to protect the patient from rupture during the rest of her life. The aim before was to prevent early re-rupture which is most common during the first few weeks after the bleed.

Open surgery for previously coiled aneurysms can be challenging as the coil ball may prevent a good closure of the aneurysm clip. It may be necessary to exclude the parent vessel temporarily, open the sac, and remove the coils before clipping the aneurysm and then remove the temporary clips from the parent vessel. These manoeuvres potentially increase the surgical morbidity.

However, despite this, the differences in aim of treatment underpin the bias toward surgery for unruptured aneurysms and towards coiling for ruptured aneurysms. Given that this woman's aneurysm had recurred despite an angiographically complete coiling, it was agreed that it should be clipped and the surgery was performed uneventfully.

Further reading

Bor AS, Koffijberg H, Wermer MJ, Rinkel GJ (2010). Optimal screening strategy for familial intracranial aneurysms: a cost-effectiveness analysis. *Neurology*; **74**: 1671–9.

Rinkel GJ (2005). Intracranial aneurysm screening: indications and advice for practice. *Lancet Neurol*; **4**: 122–8.

Schaafsma JD, Koffijberg H, Buskens E, Velthuis BK, van der Graaf Y, Rinkel GJ (2010). Cost-effectiveness of magnetic resonance angiography versus intra-arterial digital subtraction angiography to follow-up patients with coiled intracranial aneurysms. *Stroke*; **41**: 1736–42.

Shankar JJ, Lum C, Parikh N, dos Santos M (2010). Long-term prospective follow-up of intracranial aneurysms treated with endovascular coiling using contrast-enhanced MR angiography. *AJNR Am J Neuroradiol*; **31**: 1211–15.

Veznedaroglu E, Benitez RP, Rosenwasser RH (2008). Surgically treated aneurysms previously coiled: lessons learned. *Neurosurgery*; **62** (Suppl 3): 1516–24.

Waldron JS, Halbach VV, Lawton MT (2009). Microsurgical management of incompletely coiled and recurrent aneurysms: trends, techniques, and observations on coil extrusion. *Neurosurgery*; **64** (Suppl 2): 301–15.

Case 28

A 65-year-old woman presented to the neurosurgical clinic with a 2-week history of worsening left retro-orbital headache and double vision. On examination she had a left sixth nerve palsy. Seven years previously she had a similar presentation and was diagnosed to have a 15mm left carotico-ophthalmic aneurysm which was coiled at the time. On initial follow-up this had been stable with a small residual neck, but she had not been reviewed for the last 4 years.

Questions

1. What causes double vision?
2. The patient has a left sixth nerve palsy on examination. Explain how she may have double vision on looking to both the left and right.
3. Explain why a carotico-ophthalmic aneurysm might cause a sixth nerve palsy.
4. The patient underwent an MRI scan of the brain (T_2-weighted axial slice shown) and a cerebral angiogram (Fig. 28.1). Describe the important findings.
5. What is the prognosis if this condition is left untreated?
6. What are the options for treatment?

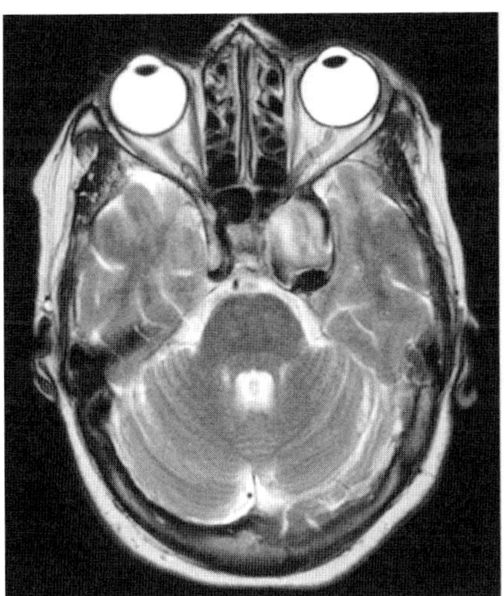

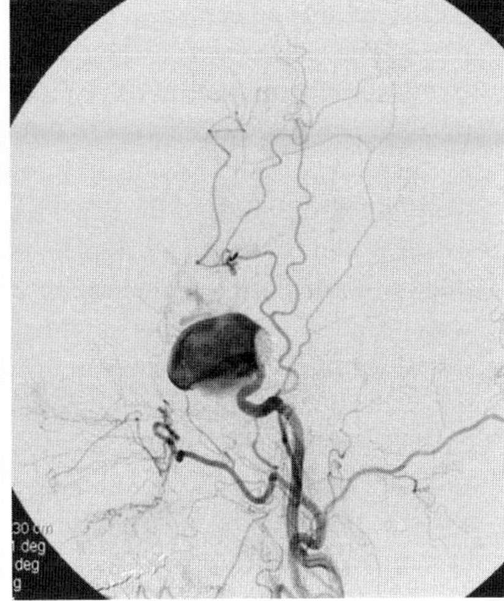

Fig. 28.1

Answers

1. What causes double vision?

Double vision can be monocular (i.e. occurs when seeing with one eye only) or binocular (occurs when seeing with both eyes). Binocular diplopia is more frequently seen in neurological disease and occurs when the two eyes do not move in synchrony. This may be due to dysfunction of the extra-ocular muscles themselves or their nerve supply, or of the central pathways involved in conjugate eye movements (see 'Assessment of eye movements', p. 140). Monocular diplopia occurs due to problems within the eye itself such as damage to the cornea, iris or lens.

2. The patient has a left sixth nerve palsy on examination. Explain how she may have double vision on looking to both the left and right.

A left sixth nerve palsy (causing paresis of the left lateral rectus muscle) leads to failure of abduction of the left eye and therefore diplopia on looking left. Diplopia on looking right may also occur in this situation because the balance of the globe is maintained by the tone of all the extra-ocular muscles. An alternative explanation is that she may also have a partial left third nerve palsy.

3. Explain why a carotico-ophthalmic aneurysm might cause a sixth nerve palsy.

If a carotid aneurysm is wholly or partially within the cavernous sinus, as it expands it can compress structures in the lateral wall of the cavernous sinus, the nearest to it being the sixth nerve (Fig. 28.2). If the aneurysm expands further it will compress more lateral structures in the lateral wall of the cavernous sinus, which are the third, fourth, and fifth nerves (ophthalmic and maxillary divisions). This would cause numbness on one side of the face (not in the jaw or lower teeth which are mandibular divisions of the trigeminal nerve) and a complete ophthalmoplegia which would consist of a complete ptosis, mid-position fixed eye, and a dilated pupil unresponsive to light. Therefore the history of a painful sixth nerve palsy with progression to compete ophthalmoplegia is very suggestive of an enlarging intracavernous carotid aneurysm. If such an aneurysm ruptured into the cavernous sinus this would cause a carotico-cavernous fistula, classically with retro-orbital headache, blurred vision in the affected eye, chemosis, and proptosis along with the sign of an audible pulsatile bruit over the eye, but if there was an intradural segment to the aneurysm a rupture of this section would lead to a subarachnoid haemorrhage, which is potentially life threatening.

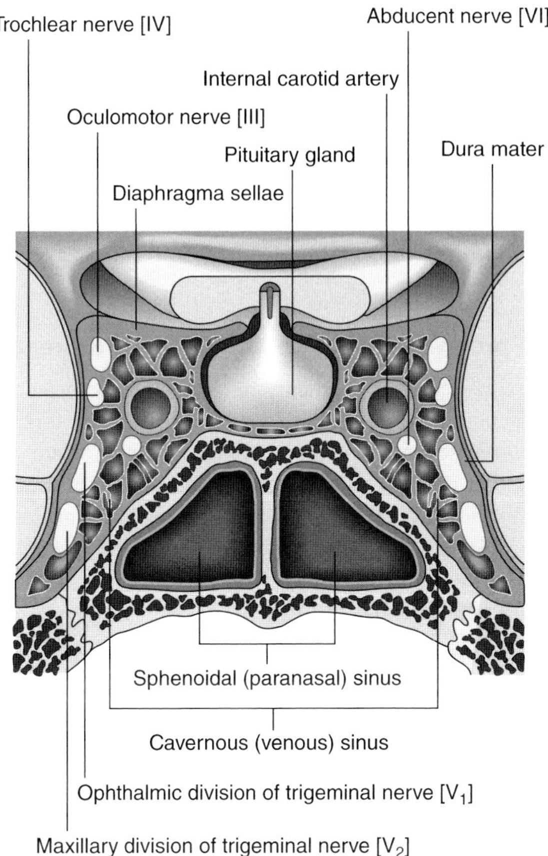

Fig. 28.2 Contents of the cavernous sinus. Reproduced with permission from Drake, R *et al., Gray's Anatomy for Students*. © Elsevier 2009.

4. The patient underwent an MRI scan of the brain (T_2-weighted axial slice shown) and a cerebral angiogram (Fig. 28.1). Describe the important findings.

The MRI shows a left-sided 30mm mass located medial to the left temporal lobe and arising in the region of the carotid artery. The angiogram confirms this to be a cerebral aneurysm arising from the proximal intradural internal carotid artery. The posterior rim of the aneurysm does not fill with intra-arterial contrast on angiography and shows low signal on the MRI where the previously inserted coils were placed.

5. What is the prognosis if this condition is left untreated?

This would be considered a giant aneurysm (maximum diameter >25mm) with the prognosis being poor even if unruptured, with the risk of rupture, death, or serious permanent neurological deficit being >50% within 1 year. Giant aneurysms can be symptomatic if they rupture, causing compression of adjacent structures (including the brainstem for posterior circulation aneurysms), or they can cause ischaemic infarction by throwing off thrombotic embolus into their distal circulatory territory.

6. What are the options for treatment?

Given the natural history, conservative management is not generally a good option but it may well have to be considered, particularly for more elderly or medically unwell patients. Operative clipping can sometimes be undertaken but often carries a higher risk of stroke and may have to be considered under cardiac bypass and hypothermic cerebral circulatory arrest. Coiling and stenting can again sometimes be an option and are not such a major procedure physiologically as open surgery, but still carry appreciable risks of stroke or death. Balloon occlusion of the feeding artery into a giant aneurysm (and hence thrombosis of the aneurysm) can often be the best option provided that it is tolerated during a test occlusion without inducing a neurological deficit. This usually allows complete occlusion of the aneurysm with no risk of recurrence and minimal physiological insult to the patient as the procedure is endovascular. If the cerebral collateral circulation is not enough to tolerate this and the patient develops a temporary deficit when performing a test occlusion, it is possible to perform a surgical extracranial to intracranial (EC–IC) bypass procedure to augment the cerebral blood flow to the affected distal circulation of the brain. Usually, the superficial temporal artery, or a segment of radial artery joined to the carotid artery in the neck, can be anastomosed onto a branch of the middle cerebral artery. This patient successfully underwent an EC–IC bypass (superficial temporal to middle cerebral) and then delayed balloon occlusion 1 month later. Her aneurysm was fully occluded.

Fig. 28.3 shows the patient's postoperative CT angiogram with the arrow indicating the presence of a superficial temporal artery branch traversing through a craniotomy defect and joining onto a vessel on the cerebral surface.

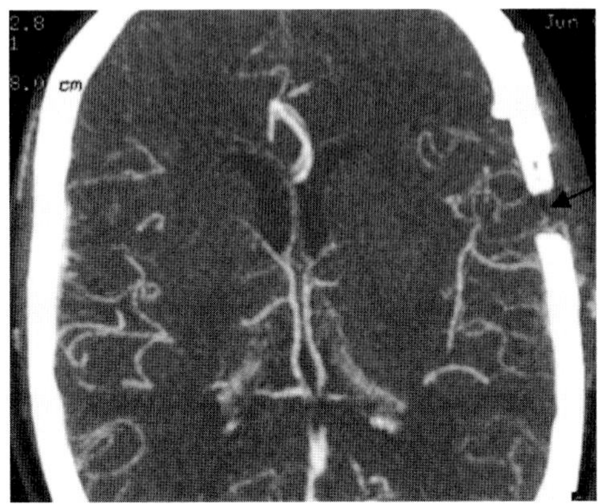

Fig. 28.3

Question

7. For what other indications can EC–IC bypass procedures be utilized?

Answer

7. For what other indications can EC–IC bypass procedures be utilized?

EC–IC procedures can be used to treat chronic cerebral haemodynamic insufficiency as a result of internal carotid artery occlusion causing haemodynamic TIAs or progressive strokes in patients with proven low blood flows in the ischaemic territory. Such patients typically develop a stereotyped neurological deficit when their cerebral perfusion might be reduced, for example when dehydrated or with a postural drop in blood pressure when standing from a sitting or lying position. Patients with a high-grade carotid stenosis (as opposed to occlusion) could have an endarterectomy or carotid stenting to help improve cerebral blood flow if they are developing haemodynamic TIAs. In modern clinical practice it is generally considered necessary to have some form of cerebral blood flow measurement to indicate ischaemia (e.g. xenon CT, PET cerebral perfusion imaging, dynamic angiography, CT perfusion) as historically these operations were done indiscriminately in patients with occluded internal carotid arteries where no proven benefit was established.

EC–IC procedures are also considered for moyamoya disease, where there is progressive intracranial cerebral arterial stenosis and occlusion of unknown aetiology, and often in children or young adult patients, which initially causes ischaemic stroke but later develops an increased risk of intracerebral bleeds as new abnormal fragile perforator arteries enlarge and attempt to supply the ischaemic regions of the brain.

Further reading

EC/IC Bypass Study Group (1985). Failure of extracranial–intracranial arterial bypass to reduce the risk of ischemic stroke. Results of an international randomized trial. *N Engl J Med*; **313**: 1191–1200.

Stiebel-Kalish H, Kalish Y, Bar-On RH, *et al.* (2005). Presentation, natural history, and management of carotid cavernous aneurysms. *Neurosurgery*; **57**: 850–7.

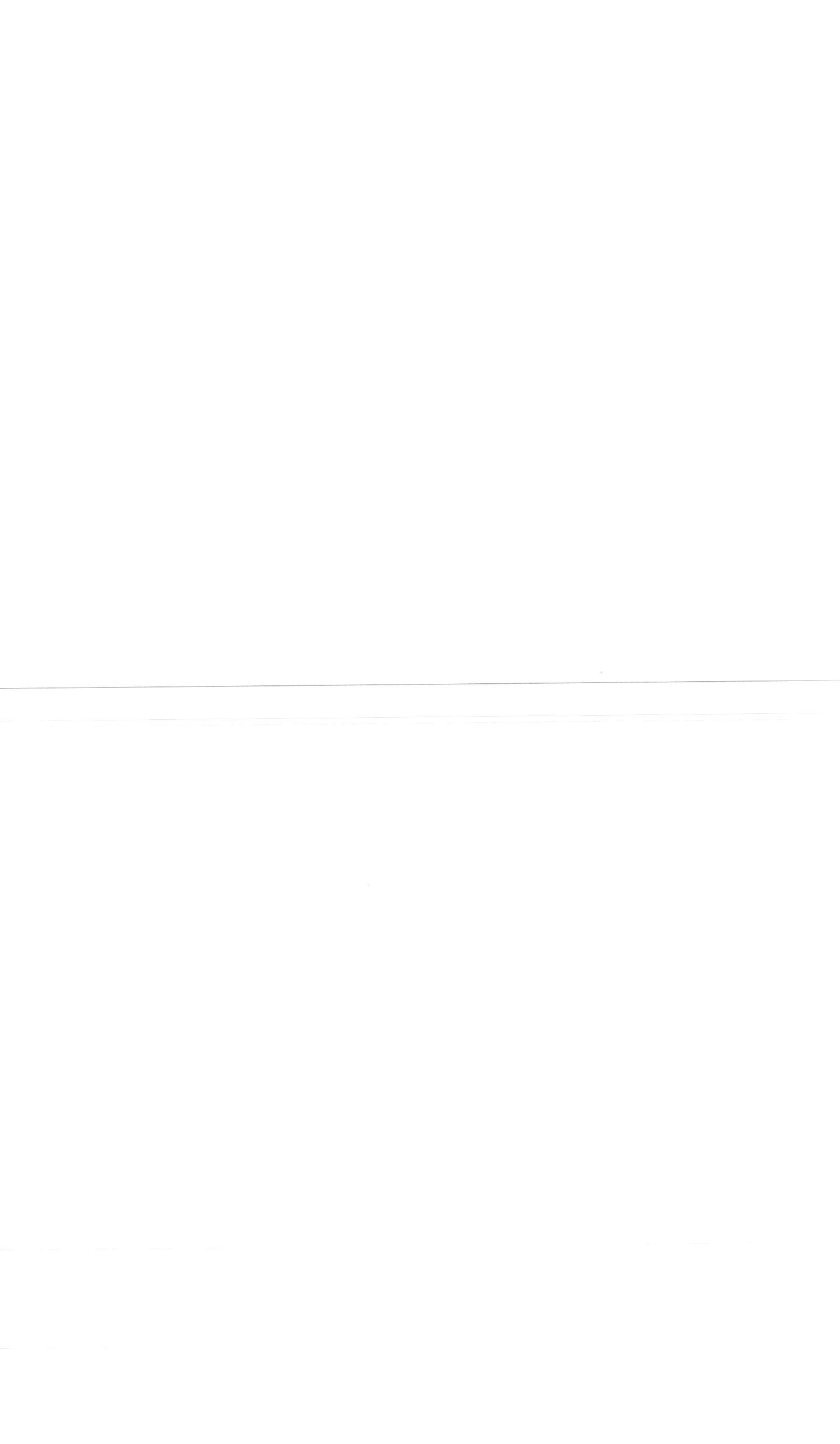

Section 4

Neuro-oncology

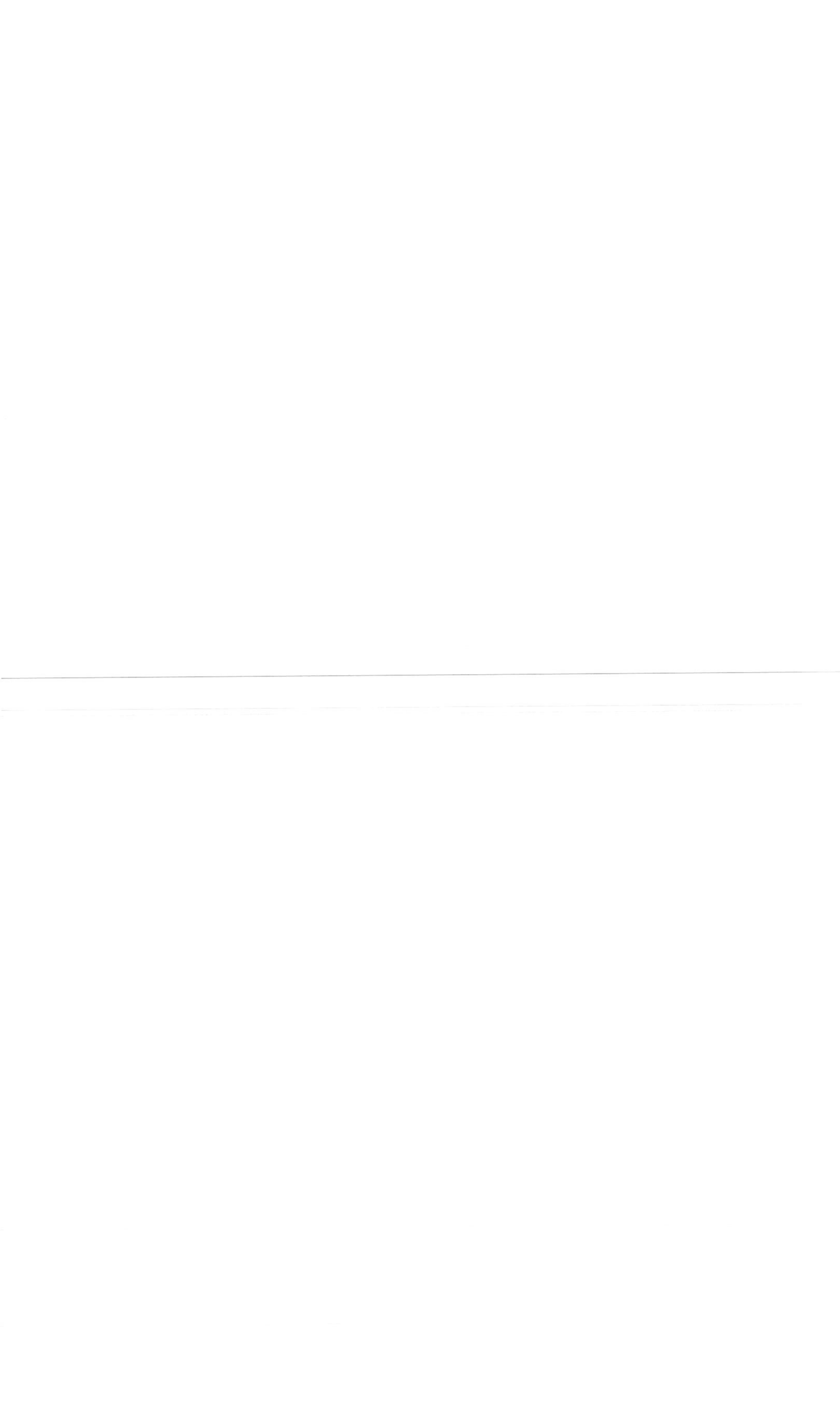

Case 29

A 68-year-old man collapsed at home. In the emergency department, he was drowsy and dysphasic, with moderate right-sided weakness (MRC grade 4/5). His left pupil was 5mm, the right was 3mm, and both reacted to light. He had attended 2 weeks earlier because of difficulties with his speech.

Questions

1. What is the neurosurgical differential diagnosis?
2. A CT scan is performed (Fig. 29.1). Describe the abnormalities seen.
3. What types of oedema occur in the brain and which does this patient have?
4. Explain the patient's drowsiness, speech problems, weakness, and pupils.

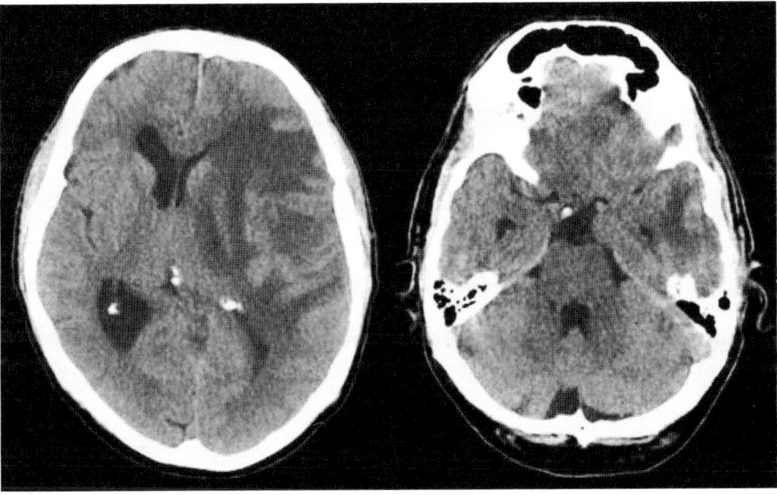

Fig. 29.1

Answers

1. What is the neurosurgical differential diagnosis?

The dysphasia and a right hemiparesis suggest a left cerebral lesion. Unequal pupils may indicate impending transtentorial herniation from mass effect. The speech difficulties two weeks earlier suggest a rapidly expanding mass lesion such as a malignant tumour or a subdural haematoma. The reasons for collapse are unclear from the limited history but he may have suffered a seizure.

2. A CT scan is performed (Fig. 29.1). Describe the abnormalities seen (Fig. 29.2).

There is a mass in the left hemisphere (A) surrounded by an extensive area of low density (B) which represents oedema. There is midline shift (C) and compartmental hydrocephalus (demonstrated by the enlarged lateral ventricles on the right (D) due to compression of the ventricular system at the foramen of Monro. There is herniation of the uncus of the left temporal lobe seen on the lower slice (E).

3. What types of oedema occur in the brain and which does this patient have?

Three main types of oedema occur in the brain.

- Cytotoxic (intracellular) oedema occurs mainly in traumatic and ischaemic brain injury. It results from defective sodium ATP-driven transmembrane channels in the affected cells, leading to sodium (and thence water) retention. It is not responsive to corticosteroids.
- Interstitial oedema occurs in hydrocephalus and is due to high CSF pressures in the ventricular system, resulting in CSF egress into the adjacent brain parenchyma.
- Vasogenic oedema is due to increased capillary permeability from breakdown of the blood–brain barrier. It is seen principally with tumours and abscesses. It is responsive to corticosteroid therapy.

Different types of oedema may coexist. In this patient it is predominantly vasogenic.

4. Explain the patient's drowsiness, speech problems, weakness, and pupils.

The drowsiness is due to raised intracranial pressure. The speech difficulties and right hemiparesis are due to involvement of the language areas and the corticospinal tract, respectively, in the left hemisphere. The dilated left pupil is due to downward displacement of the uncus of the temporal lobe compressing the third nerve that runs below it (see 'Pupillary disorders in neurosurgery', p. 220).

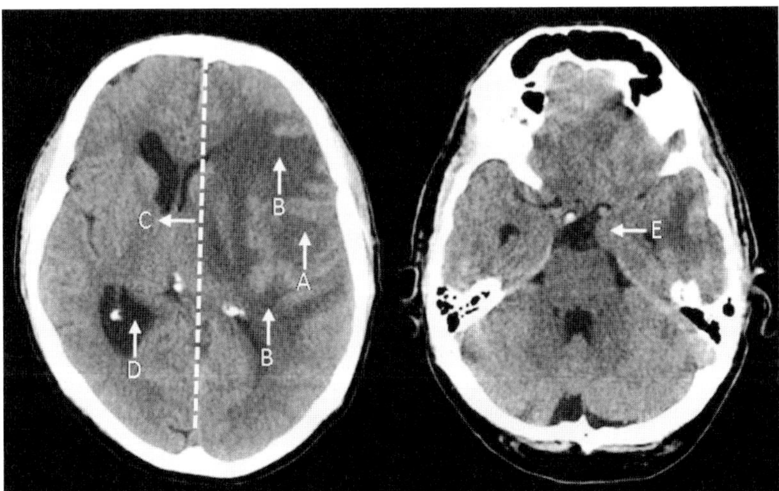

Fig. 29.2

Questions

5. A contrast-enhanced scan is performed (Fig. 29.3). What are the abnormalities and differential diagnosis?
6. How should this patient be managed?

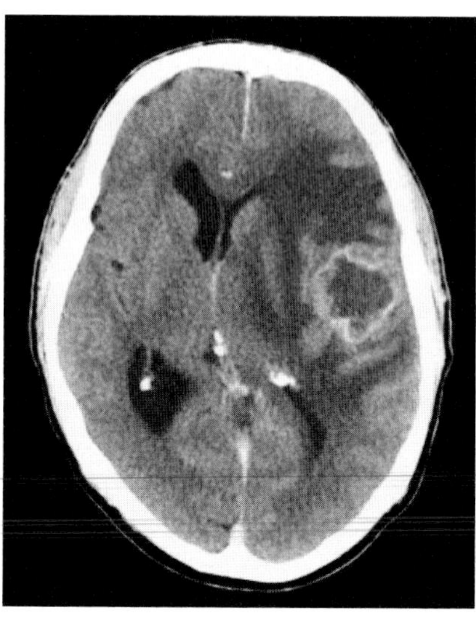

Fig. 29.3

5. A contrast-enhanced scan is performed (Fig. 29.3). What are the abnormalities and differential diagnosis?

The mass exhibits ring enhancement. The differential diagnosis is between a high-grade glioma, an abscess, and metastasis. In the absence of raised infective markers, a tumour is more likely (see 'The role of MRI in the differentiation of cerebral tumours from abscesses', p. 220).

6. How should this patient be managed?

The patient is at risk of rapid deterioration due to raised intracranial pressure. He requires corticosteroids (e.g. dexamethasone 8mg bd) to reduce vasogenic tumour oedema and decompressive surgery if he is to survive. He underwent a craniotomy and debulking of the tumour, and the histology showed a glioblastoma (WHO grade 4). Treatment for glioblastoma after surgical resection consists of radiotherapy and temozolomide for patients in good performance status. The prognosis, even with treatment, is very poor and stands at approximately a year.

Further reading

Kaal ECA, Vecht CJ (2004). The management of brain oedema in brain tumours. *Curr Opin Oncol*; **16**: 593–600.

Wen PY, Kesari S (2008). Malignant gliomas in adults. *N Engl J Med*; **359**: 492–507.

Pupillary disorders in neurosurgery

Neurosurgical residents are often called to see patients on the ward who have 'unequal pupils'. In this situation, an assessment should be made of the size of both pupils and their reactivity to light, whether the asymmetry is a new finding (anisocoria is relatively common), and whether the change has been accompanied by clinical deterioration. A unilaterally dilated pupil can be caused by pressure on the oculomotor nerve by downward displacement of the uncus of the temporal lobe in raised intracranial pressure (transtentorial herniation). The ipsilateral or contralateral (or both) may be involved, and in the context of clinical deterioration urgent action is indicated. A fixed pupil indicates that the nerve has been compressed to such an extent that neural transmission has been impeded. Frequent assessment is necessary as a fixed pupil may become reactive again with fluctuations in intracranial pressure. Always remember that pupillary disorders can represent a wide spectrum of pathology along the entire course of the sympathetic and parasympathetic pathways supplying the eye.

The role of MRI in the differentiation of cerebral tumours from abscesses (Fig. 29.4)

MRI diffusion-weighted imaging (DWI) can be used to differentiate a cystic/necrotic tumour from an abscess. The T_1 sequence with contrast in this patient demonstrates a peripherally enhancing lesion. The associated oedema is hyperintense around the lesion on T_2. DWI indicates the degree to which water molecules can diffuse out of cells. Diffusion is typically restricted in abscesses, yielding a hyperintense MRI signal on DWI. On the other hand, diffusion tends not to be restricted in tumours, which yields a hypointense signal on DWI. The pattern on the apparent diffusion coefficient (ADC) sequence is the opposite: abscesses appear hypointense, whereas cystic/necrotic tumours appear hyperintense. It should be noted that these imaging findings are not pathognomonic of the respective pathologies and the opposite findings can occasionally occur. Other imaging features which may aid in diagnosis include the shape of the ring: an irregular outline is typically seen in tumours, whereas abscesses tend to be smooth. An abscess ring may appear hypointense on T_2-weighted imaging, a feature not commonly seen in tumours. This lesion has MRI features of both a necrotic tumour and an abscess. MR spectroscopy (MRS) examines the chemical constituents of the lesion and reliably differentiates a cystic/necrotic tumour from an abscess, although this modality is not readily available in most institutions in the acute situation.

(continued)

The role of MRI in the differentiation of cerebral tumours from abscesses (Fig. 29.4) *(continued)*

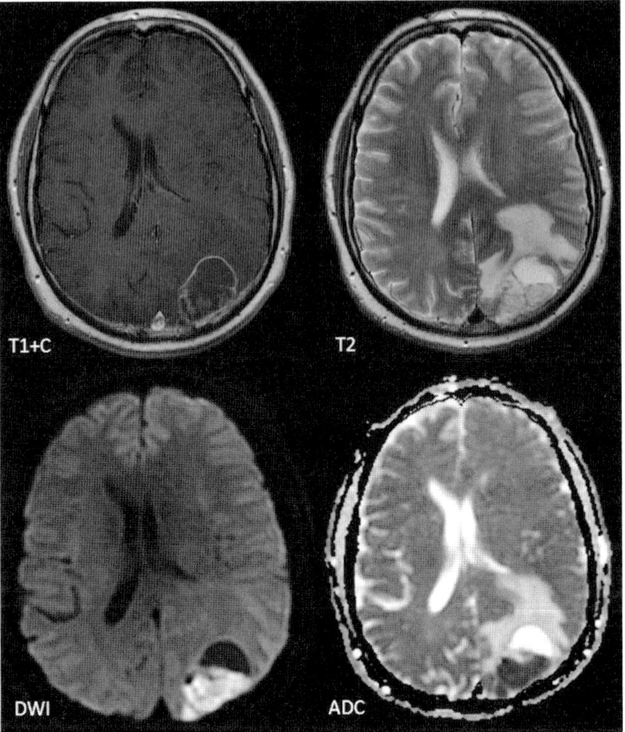

Fig. 29.4

Case 30

A previously well 53-year-old man had developed a sudden onset of severe headache 5 days previously. The headache settled within hours and he did not seek medical advice at the time. He later consulted his GP who sought a neurological referral as he was concerned about an acute vascular migraine. The headache had resolved completely by then, but he had a left-sided homonymous hemianopia.

Questions

1. Where is the lesion presumed to be?
2. What is the differential diagnosis?
3. The MRI is shown in Fig. 30.1. What is the likely diagnosis?
4. What factors influence prognosis if glioblastoma is the diagnosis?

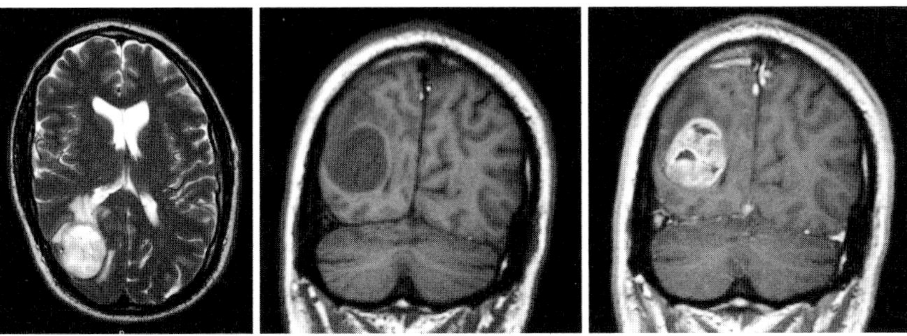

Fig. 30.1

Answers

1. Where is the lesion presumed to be?

To cause a homonymous visual field deficit the lesion must be posterior to the optic chiasm. Therefore it may be in the right optic tract, thalamus, optic radiation, visual cortex, or adjacent structures causing impingement.

2. What is the differential diagnosis?

A sudden-onset severe headache probably represents an intracranial bleed. Given the presumed location of the lesion, this is probably an intraparenchymal haemorrhage. The causes include vascular lesions such as cavernomas, arteriovenous malformations, and other lesions that can bleed including malignant tumours. Alternatively, if there is no mass lesion amyloid angiopathy, hypertension and small-vessel disease could be precipitating factors.

3. The MRI is shown in Fig. 30.1. What is the likely diagnosis?

The T_2 weighted MRI (left) shows a lesion of mixed signal intensity adjacent to the primary visual cortex of the right occipital lobe. There is surrounding oedema, represented by high signal. There is not widespread evidence of white matter disease elsewhere in the brain which, if present, would suggest underlying hypertension or vasculopathy. Therefore appearances are consistent with a tumour. Pre- and post-contrast T_1 images (centre and right) show that the abnormality enhances heterogeneously. This makes a malignant tumour likely. Metastasis is the most common malignant brain tumour, whereas glioblastoma is the most common primary brain tumour. Given the patient's previous unremarkable medical history, the latter is the likely diagnosis.

4. What factors influence prognosis if glioblastoma is the diagnosis?

Glioblastoma has a poor prognosis—median survival of 9–15 months with treatment. Prognosis is influenced by age at presentation and degree of neurological disability (Table 30.1). Younger patients with better performance status survive longer. Treatment factors affecting prognosis include extent of surgical resection (greater resection giving longer survival) and the provision of adjuvant radiotherapy and temozolomide chemotherapy, both of which prolong survival. Certain tumour attributes also influence prognosis; the best studied is *MGMT* promoter methylation status which, if present, confers additive benefits of temozolomide treatment.

This patient is relatively young with a Karnofsky score of 90. Maximal surgical resection followed by radiotherapy and temozolomide is appropriate if glioblastoma is confirmed at surgery.

The patient undergoes a macroscopic resection and glioblastoma is confirmed. He tolerated a full course of radiotherapy with concomitant temozolomide, followed by adjuvant temozolomide for 5 days a week every month. He recovered well but developed headaches a year later. They are progressive and worse in the morning. His visual field improved a little after the surgery but has returned.

Question

5. A repeat MRI is shown in Fig. 30.2. What are the management options now?

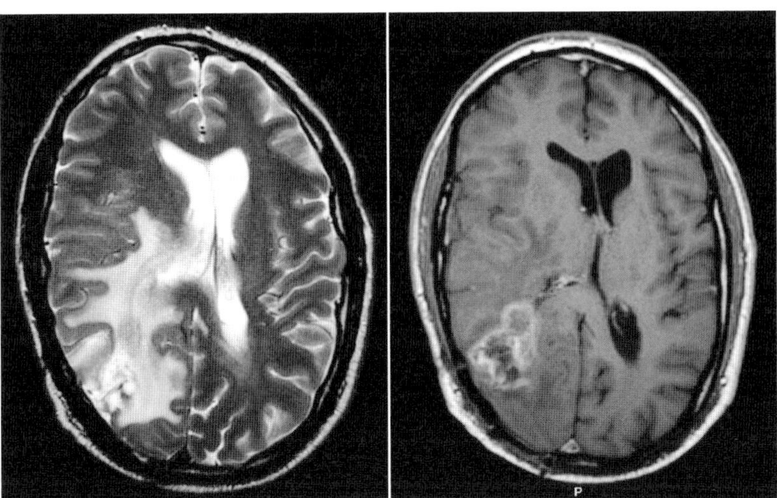

Fig. 30.2

Answer

5. A repeat MRI is shown in Fig. 30.2. What are the management options now?

There is tumour recurrence. The T_2 sequence (left) shows extensive white matter signal change in the posterior right hemisphere. This is probably vasogenic oedema, although a similar pattern follows radiotherapy. The contrast-enhanced T_1 image (right) shows midline shift and recurrent tumour at the resection site, deeper and more extensive than before.

The options are repeat surgery or chemotherapy. As he has progressed despite conventional oncological therapy (temozolomide), the oncological alternatives are PCV chemotherapy or newer agents within clinical trials. Repeat surgery may appear attractive, but if there is no further oncological management afterwards, the patient's continued decline may be rapid.

Repeat tumour debulking surgery may be contemplated if the patient has good performance status and if the pattern of regrowth suggests that surgery could remove a reasonable volume of the tumour with low neurological morbidity. The risks of the surgery should always be considered carefully and poor wound healing following previous surgery and radiotherapy may be problematic.

This patient underwent repeat debulking surgery following discussion with oncologists. He recovered well and went on to receive four cycles of PCV chemotherapy. He died 18 months after his first presentation.

Further reading

Lacroix M, Abi-Said D, Fourney DR, *et al.* (2001). A multivariate analysis of 416 patients with glioblastoma multiforme: prognosis, extent of resection, and survival. *J Neurosurg*; **95**: 190–8.

Laws ER, Parney IF, Huang W, *et al.* (2003). Survival following surgery and prognostic factors for recently diagnosed malignant glioma: data from the Glioma Outcomes Project. *J Neurosurg*; **99**: 467–73.

Stupp R, Mason WP, van den Bent MJ, *et al.* (2005). Radiotherapy plus concomitant and adjuvant temozolomide for glioblastoma. *N Engl J Med*; **352**: 987–96.

Table 30.1 Karnofsky performance status

Score	Description
100	Normal, no complaints, no evidence of disease
90	Able to carry on normal activity, minor signs or symptoms of disease
80	Normal activity with effort, some signs or symptoms of disease
70	Cares for self, unable to carry on normal activity or do active work
60	Requires occasional assistance, able to care for most needs
50	Requires considerable assistance and frequent medical care
40	Disabled, requires special care and assistance
30	Severely disabled, hospitalization indicated although death is not imminent
20	Hospitalization necessary, very sick, active supportive treatment necessary
10	Moribund, fatal processes progressing rapidly
0	Dead

Source: Karnofsky DA, Burchenal JH (1949). The clinical evaluation of chemotherapeutic agents in cancer. In: MacLeod CM (ed), *Evaluation of Chemotherapeutic Agents*. New York: Columbia University Press; p.196.

Case 31

A 27-year-old woman presents to the emergency department following a witnessed first grand mal seizure. She was working at her desk, fell to the floor, shook violently for 30 seconds, and was then unconscious. She bit her tongue but was not incontinent. In the emergency department 20 minutes later she is drowsy but responding to voice and obeying commands. Her left arm is weak.

Questions

1. What factors lower an individual's seizure threshold?
2. What is the significance of the new left arm weakness?
3. No obvious factor predisposing to a seizure is found. A CT brain is performed (Fig. 31.1). What does it show?

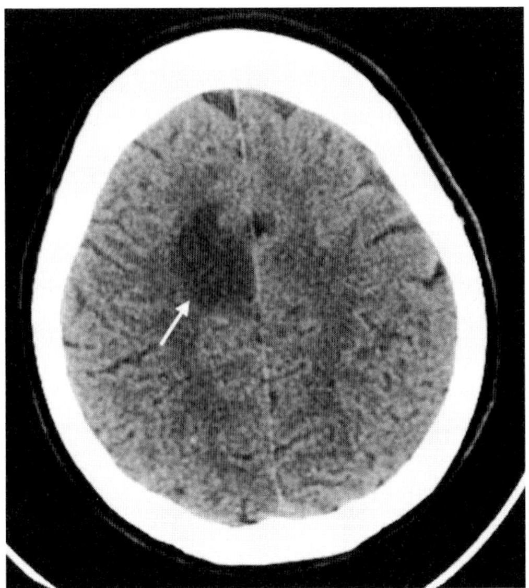

Fig. 31.1

Answers

1. What factors lower an individual's seizure threshold?

Various factors influence an individual's chance of having a seizure: the presence of a systemic inflammatory process, commonly sepsis; electrolyte imbalances, particularly of sodium; certain drugs, including some antidepressants and tramadol; sleep deprivation; rarely, flashing lights.

2. What is the significance of the new left arm weakness?

This is a potentially important focal sign which should recover (Todd's paresis). It may relate to a pre-existing mass lesion. The deficit may persist longer if it is due to an acute lesion, such as haemorrhage, commonly a cavernoma or arteriovenous malformation rather than an aneurysm, as aneurysms present with ictal headache rather than a fit with focal cortical neurological deficit. Alternatively, malignant tumours may present with a haemorrhage.

3. No obvious factor predisposing to a seizure is found. A CT brain is performed (Fig. 31.1). What does it show?

The posterior right frontal lobe low attenuation (arrow) is probably a low-grade tumour. Absent contrast enhancement will usually distinguish it from a high-grade (malignant) tumour. With clear edges, a small cortical infarct is another possibility. Diffusion-weighted MRI can help decide between infarct and tumour.

Questions

4. Sagittal T_2 (A) and coronal pre-contrast (B) and post-contrast (C) MRIs are shown in Fig. 31.2. What is the tumour location and what information does it provide?
5. What are the management options?

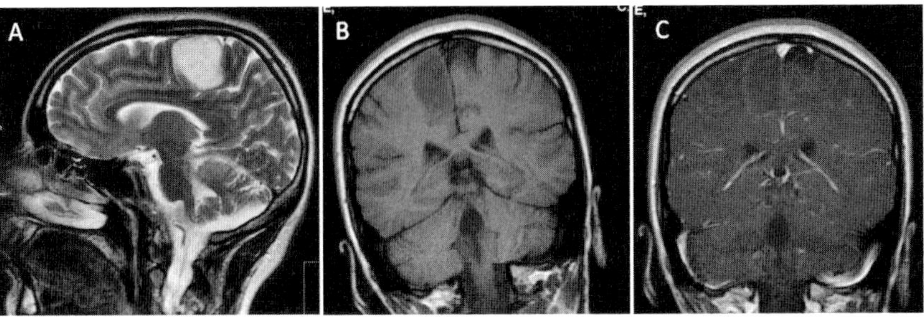

Fig. 31.2

Answers

4. Sagittal T_2 (A) and coronal pre-contrast (B) and post-contrast (C) MRIs are shown in Fig. 31.2. What is the tumour location and what information does it provide?

The tumour is in the posterior right frontal lobe, close to the motor cortex. Neither CT nor MRI show evidence of haemorrhage, so the arm weakness is likely to be Todd's palsy. Coronal sequences show no tumour contrast enhancement, so the diagnosis is low-grade glioma (probably astrocytoma).

5. What are the management options?

Anticonvulsants will be indicated to prevent further seizures (see 'Anticonvulsants in neurosurgery', p. 40).Low-grade gliomas can be treated conservatively or surgically.

Conservative management with radiological surveillance avoids surgical risk in a potentially eloquent area. However, the patient will have no histological diagnosis and hence prognosis, and the uncertainty can be difficult to manage.

Surgically, biopsy alone (for histological diagnosis) or resection of the tumour are options. Definitive histology allows for possible further non-surgical treatment (chemo- or radiotherapy), although it is not usually offered for a low-grade tumour. Biopsy may occasionally take a non-representative sample and provide erroneous information (see 'Brain biopsy', p. 233). Near the motor cortex most surgeons would use image guidance or have the patient awake during surgery for intraoperative assessment of the involved brain prior to resection. This requires a cooperative relaxed patient and an experienced anaesthetist.

Further reading

Bampoe J, Bernstein M (1999). The role of surgery in low grade gliomas. *J Neurooncol*; **42**: 259–69.

De Benedictis A, Moritz-Gasser S, Duffau H (2010). Awake mapping optimizes the extent of resection for low-grade gliomas in eloquent areas. *Neurosurgery*; **66**: 1074–84.

Duffau H (2009). Surgery of low-grade gliomas: towards a 'functional neurooncology'. *Curr Opin Oncol*; **21**: 543–9.

Ruiz J, Lesser GJ (2009). Low-grade gliomas. *Curr Treat Options Oncol*; **10**: 231–42.

Sanai N, Berger MS (2009). Operative techniques for gliomas and the value of extent of resection. *Neurotherapeutics*; **6**: 478–86.

Brain biopsy

A brain biopsy carries appreciable risk and should only be performed after other less invasive diagnostic strategies (e.g. lumbar puncture for cytology, tissue from elsewhere) and management strategies (e.g. observation if the lesion is not causing neurological compromise) have been considered. The site that carries the least risk should be chosen for biopsy. In making this decision consideration should be given to the potential trajectory and the neurological deficit that would be expected should a complication (namely haemorrhage or brain oedema) occur. Biopsy of the meninges and cortex (rather than deeper structures) should be performed if a diffuse process (such as vasculitis or progressive multifocal leuco-encephalopathy) is being investigated. Biopsy can be performed openly or stereotactically. Open biopsies are performed for superficial lesions or when there is another indication such as the relief of mass effect. Stereotaxy allows the location of an intracranial lesion to be defined in three-dimensional coordinates. This can be done using a stereotactic frame attached to the patient's head or with a computer-based image guidance system ('frameless stereotaxy'). The defined site is then accessed via a burrhole. The risks of stereotactic biopsy include haemorrhage, postoperative brain swelling, stroke, seizures, infection, and an unsuccessful biopsy (i.e. missing the lesion or obtaining an inadequate sample).

A 53-year-old woman presented with a 3-week history of dizziness, slurred speech, and numbness of the left side of her face. The MRI scan (Fig. 31.3) shows diffuse enlargement of the pons with patchy T_2 hyperintensity (A) extending to the middle cerebellar peduncle and the left cerebellar hemisphere (B). There is also a small patch of hyperintensity at the genu of the right internal capsule (C). There is patchy enhancement with gadolinium. She underwent stereotactic biopsy of the internal capsule lesion, and the histology showed a B-cell lymphoma.

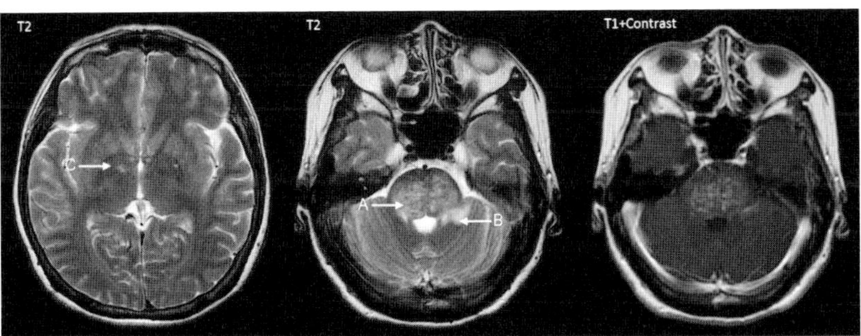

Fig. 31.3

(continued)

Brain biopsy *(continued)*

Further reading

Dorward NL, Paleologos TS, Alberti O, Thomas DGT (2002). The advantages of frameless stereotactic biopsy over frame-based biopsy. *Br J Neurosurg*; **16**: 110–18.

Feinstein B, Alberts WW, Wright EW Jr, Levin G (1960). A stereotaxic technique in man allowing multiple spatial and temporal approaches to intracranial targets. *J Neurosurg*; **17**: 708–20.

Awake neurosurgery

Neurosurgery is sometimes performed with the patient awake. These contexts are, first, when intraoperative assessment of neurological function is required and, secondly, when the patient requires an operation but is not a suitable candidate for general anaesthesia. The first context includes cortical mapping in epilepsy surgery, resection of tumours in eloquent brain areas (e.g. near language areas), and deep brain stimulation for Parkinson's disease or pain. The second context is usually seen in elderly patients for procedures that can be performed under local anaesthetic such as burrhole drainage of a chronic subdural haematoma or insertion of an external ventricular drain. The key is an effective anaesthetic regimen. Methods vary, but in general local anaesthetic is applied to the scalp incision and all or part of the operation is performed with varying degrees of sedation, analgesia, and/or anaesthesia so that the patient is conscious (and able to respond) during the desired stages of the operation whilst remaining comfortable. The brain and skull do not contain nociceptors, although the scalp and meninges do and are potential sources of pain.

Case 32

A 3-year-old boy has a 6-week history of motor decline. His parents report that previously he was running and playing normally but now is walking slowly and holding on to objects or people to support himself. His GP arranged a non-urgent paediatric outpatient appointment. However, for the past 2 days the child has been irritable and holding his head. This morning he vomited and so came to hospital.

Question

1. What typical diagnosis does the history suggest?

Answer

1. What typical diagnosis does the history suggest?

Motor decline can be non-specific, but the poor balance points to a cerebellar problem. Holding the head, being irritable, and vomiting suggest raised intracranial pressure. These are typical features of a posterior fossa mass lesion compressing the fourth ventricle and causing hydrocephalus. Although any mass lesion can cause this picture, a tumour is the likely diagnosis given the progressive symptoms and age.

Questions

2. What are the clinical findings in a patient with a posterior fossa mass lesion?
3. Explain why a cerebellar lesion causes incoordination ipsilaterally.
4. On examination this patient is alert but miserable. Examination of coordination and fundoscopy are not possible. How should he be investigated?

Answers

2. What are the clinical findings in a patient with a posterior fossa mass lesion?

A cerebellar hemispheric lesion causes loss of coordination ipsilaterally. If the lesion involves the cerebellar vermis (midline), there may be truncal ataxia with a broad-based gait. Hydrocephalus in children can cause downward deviation of the eyes ('sun-setting'), bilateral sixth nerve palsies (see 'False localizing signs', p. 298), and under the age of 18 months bulging of the anterior fontanelle if it is open. Fundoscopy may be difficult to perform in children, but will show papilloedema in most patients with raised intracranial pressure. Visual acuity may be reduced.

3. Explain why a cerebellar lesion causes incoordination ipsilaterally.

Efferent outputs from the cerebellum to the limbs either 'double cross' (the dentato-rubro-thalamic tract and the globose-emboliform-rubral tract) or do not cross (the fastigial-vestibular and fastigial-reticular tracts). Hence cerebellar lesions cause ipsilateral symptoms.

4. On examination this patient is alert but miserable. Examination of coordination and fundoscopy are not possible. How should he be investigated?

He requires urgent imaging of the brain. MRI is preferable as it will delineate the pathology, but if there is neurological compromise due to presumed hydrocephalus a CT scan could be performed if more readily available.

Questions

5. An MRI is performed (Fig. 32.1).
   (a) What sequences are shown?
   (b) Describe the abnormalities.
   (c) What are the possible diagnoses?
6. How should the patient be treated in the emergency setting?

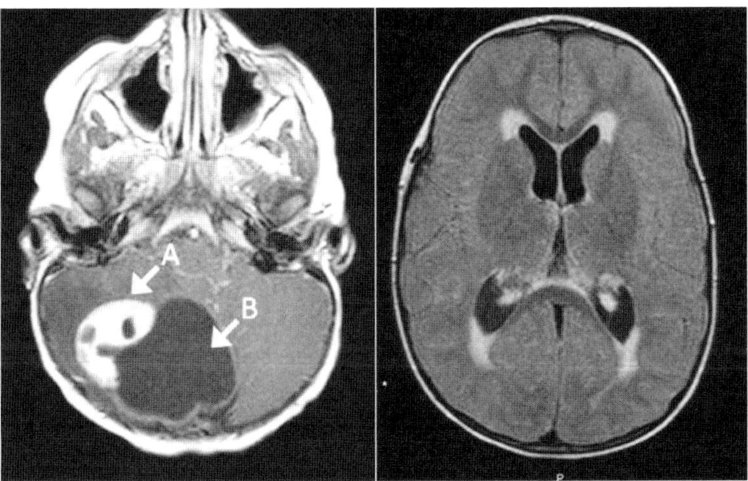

Fig. 32.1

Answers

5. An MRI is performed (Fig. 32.1).

(a) What sequences are shown?

These are axial T_1 post-contrast (left) and axial FLAIR (right) sequences.

(b) Describe the abnormalities.

The T_1 image shows a large mass lesion with a solid component (A) and large cystic component (B) arising from the right cerebellar hemisphere and extending across the midline. The solid component has a strong uniform enhancement pattern with some discrete non-enhancing spots in it as compared with the non-contrast scan (not shown). The fourth ventricle cannot be seen and is effaced by the mass. The FLAIR sequence shows lateral ventricular enlargment, and the whiter areas around the tips of the ventricles are indicative of 'trans-ependymal flow' of CSF indicating high pressure.

(c) What are the possible diagnoses?

This is a posterior fossa tumour with obstructive hydrocephalus. An avidly enhancing solid component with a cyst suggests pilocytic astrocytoma. Other childhood tumours are ependymoma and medulloblastoma (primitive neuroectodermal tumour (PNET)). Pilocytic astrocytoma is benign and often curable with surgery. Ependymoma and medulloblastoma are malignant and require adjuvant chemoradiotherapy. Table 32.1 summarizes the typical imaging findings, although these tumours can be indistinguishable radiologically.

Table 32.1 Radiological features of posterior fossa tumours in children

Tumour	Location	Features	Enhancement
Pilocytic astrocytoma	Lateral	Solid portion low density on unenhanced CT Solid nodule with large associated cyst	Enhancing nodule with non-enhancing cyst
Ependymoma	Fourth ventricle	Often heterogeneous and calcified Grows through fourth ventricle foramina	Variable
Medulloblastoma	Usually midline, fourth ventricle	High density on non-contrast CT May have calcification	Variable

6. How should the patient be treated in the emergency setting?

Within 24 hours, dexamethasone helps reduce the peritumoural oedema, usually allowing CSF flow through the fourth ventricle to alleviate the hydrocephalus. If the headache does not resolve or the GCS worsens, treating the hydrocephalus with an external ventricular drain or endoscopic third ventriculostomy is required.

Even with improvement on steroids, most paediatric neurosurgeons would consider a third ventriculostomy a few days after presentation and plan tumour resection thereafter. This often facilitates the definitive surgery. Spinal MRI is also required to exclude CSF metastases which are harder to identify postoperatively because of the presence of CSF blood products.

In this case, clinically there is raised intracranial pressure but the hydrocephalus is not severe on imaging. The patient does not require emergency CSF drainage but is commenced on dexamethasone. Radiologically this is pilocytic astrocytoma and excision should be curative. If the tumour were malignant, surgery with maximal resection would be followed by adjuvant chemoradiotherapy.

Further reading

Schijman E, Peter JC, Rekate HL, Sgouros A, Wong TT (2004). Management of hydrocephalus in posterior fossa tumours: how, what, when? *Childs Nerv Syst*; **20**: 192–4.

Case 33

An 82-year-old woman with 6 weeks of progressive right hemiparesis is referred from the medical team. She denies headaches or seizures, and is self-caring and independent, although widowed last year. Her medical history includes type 2 diabetes and hypertension, and she is on aspirin.

On examination she walks well with a stick in her left hand. Her right arm is weak and she is unable grasp a pen. She has brisk biceps, supinator, and triceps jerks in her right arm. Her left arm and both legs are normal.

Questions

1. Damage to which tract typically leads to an inability to grasp a pen or hold small objects?
2. What is the abnormality on her brain MRI (Fig. 33.1)?
3. Where is this lesion in relation to the motor cortex?
4. Does the location suggest any further clinical signs?
5. Which treatment option would you prefer for this patient?
6. Are there any preoperative considerations?

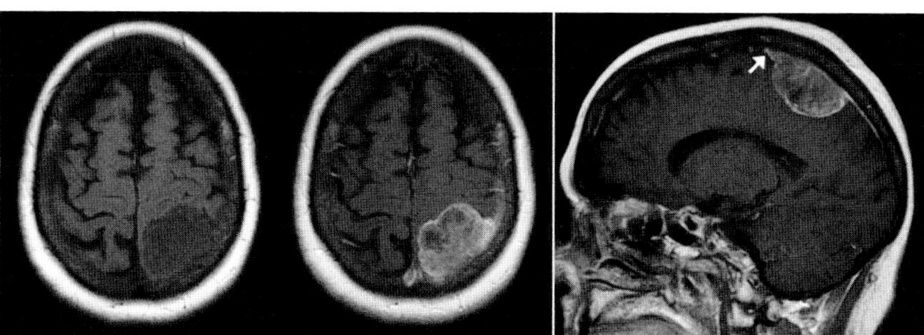

Fig. 33.1

Answers

1. Damage to which tract typically leads to an inability to grasp a pen or hold small objects?

Impairments of fine motor movements typically arise from lesions of the pyramidal (corticospinal) tract.

2. What is the abnormality on her brain MRI (Fig. 33.1)?

An enhancing extra-axial mass overlies the left parietal lobe. It is durally based with a dural 'tail.' (arrow), suggesting a meningioma.

3. Where is this lesion in relation to the motor cortex?

The motor cortex can be identified as follows (Fig. 33.2).

- Superior frontal sulcus—pre-central sulcus method: the superior frontal sulcus (A) joins the precentral sulcus (B) (in 85%) and hence the central sulcus (C) and the motor cortex (D) can be determined.
- Midline sulcus sign: the most prominent sulcus approaching the interhemispheric fissure (E) is the central sulcus (in 70%).

This tumour overlies sensory areas, behind the post-central gyrus (F). The motor symptoms are due to mass effect on the pre-central gyrus.

Table 33.1 Simpson classification of meningioma removal

Grade I	Macroscopically complete tumour removal, with excision of its dural attachment and of abnormal bone Resection of the sinus where tumour arises from the wall of a dural venous sinus
Grade II	Macroscopically complete tumour removal with endothermy coagulation of its dural attachment
Grade III	Macroscopically complete tumour removal without resection or coagulation of its dural attachment or its extradural extension
Grade IV	Partial tumour removal
Grade V	Biopsy only

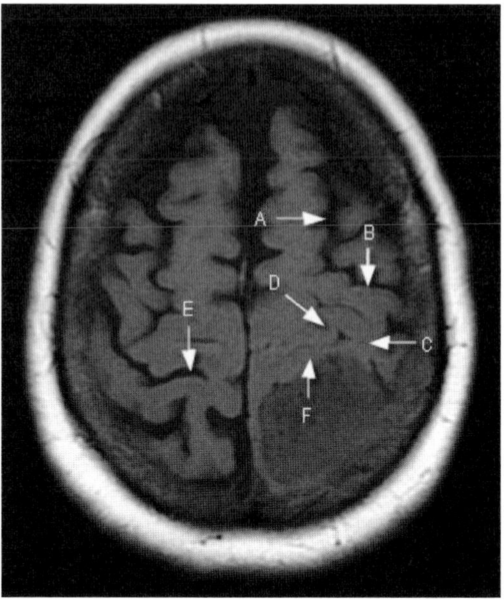

Fig. 33.2

4. Does the location suggest any further clinical signs?

Whilst initial sensory examination may be normal, cortical sensory loss may be elicited by asking the patient to carry out tasks of sensory discrimination such as naming a number drawn on her palm or asking her to remove objects from a pocket. These tasks require cortical integration of somatosensory stimuli with spatial awareness and decision-making.

5. Which treatment option would you prefer for this patient?

Management of meningiomas may be expectant (observation with treatment of seizures if required), surgery, or radiosurgery. This patient has a partial deficit and treatment is appropriate. Radiosurgery is valuable to control small (<3cm) tumours that are surgically inaccessible. It will prevent progression of the tumour but will not remove it. Open surgery has a high cure rate, related to the Simpson grade (Table 33.1) which is highest for meningiomas of the cranial convexity. Therefore, despite her age, surgery was undertaken.

6. Are there any preoperative considerations?

Meningiomas may bleed considerably during surgery. They derive their blood supply principally from the dura but also recruit vessels from the adjacent brain. Neurovascular embolization may be performed preoperatively for large tumours. This is rarely necessary for tumours of the convexity as the dural blood supply will be encountered early on in the operation and is readily dealt with. Preoperative embolization has a stronger role for skull base tumours or those where the blood supply will be encountered late in the surgery.

Question

7. The patient undergoes surgery and recovers with a slow improvement in her hemiparesis. The histology shows an atypical meningioma, WHO grade 2. What implications does this have?

Answer

7. The patient undergoes surgery and recovers with a slow improvement in her hemiparesis. The histology shows an atypical meningioma, WHO grade 2. What implications does this have?

Atypical meningiomas are not malignant but have a higher recurrence rate, even after complete excision. Patients should be followed closely with a view to early treatment of recurrence if necessary. Treatment could involve further surgery or radiotherapy.

Further reading

Aghi MK, Carter BS, Cosgrove GR, *et al.* (2009). Long-term recurrence rates of atypical meningiomas after gross total resection with or without postoperative adjuvant radiation. *Neurosurgery*; **64**: 56–60.

Dowd CF, Halbach VV, Higashida RT (2003). Meningiomas: the role of preoperative angiography and embolization. *Neurosurg Focus*; **15**: E10.

Naidich TP, Brightbill TC (1996). Systems for localizing fronto-parietal gyri and sulci on axial CT and MRI. *Int J Neuroradiol*; **2**: 313–38.

Simpson D (1957). The recurrence of intracranial meningiomas after surgical treatment. *J Neurol Neurosurg Psychiatry*; **20**: 22–39.

Case 34

A 71-year-old man presents to his GP with a worsening headache which started suddenly 6 days previously. He became very dizzy and his wife noticed him staggering as if drunk. His balance has been poor since then and he has spent the week in bed.

His past medical history includes a stroke 6 years previously from which he recovered fully. He is a previous heavy smoker. He takes aspirin and a statin.

Question

1. What is the differential diagnosis?

Answer

1. What is the differential diagnosis?

The differential diagnosis for a sudden-onset headache includes any type of intracranial bleed or migraine. Subsequent problems with balance indicate pyramidal motor pathway or cerebellar involvement. A bleed causing hydrocephalus would also lead to unsteadiness.

Questions

2. The patient's GP arranges a CT scan and he is then referred to neurosurgery
   (a) What are the findings on the scans (Fig. 34.1) (left, pre-contrast; right, post-contrast)?
   (b) What is the likely diagnosis?
3. How should this patient be managed acutely?
4. He undergoes a chest X-ray and a CT of his body (Fig. 34.2). What is seen? How would you manage him now?

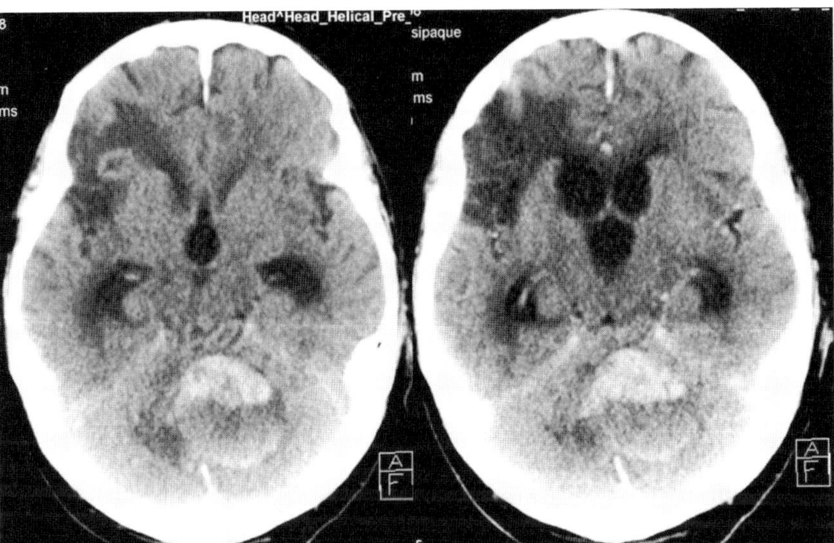

Fig. 34.1

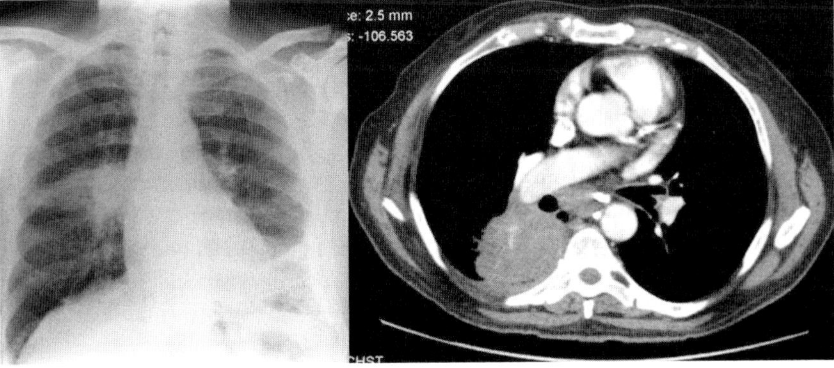

Fig. 34.2

Answers

2. The patient's GP arranges a CT and he is then referred to neurosurgery.

(a) What are the findings on the scans (Fig. 34.1) (left, pre-contrast; right, post-contrast)?

a) There is a well-defined weakly enhancing mass in the left cerebellar hemisphere crossing the midline. It is heterogeneous on the non-contrast CT, but high density suggests recent haemorrhage. The fourth ventricle is occluded, causing hydrocephalus. There is an old area of right frontotemporal encephalomalacia indicating his previous stroke.

(b) What is the likely diagnosis?

The most common cause of a posterior fossa tumour in adults is metastasis. Malignant tumours can present with intra-tumoural haemorrhage. Malignant primary brain tumours (glioblastoma) of the cerebellum are most uncommon.

3. How should this patient be managed acutely?

There is hydrocephalus but the patient is alert and does not need immediate surgery. He receives dexamethasone 8mg bd to reduce vasogenic oedema around the tumour; this will improve his headaches and may improve the hydrocephalus. His aspirin is stopped in anticipation of surgery. An urgent effort should be made to locate a primary tumour and the extent of the metastatic disease for the following reasons.

1) If prognosis is especially poor, cranial surgery may not be in his best interests.
2) This information will inform discussion with oncologists, the patient, and the family. If a histological diagnosis is needed tissue may be obtained more easily from other sites (e.g. via a CT-guided biopsy) than from a posterior fossa craniotomy.

4. He undergoes a chest X-ray and a CT of his body (Fig. 34.2). What is seen? How would you manage him now?

There is a right hilar mass posteriorly situated on the CT, consistent with a primary lung tumour. Metastatic lung cancer has a poor prognosis. If the patient does not undergo surgery, he will probably die of hydrocephalus in the next few days or weeks. Surgery may extend his life by a few weeks but little more.

Staging requires an MRI of the brain to look for small metastases, and CT of the chest, abdomen, and pelvis. Tissue should be sampled from wherever is most convenient to inform a multidisciplinary discussion between oncologists, neurosurgeons, thoracic surgeons, and palliative care specialists to decide whether or not to treat the patient aggressively. In practice, when the first presentation of malignancy is with metastatic disease, it is difficult to offer only palliative care without a tissue diagnosis. He underwent a posterior fossa craniotomy which confirmed a secondary tumour from lung adenocarcinoma. He recovered well from the operation and after 6 days was discharged to a hospice before going home. He subsequently only survived a further 4 weeks.

Further reading

Kalkanis SN, Kondziolka D, Gaspar LE, *et al.* (2010). The role of surgical resection in the management of newly diagnosed brain metastases: a systematic review and evidence-based clinical practice guideline. *J Neurooncol*; **96**: 33–43.

Mintz A, Perry J, Spithoff K, Chambers A, Laperriere N (2007). Management of single brain metastasis: a practice guideline. *Curr Oncol*; **14**: 131–43.

Thomas SS, Dunbar EM (2010). Modern multidisciplinary management of brain metastases. *Curr Oncol Rep*; **12**: 34–40.

Case 35

A 44-year-old nurse is referred by ENT with a 6-month history of right ear tinnitus. Audiography revealed high-frequency hearing loss on this side. She has useful hearing in the right ear and can repeat words whispered to her when the left ear is occluded. There is no other neurological deficit.

Questions

1. Three images from the MRI scan are shown in Fig. 35.1.
   (a) What is the finding?
   (b) What is the differential diagnosis?
2. What are the management options? What are the risks and benefits of each?

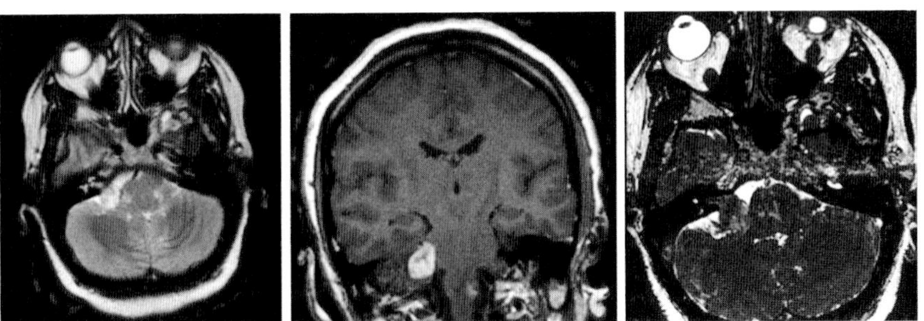

Fig. 35.1

Answers

1. Three images from the MRI scan are shown (Fig. 35.1).

(a) What is the finding (Fig. 35.2)?

There is a mass lesion in the right cerebellopontine angle (A). It enhances with contrast and appears to be partly within the internal acoustic meatus (B). There is a little distortion of the brainstem (C) but the fourth ventricle (D) is open and there is no hydrocephalus.

(b) What is the differential diagnosis?

The mass is enhancing and extra-axial. The three most likely possibilities are acoustic neuroma (vestibular schwannoma), meningioma, and metastasis. The long history and absence of systemic disease symptoms make metastasis unlikely. Acoustic neuroma is the more likely of the benign tumours as it is more common in this location, and this tumour has an intracanalicular (within the internal acoustic meatus) component which has spilled out into the CP angle—the so-called 'ice-cream cone' appearance. A meningioma often has a dural tail on imaging.

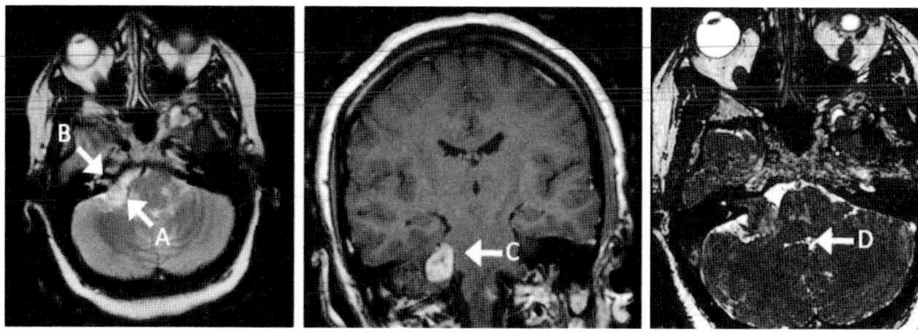

Fig. 35.2

2. What are the management options? What are the risks and benefits of each?

The three management options are observation, surgery, and radiosurgery. Treatment will not improve the patient's symptoms and therefore it should be offered for progression of the tumour (and its associated problems). There is evidence to suggest that hearing loss can be minimized with early surgery for small acoustic neuromas, but this is insufficient to justify surgery unless the patient has a very strong preference.

Observation

This will involve interval MRI scanning (at intervals of 6 months to a year). If tumour growth is demonstrated, treatment will need to be considered.

Radiosurgery

This involves image-guided accurate delivery of radiation to small volumes of brain with the use of collimation (multiple intersecting beams) to reduce the dose to surrounding structures. Complex volumes can be treated, usually in a single session. Unlike conventional radiotherapy for tumours, which relies on DNA damage to induce cell death, radiosurgery gives higher doses per unit volume and causes focal vascular changes that slowly result in intimal thickening and vascular occlusion of a region of interest. In the case of tumours, benign or malignant, this is intended to control (i.e. to slow growth or to shrink) a lesion: it may also be employed for arteriovenous malformations and other vascular lesions. If it fails, surgery may still be undertaken later. High rates of control for small (<3cm diameter) acoustic neuromas are reported. There are concerns over rare malignant transformation of benign tumours. Radiosurgery will usually preserve the residual hearing function, which may remain useful.

Open surgery

Open surgery has the advantage of usually being curative. This may be psychologically preferable for the patient. The risks relate principally to the lower cranial nerves, particularly the eighth and seventh nerve. Facial weakness can be minimized by the use of intraoperative facial nerve monitoring. The risks of facial nerve injury increase with the size of the tumour. This has resulted in an interest in subtotal removal of large acoustic neuromas with the aim of preserving facial nerve function; the remainder can then be observed for growth or treated up front with stereotactic radiotherapy.

This patient opts for surgery. This is performed via a retrosigmoid approach in the prone position. Facial nerve monitoring is used to identify and spare the seventh nerve which is seen to be well preserved at the end of the operation which completely removes the tumour. Her facial nerve function is unaffected.

Questions

3. The patient returns to the emergency department after 3 days having noticed drooping of the right side of her mouth which has come on gradually over the previous 24 hours. When she blinks, her right eye is slow to close. What is the likely diagnosis and how should it be managed?
4. Are there any objective tools for the measurement of facial weakness?
5. An MRI is performed (Fig. 35.3). Describe the findings.
6. What is the management?

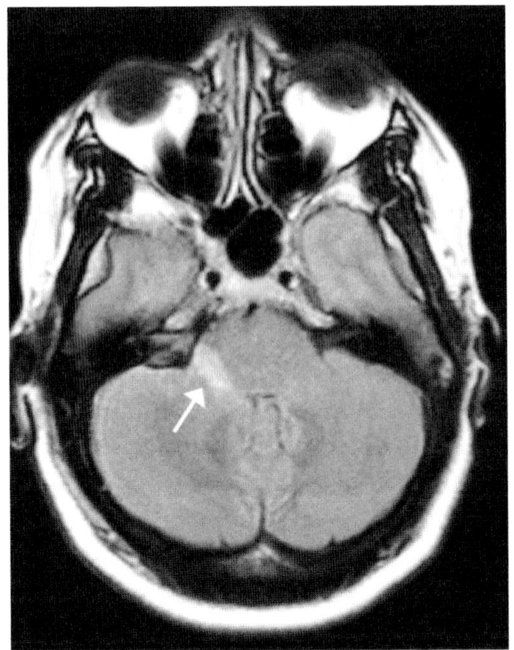

Fig. 35.3

Answers

3. The patient returns to the emergency department after 3 days having noticed drooping of the right side of her mouth which has come on gradually over the previous 24 hours. When she blinks, her right eye is slow to close. What is the likely diagnosis and how should it be managed?

The patient has a right lower motor neuron facial nerve palsy. The facial nerve was known to be intact at the end of the operation. The diagnosis is of delayed swelling of the nerve. She requires imaging to exclude a delayed postoperative haematoma.

4. Are there any objective tools for the measurement of facial weakness?

There are several grading scales for facial weakness. The House–Brackmann scale (Table 35.1) is commonly employed for this purpose.

Table 35.1 House–Brackmann scale

Grade	Description
1	Normal symmetrical function in all areas
2	Slight weakness noticeable only on close inspection Complete eye closure with minimal effort Slight asymmetry of smile with maximal effort Synkinesis barely noticeable; contracture or spasm absent
3	Obvious weakness, but not disfiguring May not be able to lift eyebrow Complete eye closure and strong but asymmetrical mouth movement with maximal effort Obvious, but not disfiguring, synkinesis, mass movement, or spasm
4	Obvious disfiguring weakness Inability to lift brow Incomplete eye closure and asymmetry of mouth with maximal effort Severe synkinesis, mass movement, spasm
5	Motion barely perceptible Incomplete eye closure, slight movement of corner mouth Synkinesis, contracture, and spasm usually absent
6	No movement, loss of tone, no synkinesis, contracture, or spasm

5. An MRI is performed (Fig. 35.3). Describe the findings.

There is a small area of high FLAIR signal in the lateral pons (arrow). This is consistent with postoperative oedema.

6. What is the management?

The facial nerve palsy should improve with conservative management; a short course of steroids is sometimes given. The ipsilateral eye must also be addressed. If the corneal reflex is absent, the patient is at risk of corneal ulceration. If the facial weakness prevents full eye closure (the key distinction between House–Brackmann grades 3 and 4), the risk is greater. Eye care involves the application of artificial tears or lubricant several times a day. She should also be shown how to keep the eye taped shut, particularly at night. If eye closure remains a problem, it can be sutured shut with a fine nylon stitch, or a lateral tarsorrhaphy can be performed, or a gold weight can be attached to the upper eyelid to facilitate closure.

Further reading

House JW, Brackmann DE (1985). Facial nerve grading system. *Otolaryngol Head Neck Surg*; **93**: 146–7.

Pollock BE (2008). Vestibular schwannoma management: an evidence-based comparison of stereotactic radiosurgery and microsurgical resection. *Prog Neurol Surg*; **21**: 222–7.

Pollock BE (2009). Stereotactic radiosurgery of benign intracranial tumors. *J Neurooncol*; **92**: 337–43.

Wackym PA (2005). Stereotactic radiosurgery, microsurgery, and expectant management of acoustic neuroma: basis for informed consent. *Otolaryngol Clin North Am*; **38**: 653–70.

Yamakami I, Uchino Y, Kobayashi E, Yamaura A (2003). Conservative management, gamma-knife radiosurgery, and microsurgery for acoustic neurinomas: a systematic review of outcome and risk of three therapeutic options. *Neurol Res*; **25**: 682–90.

Yang I, Sughrue ME, Han SJ, *et al.* (2010). A comprehensive analysis of hearing preservation after radiosurgery for vestibular schwannoma. *J Neurosurg*; **112**: 851–9.

Surgical approaches for acoustic neuroma

The three surgical approaches used are translabyrinthine, subtemporal, and retrosigmoid. Facial nerve monitoring is considered mandatory with all approaches to minimize the risk of facial nerve injury.

The translabyrinthine approach uses a curved incision behind the ear and drills through the petrous temporal bone and semicircular canal towards the triangle of dura between the sigmoid sinus, petrous apex, and jugular bulb inferiorly. The acoustic nerve is identified early where it is distinct from the facial nerve. It is considered preferable for small tumours lateral in the internal acoustic meatus. It results in complete sensorineural hearing loss but good rates of facial nerve preservation.

The subtemporal, or middle fossa approach, involves elevating the dura of the middle fossa from anterior to posterior and then drilling the medial part of the petrous apex to expose the internal acoustic meatus. It offers the highest rates of hearing preservation for small intracanalicular acoustic neuromas. However, it does pose risks to the posterior temporal lobe and the vein of Labbe with consequent venous infarction.

The retrosigmoid approach provides access to the CP angle for acoustic neuromas as well as for other tumours. Access to the intracanalicular component of tumours is more difficult. It involves a posterior fossa craniotomy or craniectomy behind the sigmoid sinus with retraction of the cerebellum medially. It allows CSF drainage via fenestration of the cisterna magna to improve brain relaxation and hence operating conditions.

Further reading

Bennett M, Haynes DS (2007). Surgical approaches and complications in the removal of vestibular schwannomas. *Otolaryngol Clin North Am*; **40**: 589–609.

Gharabaghi A, Samii A, Koerbel A, Rosahl SK, Tatagiba M, Samii M (2007). Preservation of function in vestibular schwannoma surgery. *Neurosurgery*; **60**: ONS124–8.

Sameshima T, Fukushima T, McElveen JT **Jr**, Friedman AH (2010). Critical assessment of operative approaches for hearing preservation in small acoustic neuroma surgery: retrosigmoid vs middle fossa approach. *Neurosurgery*; **67**: 640–4.

Case 36

A 27-year-old hairdresser presents to her local emergency department with progressive headaches, vomiting, and blurred vision over 2 weeks. She has been waking up at night and vomiting profusely in the mornings. Over the past 24 hours her headaches have been unremitting. She is alert and orientated. Her power is preserved throughout and coordination is normal. She is not photophobic or meningitic. She has reduced visual acuity at 6/12 in the right eye and 6/18 in the left. On fundoscopy there is gross papilloedema.

Question

1. This patient has features of increasing intracranial pressure without focal neurological signs or symptoms. What is the differential diagnosis?

Answer

1. This patient has features of increasing intracranial pressure without focal neurological signs or symptoms. What is the differential diagnosis?

The differential diagnosis is a large space-occupying lesion in a non-eloquent area such as the right frontal or temporal lobe. The short history makes a malignant tumour more likely than a benign tumour. The second possibility is hydrocephalus. There are many causes of hydrocephalus presenting in adulthood; most will also have symptoms of the causative condition, such as meningitis, subarachnoid haemorrhage, or cerebellar tumour. Presentation with hydrocephalus alone suggests small mass lesions around the third ventricle, cerebral aqueduct, and fourth ventricle. These include colloid cysts of the third ventricle, pineal region tumours, and fourth ventricular tumours including choroid plexus tumours and ependymoma. Aqueduct stenosis commonly presents in the neonatal period, but may present in a delayed manner in older patients.

Questions

2. Describe the abnormalities on the MRI scan (Fig. 36.1).
3. What is the differential diagnosis?
4. How should she be managed?

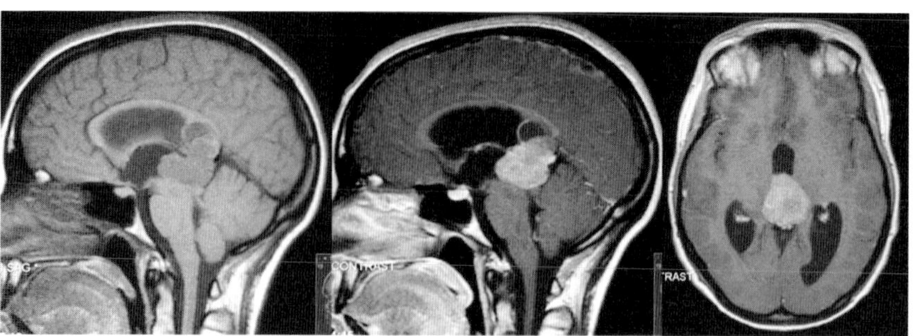

Fig. 36.1

Answers

2. Describe the abnormalities on the MRI scan (Fig. 36.1).

There is a well defined homogenously enhancing mass in the posterior aspect of the third ventricle, with a small cyst superiorly. There is marked associated hydrocephalus. The basal CSF cisterns, including the prepontine cistern, are patent.

3. What is the differential diagnosis?

This is a pineal region tumour; germinomas and teratomas are most common. Other pineal region tumours include pineocytoma or its malignant counterpart pineoblastoma, astrocytomas, and meningiomas. In an older patient one might suspect a metastasis.

4. How should she be managed?

Steroids should be given, but there is no visible perilesional oedema and improvement with steroids may be minimal. The hydrocephalus should be treated with either an EVD or an endoscopic third ventriculostomy (ETV). ETV allows physiological CSF resorption and avoids external hardware with attendant risk of infection. Depending on the angle of approach, it may also allow biopsy of the tumour if positioned posteriorly in the third ventricle after creating the ventriculostomy.

Questions

5. What is the value of tumour markers in pineal region tumours?
6. How may surgery be performed? Which anatomical structures are at risk? Should she have any special preoperative investigations?

Answers

5. What is value of tumour markers in pineal region tumours?

Tumour markers in the serum and CSF can aid diagnosis although they do not provide a definitive diagnosis. They are also important in monitoring response to treatment (Table 36.1).

An ETV produced good resolution of her symptoms. Her tumour marker studies are negative and therefore she is scheduled for surgery.

Table 36.1 Characteristics of pineal region tumours

	α-fetoprotein (AFP)	β-human chorionic gonadotrophin (β-HCG)	Placental alkaline phosphatase (P-ALP)	Melatonin
Germinoma	–	+	+	–
Teratoma	+	–	–	–
Yolk sac tumour	+	–	+/–	–
Embryonal carcinoma	+	+	+	–
Choriocarcinoma	–	+	+/–	–
Pinealocytoma	–	–	–	+
Pinealoblastoma	–	–	–	+

Adapted from Rengachary and Ellenbogen (2005). Reproduced with permission from Elsevier.

6. How may surgery be performed? Which anatomical structures are at risk? Should she have any special preoperative investigations?

The pineal region is surgically challenging. The most common approach is the supracerebellar infratentorial approach, which was used here. With the patient in a sitting position a craniotomy was performed over the cerebellum to allow it to fall away from the tentorium. Access to the pineal region is then through the corridor above the cerebellum and below the tentorium. The pineal region contains a number of large veins, including the internal cerebral veins that join to form the vein of Galen which feeds into the straight sinus in the tentorium. During the approach the craniotomy will be near the transverse sinus which can bleed torrentially if opened.

Because of the patient's sitting position and the chance of inadvertent opening of dural venous sinuses, there is a risk of intraoperative air embolism. Cerebral venous pressure in the sitting position is lower than atmospheric pressure and hence open veins may suck air in. The anaesthetist must be prepared: the treatment involves emergency repositioning of the patient or a central venous line in the right atrium to evacuate air with a syringe. Before surgery, a bubble echo study should be performed to look for an atrial septal defect, the presence of which would increase the chances of a systemic air embolism.

Further reading

Banks KP, Brown SJ (2006). AJR teaching file: solid masses of the pineal region. *Am J Roentgenol*; **186**: S233–5.

Edwards MS, Hudgins RJ, Wilson CB, Levin VA, Wara WM (1988). Pineal region tumors in children. *J Neurosurg*; **68**: 689–97.

Lee JY, Wakabayashi T, Yoshida J (2005). Management and survival of pineoblastoma: an analysis of 34 adults from the brain tumor registry of Japan. *Neurol Med Chir (Tokyo)*; **45**: 132–41.

Macfarlane R, Marks PV (1989). Tumours of the pineal region. *Br J Hosp Med*; **41**: 548–53.

Rengachary SS, Ellenbogen RG (2000). *Principles of Neurosurgery* (2nd edn). St Louis, MO: Mosby.

Smirniotopoulos JG, Rushing EJ, Mena H (1992). Pineal region masses: differential diagnosis. *Radiographics*; **12**: 577–96.

Case 37

Case 37 A

A 48-year-old man was referred to the neurosurgical service by the neurologists with a 3-year history of intermittent headaches. He denies any other symptoms.

Question

1. A CT scan is obtained (Fig. 37.1). What are the abnormalities?

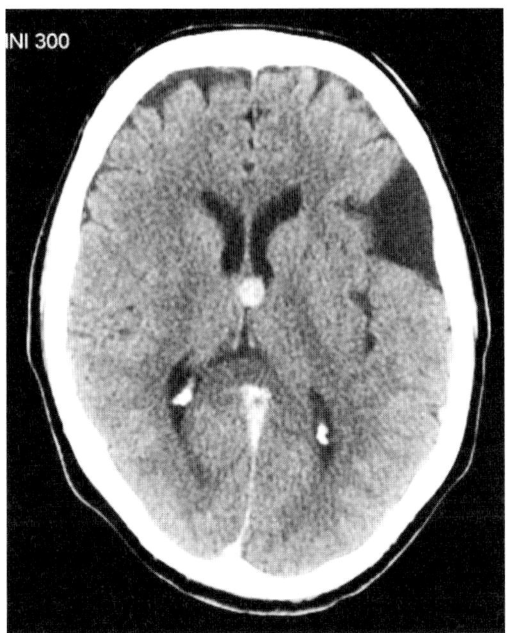

Fig. 37.1

Answer

1. A CT scan is obtained (Fig. 37.1). What are the abnormalities (Fig. 37.2)?

There is a small well-circumscribed mass within the third ventricle abutting the left foramen of Monro (A). It is hyperdense on this non-contrast CT scan. This is a colloid cyst of the third ventricle. There is no associated hydrocephalus. There is also an incidental left temporal arachnoid cyst (B) and scalloping of the bone (C). This is a developmental anomaly which manifests as a widened cortical CSF space.

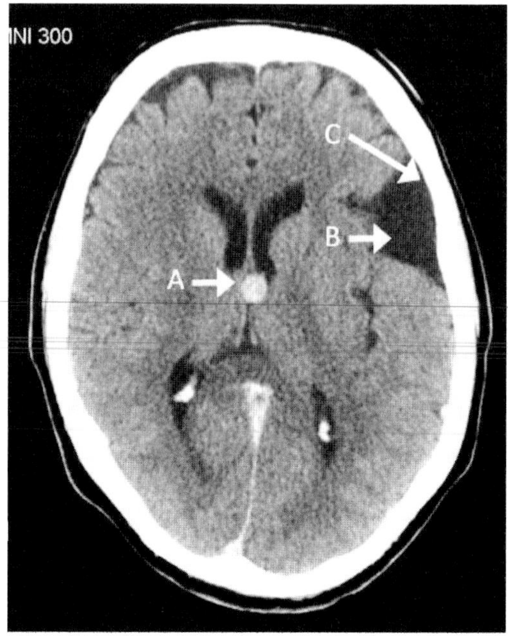

Fig. 37.2

Questions

2. An MRI scan is performed (Fig. 37.3). What are the properties of the cyst and why?
3. How should this patient be managed?

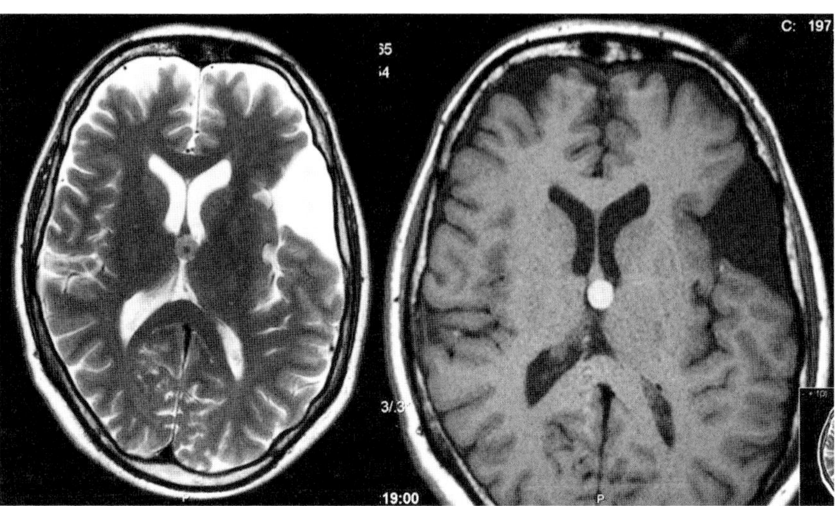

Fig. 37.3

Answers

2. An MRI scan is performed (Fig. 37.3). What are the properties of the cyst and why?

The T_2 (left) and T_1 (right) scans are shown. The cyst is hypointense on T_2 and hyperintense on T_1. This is due to the presence of protein within the cyst which also gives it high density on CT.

3. How should this patient be managed?

The concern with colloid cysts is that they can cause rapid deterioration from acute hydrocephalus and potentially death. This is usually preceded by a period of headaches which may last for weeks and months or for a few hours only. Therefore treatment is conservative unless the patient has headaches, hydrocephalus, or a cyst of diameter >10mm. Sudden death is only reported in patients with cysts of this size. Surgery to remove the cyst is performed transcallosally or transcortically via the lateral ventricle. Endoscopes may be used for surgical assistance. A third option for patients with large cysts that are higher intensity on T_2, and therefore suspected to be liquid, is stereotactic aspiration.

This man's colloid cyst is 8mm in diameter and there is no associated hydrocephalus. He does have headaches, although they are not particularly progressive. Conservative management is justified with repeat imaging to monitor for increases in size. However, he should be counselled about attending the emergency department promptly if he develops new or worsening headaches. In view of this advice he may opt for early surgery.

Case 37 B

A second patient is referred with a similar problem which presented in a different manner. She is a 34-year-old woman who is otherwise well. One afternoon she developed headaches which prevented her from sleeping after lunch. She started vomiting shortly afterwards and became confused. By the time she arrived at the emergency department she was grunting occasionally, localizing to pain, and not opening her eyes. Her blood pressure was 180/110mmHg and she was intubated.

Questions

4. An urgent CT scan is performed (Fig. 37.4). What does it show?
5. What is the correct emergency management for this patient?

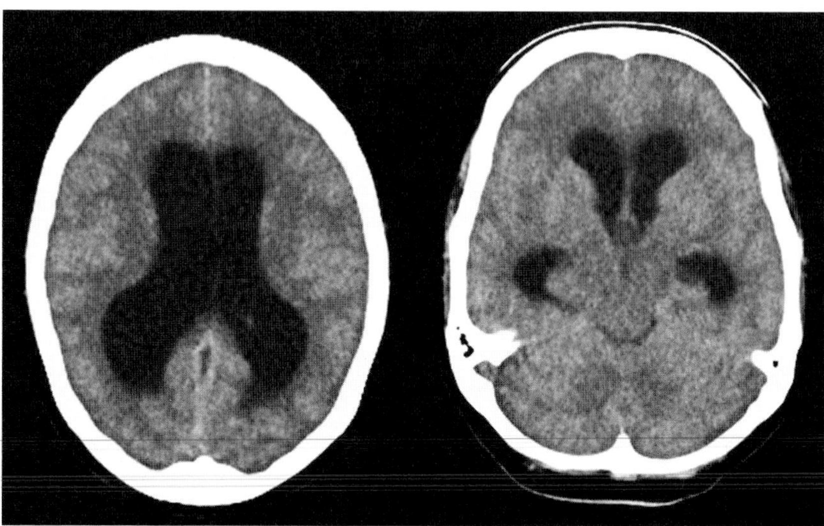

Fig. 37.4

Answers

4. An urgent CT scan is performed (Fig. 37.4). What does it show?

This is a colloid cyst of the third ventricle with acute hydrocephalus. This is the acute presentation of colloid cysts and is life threatening without immediate management.

5. What is the correct emergency management for this patient?

She should be transferred immediately to theatre for CSF drainage. The priority is to relieve the hydrocephalus rather than to remove the cyst itself. It would be reasonable to administer mannitol.

On arrival in the neurosurgery theatre, both her pupils were 5mm and unreactive. She underwent immediate bilateral EVD insertion.

Question

6. Following surgery the patient returns to the ITU. Her pupils are smaller and sluggishly reactive. She remains sedated and intubated. Twelve hours later her EVDs stop draining and a repeat CT scan is performed (Fig. 37.5). What has happened and should the drains be changed?

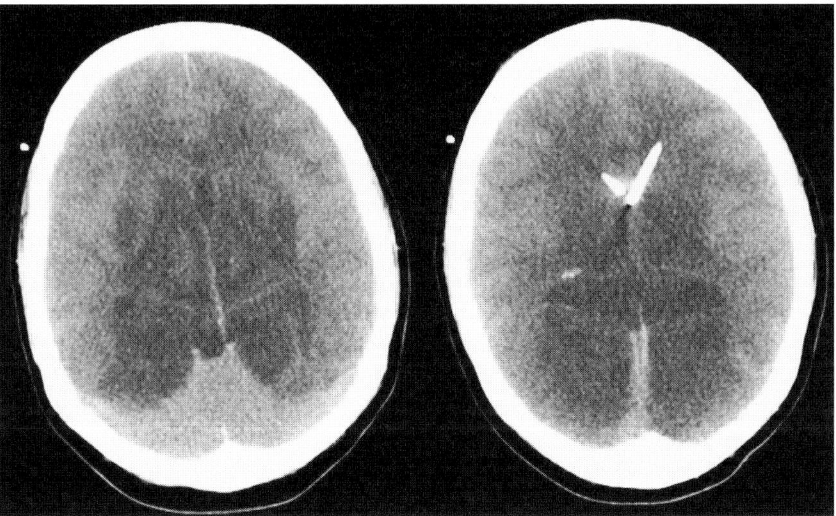

Fig. 37.5

Answer

6. Following surgery the patient returns to the ITU. Her pupils are smaller and sluggishly reactive. She remains sedated and intubated. Twelve hours later her EVDs stop draining and a repeat CT scan is performed (Fig. 37.5). What has happened and should the drains be changed?

There is widespread supratentorial cerebral infarction and generalized brain swelling as a result of the severe raised intracranial pressure. The EVDs are appropriately positioned on both sides and the ventricles are obliterated. Changing the drains at this stage will be futile as brainstem death will soon ensue (see 'Brainstem testing').

Brainstem testing

Brainstem testing is a series of reproducible bedside tests that can be used to confirm brain death. Brain death is an important diagnosis as an ethical and legal definition as it changes the status of a patient and allows clarification of the end-of-life processes for patients' relatives and clinicians.

Counselling of patients' relatives before brainstem testing is very important. Many hospitals will have experienced specialist nurses, but medical input is important.

The diagnosis of brainstem death differs according to the country of practice. However, the implication of the diagnosis is universal: neurological damage to the brain is complete and irreversible. In the UK brainstem death is confirmed on purely clinical criteria by two clinicians, both of whom must have at least 5 years' specialist experience, and one of whom is a consultant. Neither should be members of the transplant service. These two clinicians must perform the clinical tests independently of each other. If the patient satisfies the criteria according to both clinicians they are certified brain dead at the time the first set of tests were performed. If not, then the patient is not brain dead and management must continue as indicated clinically.

Before brainstem testing can be performed the following series of criteria must be satisfied to make the testing valid.

- The aetiology of the event causing brain death should be known. Massive intracranial haemorrhage and severe raised intracranial pressure due to trauma or stroke are the most common aetiologies. Hypoxic injury after cardiac arrest and other medical illnesses is also acceptable; however, a longer period of expectant management is often reasonable in such cases to allow any prospect of recovery to declare itself.

(continued)

Brainstem testing *(continued)*

- The unconscious state should not be attributable to drugs, whether taken before the illness or given in hospital. This particularly applies to anaesthetic drugs given in the intensive care setting; short-acting agents such as fentanyl may be judged to have worn off after a few hours, whereas larger doses of thiopental may take a few days to be confidently excluded.
- Hypothermia and metabolic, chemical, and respiratory imbalance must be corrected to give the injured brain the optimum conditions to demonstrate some response.

Brainstem testing involves the examinations listed in Table 37.1.

Table 37.1 Brainstem testing

Test	Response consistent with brainstem death
Pupillary response	Pupils fixed and dilated No light reflex
Corneal reflex	Absent
Vestibulo-ocular reflex: 50mL ice-cold water instilled to external auditory meatus (confirmed no wax in canal)	No eye movements are seen
Painful stimulus	No motor response of any form by any cranially innervated muscle or limbs
Gag reflex	Absent to tracheal/endobronchial suction
Respiratory response: preventilate with 100% O_2 and then disconnect from ventilator to allow CO_2 to rise without associated hypoxia; measure blood gas to confirm raised PCO_2	No respiratory effort at $PaCO_2$ >6.65kPa

Pitfalls in brainstem testing

Limb and trunk movements may be seen in brainstem dead patients as part of an exaggerated series of spinally mediated reflexes. They may occur in response to light touch, turning, or other minor stimuli. Relatives may consider them a sign associated with consciousness. Therefore painful stimuli to diagnose brainstem death should be applied to a cranially innervated region, typically the supraorbital ridge.

Differences exist in the diagnosis of formal brain death in the USA. UK brainstem testing does not test whole brain activity, and there is potentially the prospect of there being viable cortical function although without input from the external world via the brainstem and cranial nerves. This is not the same as 'locked-in' syndrome which requires some brainstem and cranial nerve function. To reflect this issue in UK brainstem testing, the phrase used is 'brainstem death' rather than brain death (which was used until 1995, when it was formally abandoned). There is no recognition of brainstem death in the USA; however, brain death is recognized. It requires clinical testing as in the UK but in addition either an EEG showing no cortical activity or a radionuclide scan showing complete absence of cerebral blood flow is required to confirm complete brain death.

Further reading

Academy of Medical Royal Colleges (2008). *A Code of Practice for the Diagnosis and Confirmation of Death*. Available online at: http://www.aomrc.org.uk/publications/reports-guidance.html

Conference of Medical Royal Colleges and their Faculties in the UK (1976). Diagnosis of brain death. *BMJ*; **ii**: 1187–8.

Conference of Medical Royal Colleges and their Faculties in the UK (1995). Criteria for the diagnosis of brain stem death. *J R Coll Physicians* (London); **29**: 381–2.

Case 38

A 31-year-old man presents via the ophthalmology department. He has a 2-week history of progressive difficulty with his vision, particularly bumping into things that he did not realize were next to him and having to turn excessively to either side to see people that are talking to him. The events culminated in a car accident when he drove into a parked car on his side of the road.

Questions

1. What type of visual problem does he have?
2. What is the likely diagnosis from the history? Should any other questions be asked?
3. A pre- and post-contrast CT scan is performed (Fig. 38.1). What does it show? What is the differential diagnosis?
4. What are the next steps in the management of this patient?
5. The prolactin level in this patient is moderately elevated (93ng/mL, normal range <20ng/mL). What is the relevance of this result, and how would it affect management?
6. How would you manage the patient's hormonal replacement in the perioperative period?
7. He undergoes trans-sphenoidal surgery which is uneventful. Immediately afterwards he feels that his vision has improved. However, the evening after surgery his urine output increases to a steady 300 mL/hour. What is the differential diagnosis for the increased urine output and the management of each possibility?

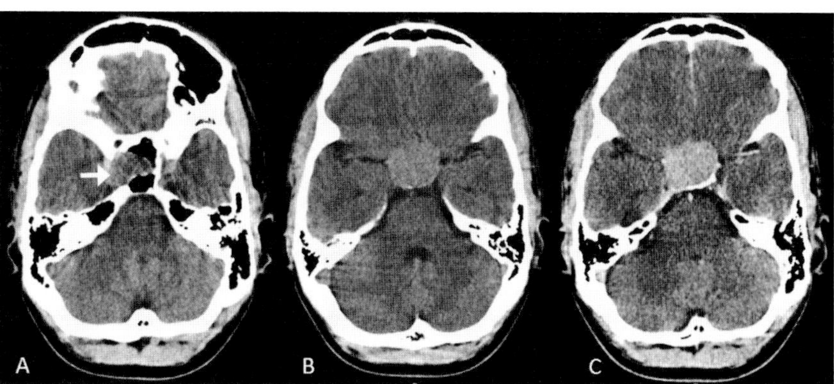

Fig. 38.1

Answers

1. What type of visual problem does he have?

Bumping into objects in the periphery and needing to turn excessively to see people points to a visual field defect affecting the temporal fields of vision.

2. What is the likely diagnosis from the history? Should any other questions be asked?

A bitemporal visual field defect is caused by compression of the central part of the optic chiasm and is the typical finding in patients with large pituitary tumours. Features of pathological hormonal secretion by the tumour should be sought. Constant lethargy, loss of sex drive, and impotence should raise the possibility of pituitary failure. In men, galactorrhoea, loss of body hair, and impotence may suggest excessive prolactin secretion from a prolactinoma. Most pituitary tumours large enough to present with visual failure will be non-functioning.

3. A pre- and post-contrast CT scan is performed (Fig. 38.1). What does it show? What is the differential diagnosis?

There is a well-defined mass eroding the right side of the sella turcica (A, arrow), from which it arises into the suprasellar region (B). It enhances uniformly (C). The most likely diagnosis is a large pituitary tumour. The differential diagnosis (of other tumours in this location) includes craniopharyngioma and meningioma. However, in this case the bony erosion suggests that the mass has arisen in the pituitary fossa and therefore this is almost certainly a pituitary tumour.

4. What are the next steps in the management of this patient?

This patient has visual failure due to the tumour and requires treatment before his vision deteriorates. Further assessment is required.

1. A formal visual field examination (Goldmann fields) to document the extent of his visual failure.
2. Definitive imaging in the form of an MRI of the pituitary fossa. This will clarify the diagnosis and show the relationship of the tumour to the optic chiasm.
3. A full pituitary hormone screen. Pituitary function should be assessed by an early-morning cortisol, follicle-stimulating hormone, luteinizing hormone, thyroid-stimulating hormne, growth hormone, and prolactin levels. The three hormones commonly secreted by pituitary tumours are cortisol, growth hormone, and prolactin. Cortisol and growth hormone cause Cushing's disease and acromegaly, respectively. An urgent prolactin level is vital in this patient to exclude a prolactinoma as the initial treatment is then medical (with cabergoline or bromocriptine).

In this patient, the MRI (Fig. 38.2) confirms sellar expansion due to the pituitary tumour. On the T_2 images the optic chiasm (arrow) can be seen stretched over the tumour, accounting for the visual failure.

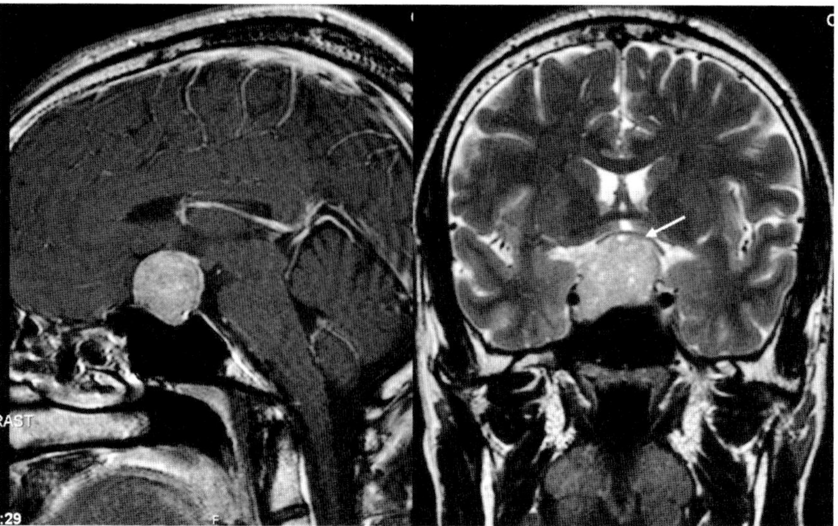

Fig. 38.2

5. The prolactin level in this patient is moderately elevated (93ng/mL, normal range <20ng/mL). What is the relevance of this result, and how would it affect management?

This is probably due to compression of the pituitary stalk by the tumour, resulting in loss of hypothalamic dopamine-mediated inhibition of prolactin release from the pituitary gland. The result is a prolactin level elevated to that of a few times normal. This level is also seen with small prolactin-secreting tumours (microprolactinomas). If a large tumour causing visual failure is a macroprolactinoma the serum prolactin level is typically increased a few hundredfold.

The prolactin level is not grossly elevated, the diagnosis is a non-functioning pituitary macro-adenoma, and the patient should undergo surgery. In the context of sellar expansion and an optic chiasm which is clearly elevated, the surgical approach should be trans-sphenoidal.

6. How would you manage the patient's hormonal replacement in the perioperative period?

This depends on his preoperative status. If he has been shown biochemically or clinically to have impaired pituitary function preoperatively, he will have been started on steroid replacement and this should continue postoperatively. The dose should be increased on the day of surgery and for the subsequent days and then returned to maintenance around day 4. If he has normal preoperative pituitary function, perioperative steroid replacement should still be given. However, in this case it is reasonable to measure the morning cortisol level prior to giving steroid replacement on days 4 and 5 postoperatively; if it is normal, steroid replacement is stopped.

7. He undergoes trans-sphenoidal surgery which is uneventful. Immediately afterwards he feels that his vision has improved. However, the evening after surgery his urine output increases to a steady 300 mL/hour. What is the differential diagnosis for the increased urine output and management of each possibility?

There are two possibilities. First, the perioperative intravenous fluid regimen may have been excessive and he is offloading fluid physiologically. The management of this is expectant. The second more important diagnosis is diabetes insipidus (DI) due to loss of antidiuretic hormone (ADH). This is a common transient complication of pituitary surgery and may result in severe dehydration and hypernatraemia. If he is developing DI, he will be clinically dehydrated and thirsty. The serum sodium level should be checked urgently.

If the diagnosis is DI, the patient should be given a supply of water and instructed to drink according to his thirst. He may be given synthetic ADH (desmopressin, DDAVP) as a subcutaneous injection.

The sodium level should be monitored and fluid balance charts maintained until at least day 3 postoperatively.

Further reading

Elhateer H, Muanza T, Roberge D, *et al.* (2008). Fractionated stereotactic radiotherapy in the treatment of pituitary macroadenomas. *Curr Oncol*; **15**: 286–92.

Jaffe CA (2006).Clinically non-functioning pituitary adenoma. *Pituitary*; **9**: 317–21.

Nemergut EC, Zuo Z, Jane JA Jr, Laws ER Jr (2005). Predictors of diabetes insipidus after transsphenoidal surgery: a review of 881 patients. *J Neurosurg*; **103**: 448–54.

Youssef AS, Agazzi S, van Loveren HR (2005). Transcranial surgery for pituitary adenomas. *Neurosurgery*; **57** (Suppl): 168–75.

Case 39

A 31-year-old man is referred by endocrinologists. His GP had found hypertension. He was referred for investigation of the underlying cause and was found to have coarse facial features, thickening of the skin around the hands, and a large jaw. After direct questioning he admitted that his appearance had changed somewhat over the last few years but he assumed that he was ageing normally.

Questions

1. What is the diagnosis?
2. What are the other clinical features of the condition?
3. How can the diagnosis be confirmed?

Answers

1. What is the diagnosis?

These clinical features are suggestive of acromegaly.

2. What are the other clinical features of the condition?

The features of acromegaly are due to excessive growth hormone secretion and include a prominent supraorbital ridge, protrusion of the lower jaw (prognathism), increased interdental spaces, enlargement of the nose, ears, tongue, hands, and feet, and coarse skin. Untreated acromegaly may lead to hypertension, diabetes, carpal tunnel syndrome, obstructive sleep apnoea, and visual failure. The risk of bowel cancer is increased. Patients may have noticed that they have outgrown their shoes or gloves, or that their appearance has changed in photographs.

3. How can the diagnosis be confirmed?

The diagnosis is confirmed by an oral glucose tolerance test (with serial glucose and growth hormone measurements). Oral glucose (100g) should suppress growth hormone levels to below 1ng/mL. Failure for this to occur suggests acromegaly. Isolated growth hormone levels fluctuate during the day. However, the serum insulin-like growth factor 1 (IGF-1) level remains relatively constant throughout the day and can be used as a reliable marker of acromegaly.

Questions

4. What are the causes of excess growth hormone secretion?
5. The patient undergoes a glucose tolerance test and associated blood tests. Comment on the results (Table 39.1). What further investigations are now required?

Table 39.1

Time (min)	0	30	60	90	120
Glucose (mmol)	6.6	10.4	11.8	8.8	5.5
GH (mU/L)	9.4	26.2	29.8	16.6	12.6
IGF-1 (nmol/L)	98.6 (range 15.2–42.8)				

Answers

4. What are the causes of excess growth hormone secretion?

The most common cause is a pituitary adenoma. However, ectopic growth hormone secretion can also occur from breast, lung, and ovarian tumours as well as from carcinoid and hypothalamic tumours.

5. The patient undergoes a glucose tolerance test and associated blood tests. Comment on the results (Table 39.1). What further investigations are now required?

These results confirm failure to suppress growth hormone in response to oral glucose loading. The IGF-1 level is also markedly elevated. The results are consistent with acromegaly, and an MRI scan of the pituitary is required to look for a pituitary adenoma.

Questions

6. The MRI images are shown in Fig. 39.1 (left, pre-contrast; right, post-contrast). What are the key findings?
7. What are the treatment options?
8. The endocrinologists wish for a surgical opinion. How should surgery be performed and what are the associated risks?

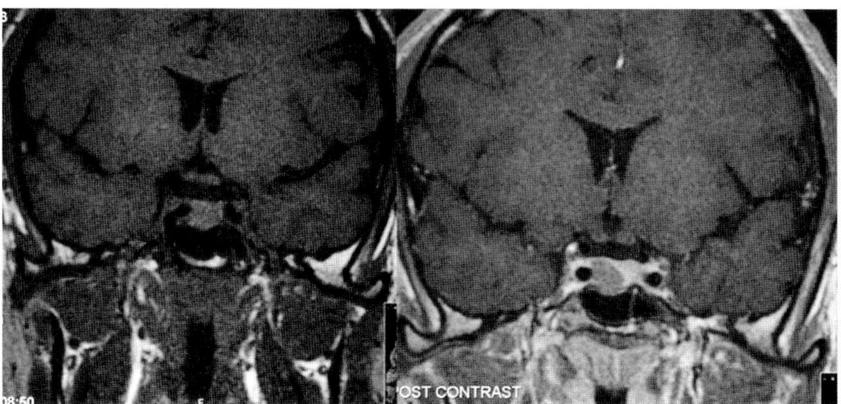

Fig. 39.1

Answers

6. The MRI images are shown in Fig. 39.1 (left, pre-contrast, right, post-contrast). What are the key findings (Fig. 39.2)?

The post-contrast image shows diffuse enhancement of the pituitary gland (A) and a non-enhancing nodule within it on the right side of the gland (B), which is the adenoma. Pituitary adenomas are opposite to most cranial and spinal tumours as the normal pituitary enhances whilst tumour does not. The scan shows the relationship of the pituitary gland to the optic chiasm (C), confirming their separation. Hence visual failure is not imminent.

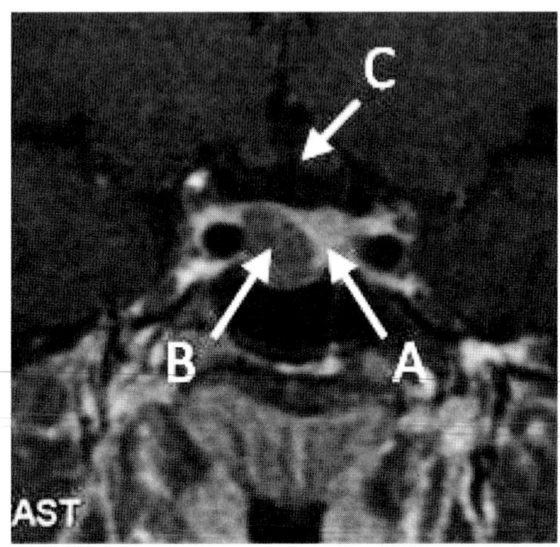

Fig. 39.2

7. What are the treatment options?

Medical treatment consists of somatostatin analogues to suppress growth hormone production. These require repeated injections every 2–4 weeks and although they may be used for long-term control the usual treatment is surgical. Radiotherapy will be an option in the future if medical and surgical treatment fail.

8. The endocrinologists wish for a surgical opinion. How should surgery be performed and what are the associated risks?

This is a small tumour confined to the sella and therefore surgery should be trans-sphenoidal, either open or endoscopically assisted depending on local preference. The main risks of surgery are haemorrhage, CSF leak, visual deficit, and recurrence. Patients with acromegaly have by definition swollen soft tissues, making them prone to surgical bleeding. The risk of postoperative CSF leak should be low given that the diaphragma sellae should be of normal thickness and location. Equally, the risk of optic chiasm injury should be low as the chiasm is some way from the tumour.

There is risk of injury to the cranial nerves running in the cavernous sinus. Surgery may not be curative and he may require continued medical therapy despite the operation.

Further reading

Bates PR, Carson MN, Trainer PJ, Wass JA (2008). UK National Acromegaly Register Study Group (UKAR-2). Wide variation in surgical outcomes for acromegaly in the UK. *Clin Endocrinol (Oxf)*; **68**: 136–42.

Cazabat L, Souberbielle JC, Chanson P (2008). Dynamic tests for the diagnosis and assessment of treatment efficacy in acromegaly. *Pituitary*; **11**: 129–39

Losa M, Gioia L, Picozzi P, *et al.* (2008). The role of stereotactic radiotherapy in patients with growth hormone-secreting pituitary adenoma. *J Clin Endocrinol Metab*; **93**: 2546–52.

Sherlock M, Aragon Alonso A, Reulen RC, *et al.* (2009). Monitoring disease activity using GH and IGF-I in the follow-up of 501 patients with acromegaly. *Clin Endocrinol (Oxf)*; **71**: 74–81.

Case 40

A 65-year-old man presents with sudden-onset headache, nausea, and visual disturbance. He reports loss of libido for the last 4 years, but otherwise has no previous medical history. He is in quite severe distress due to the headache but is alert and orientated, with no focal neurological deficits.

Question

1. A CT scan is performed (Fig. 40.1). What does it show?

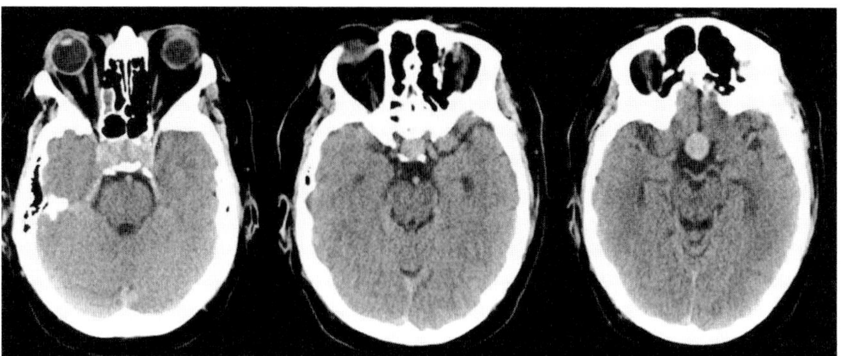

Fig 40.1

Answer

1. A CT scan is performed (Fig. 40.1). What does it show?

There is a mixed-density mass situated in the sella turcica with extension into the cavernous sinuses laterally and the chiasmatic cistern above. The diagnosis is pituitary apoplexy. An MRI scan is performed (Fig. 40.2). The optic chiasm is displaced superiorly (A). There is mixed high- and low-intensity signal within the tumour indicating recent haemorrhage. The high density on the CT scan supports the diagnosis of a haemorrhagic lesion, confirmed as a tumour on MRI (B).

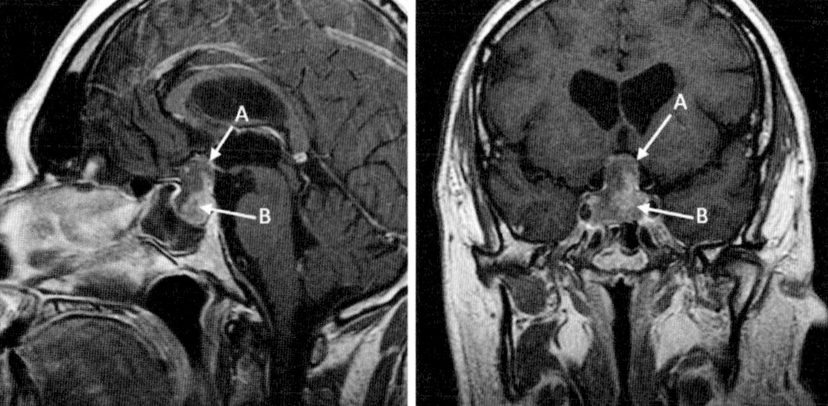

Fig 40.2

Questions

2. What is the definition of pituitary apoplexy?
3. How should this patient be managed?

Answers

2. What is the definition of pituitary apoplexy?

Pituitary apoplexy is a clinical syndrome characterized by sudden-onset headache, vomiting, visual disturbance, and reduced consciousness caused by haemorrhage and/or infarction of the pituitary gland. Compression of the optic chiasm above may lead to reduced visual acuity and fields. Involvement of the cavernous sinuses laterally may lead to ocular palsies.

3. How should this patient be managed?

Cranial nerve function should be carefully documented, particularly the visual acuity, visual fields, and eye movements. Serum electrolytes and a pituitary function screen should be performed. Secondary adrenal insufficiency is the major source of mortality associated with pituitary apoplexy, and haemodynamic function must be closely monitored. Corticosteroid replacement is recommended if the presentation is severe (Rajasekaran *et al.* 2011). Some studies have shown that early surgery leads to a greater improvement in visual function, whilst others have shown no difference in outcome between surgically and conservatively managed cases.

In general, patients with severe or deteriorating neuro-ophthalmic symptoms are surgical candidates and other cases are managed conservatively.

This patient underwent surgery due to deteriorating visual fields and a progressive right third nerve palsy.

Further reading

Rajasekaran S, Vanderpump M, Baldeweg S, *et al.* (2011). UK guidelines for the management of pituitary apoplexy. *Clin Endocrinol*; **74**: 9–20.

Case 41

A 12-year-old boy was referred by his paediatrician following 5 weeks of visual deterioration, particularly in the right eye. He kept bumping into things at home. He had experienced no headaches or vomiting. He had a visual acuity of 6/36 on the left and 6/12 on the right, and a bitemporal visual field loss to confrontation. The optic fundi were normal.

Question

1. Where would you localize the lesion, what is the differential diagnosis, and what investigations need to be organized?

Answer

1. Where would you localize the lesion, what is the differential diagnosis, and what investigations need to be organized?

The bitemporal hemianopia means that the optic chiasm is affected. In theory, a lesion compressing from below the chiasm would affect the upper quadrants first and a lesion compressing from above would cause a lower bitemporal quadrantanopia first. In practice, this is only occasionally seen. The most likely diagnosis at this age is a craniopharyngioma, followed by a pituitary tumour (rare in children). In adults, a suprasellar aneurysm and meningioma are also possibilities. Imaging with CT or preferably MRI would be appropriate as well as endocrine pituitary investigation. Formal visual field and acuity assessment should be undertaken by an ophthalmologist.

Question

2. Two of the relevant MRI axial slices are shown in Fig. 41.1. Comment on the findings.

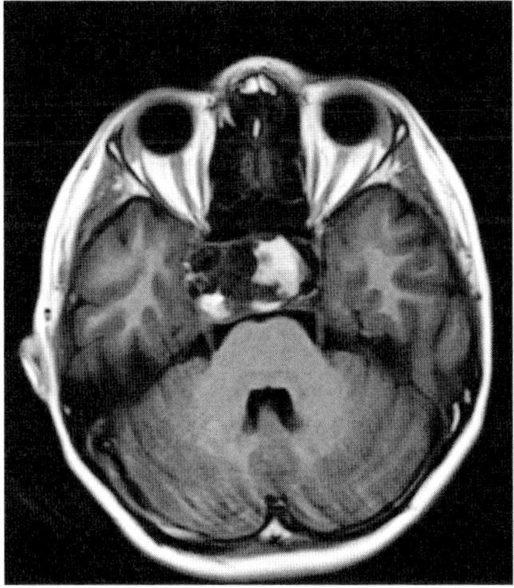

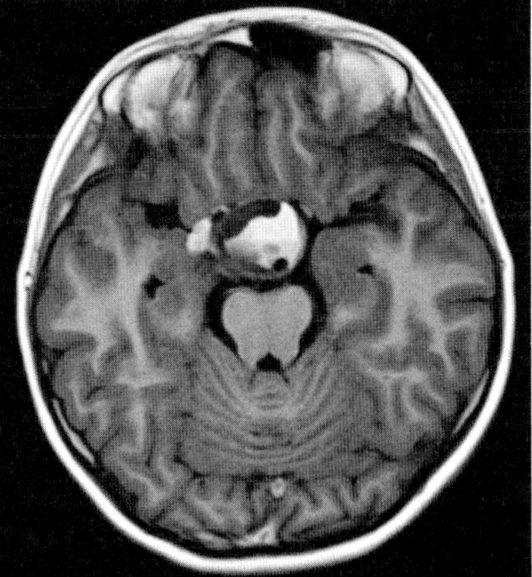

Fig. 41.1

Answer

2. Two of the relevant MRI axial slices are shown in Fig. 41.1. Comment on the findings (Fig. 41.2).

T_1 axial slices are shown. There is a partly cystic (A), partly solid (B) loculated suprasellar lesion in close proximity to the optic nerves and chiasm, although the exact position is not determined. The temporal horns of both lateral ventricles are just visible (C) and do not appear enlarged. This is consistent with the patient's presentation, as headaches were not a feature. Within the wall of the cyst, areas of hypointensity (D) represent calcification (this could also be seen on CT) and are typical of craniopharyngiomas. The carotid arteries are partly encapsulated by the cyst and displaced laterally (E).

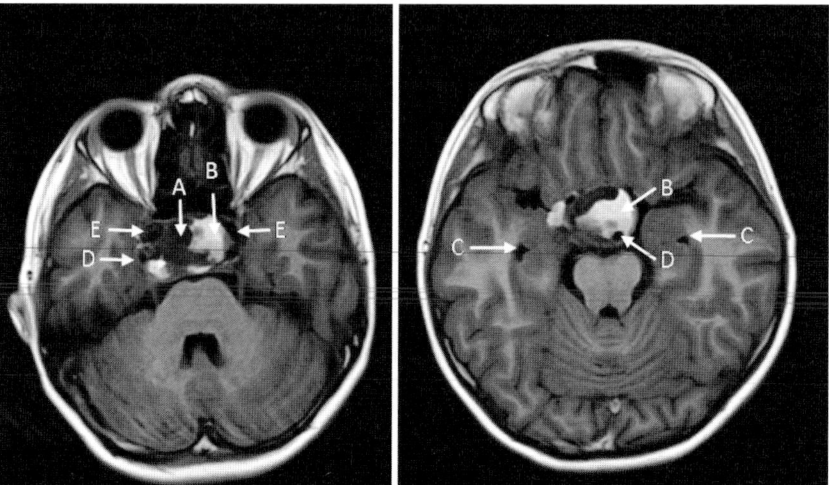

Fig. 41.2

Questions

3. What operative options exist for treating craniopharyngiomas?
4. Outline the main concerns in the immediate postoperative period.

Answers

3. What operative options exist for treating craniopharyngiomas?

The general approach is to debulk solid elements and drain the cystic areas, taking care not to disturb the superior aspect which can be stuck to the hypothalamus. Macroscopic excision has fallen out of favour because of the hypothalamic damage caused which could leave children with short stature, hyperphagia, morbid obesity, polydipsia, sleep disturbance, cognitive problems, or, in more severe cases, persistent coma. Postoperative radiotherapy is usually effective in preventing regrowth and long-term control is generally achievable.

Hydrocephalus may need ventriculoperitoneal shunting and it is also possible to place a catheter and subcutaneous reservoir into a cystic cavity to allow repeated aspiration of recurrent cystic areas. This most commonly occurs after radiotherapy.

A number of different operative approaches can be used for the craniotomy depending on the anatomical localization of the craniopharyngioma: laterally via a pterional craniotomy and splitting the sylvian fissure, a subfrontal or lateral subfrontal approach coming from underneath the frontal lobe, and an anterior interhemispheric or even transcallosal approach from superiorly if the tumour extends upwards significantly into the third ventricle. If there is a significant component in the pituitary fossa (sellar extension) a trans-sphenoidal approach can be used.

In removing tumour from around the optic nerves or chiasm, care has to be taken not to completely strip the vascular supply to the optic apparatus from above and below the chiasm as this can result in blindness.

4. Outline the main concerns in the immediate postoperative period.

In addition to the usual neurological observations of the GCS, limb or focal deficit, and pupil responses, the visual fields and acuity need to be closely observed in case of deterioration from postoperative haematoma or swelling of the optic nerves. Diabetes insipidus is usually transient but can last several days or weeks. Steroid replacement with hydrocortisone may be required to avoid an Addisonian crisis with systemic hypotension, abdominal pains, vomiting, diarrhoea, low sodium levels, and high potassium or calcium levels.

Further reading

Puget S, Grill J, Habrand JL, Sainte-Rose C (2006). Multimodal treatment of craniopharyngioma: defining a risk-adapted strategy. *J Pediatr Endocrinol Metab*; **19** (Suppl 1): 367–70.

Spoudeas HA, Saran F, Pizer B (2006). A multimodality approach to the treatment of craniopharyngiomas avoiding hypothalamic morbidity: a UK perspective. *J Pediatr Endocrinol Metab*; **19** (Suppl 1): 447–51.

Case 42

A 47-year-old accountant is referred by his GP with 3 months of ascending numbness that began in his toes and spread upwards towards his umbilicus. He was initially investigated for diabetes and presumed peripheral neuropathy, but fasting blood glucose was normal (4.7 mmol/l). He has had stiffness in his legs which is troublesome first thing in the morning. His bladder and bowel function are normal and he reports no symptoms in his upper limbs.

On examination he is thin but denies recent weight loss. Tone is increased in the legs and power is reduced (4/5). His knee and ankle jerks are very brisk and there is ankle clonus on both sides. One plantar reflex is upgoing and the other is equivocal. He has subjective numbness throughout his legs up to the level of the umbilicus but preserved pinprick sensation. He has no spinal tenderness.

Questions

1. What is the differential diagnosis?
2. Explain how ascending numbness results from extrinsic spinal cord compression.
3. The GP has arranged an MRI (Fig. 42.1). What is the radiological diagnosis?
4. The patient has numbness up to the umbilicus which corresponds to the T10 dermatome. Why is there a discrepancy between the level of the lesion (in this case T7) and the sensory level (at T10)?
5. How should the patient be counselled? If surgery is to be offered, how should it be done?

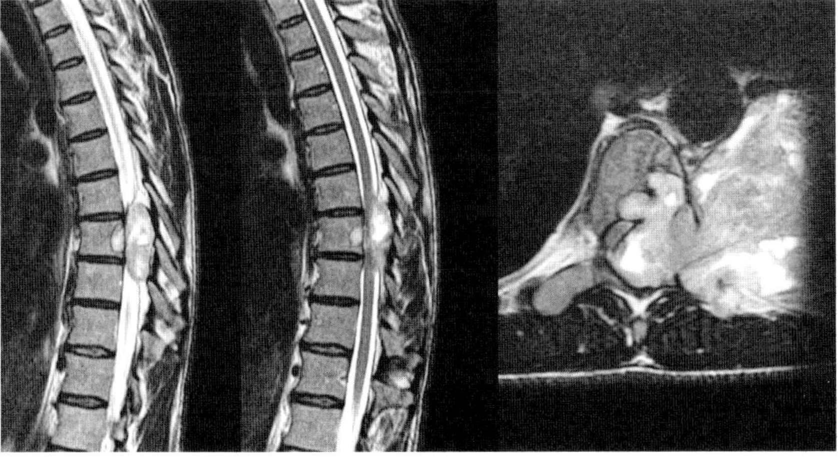

Fig. 42.1

Answers

1. What is the differential diagnosis?

The patient clinically has a spastic paraparesis (see 'Types of spinal cord lesions', p. 299). Sparing of the upper limb suggests that the pathology lies below the cervical region. The two most common causes of spinal cord compression are degenerative disease and bony metastases. Spinal metastases causing cord compression usually cause pain. The next most common cause, especially in the absence of back pain, is a progressively enlarging thoracic disc prolapse. This is far less common than lumbar disc prolapse and many thoracic disc fragments are calcified. The third possibility is a benign tumour, of which neurofibroma and meningioma are the most common.

2. Explain how ascending numbness results from extrinsic spinal cord compression.

The sensory and motor tracts in the spinal cord are somatotopically arranged (Fig. 42.2). In the lateral spinothalamic tract, sacral fibres are situated most laterally followed by lumbar, thoracic, and cervical fibres more medially. Therefore sensory disturbance due to extrinsic spinal cord compression is typically perceived to begin in the lower limbs and progresses upwards.

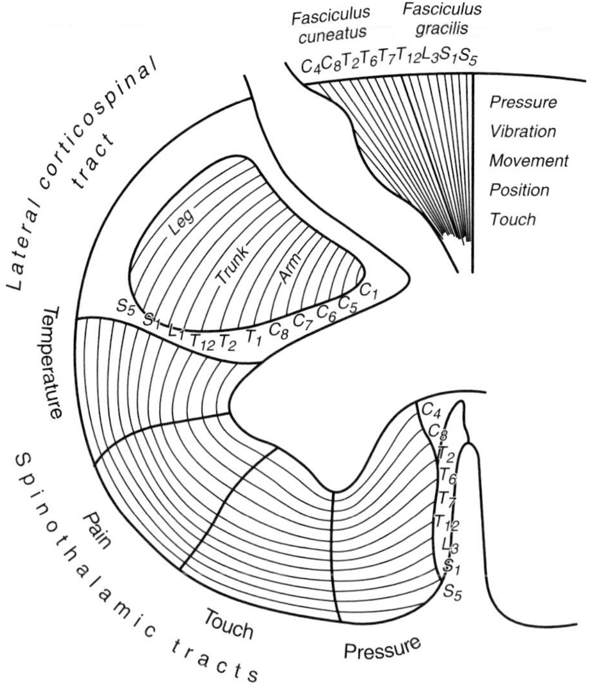

Fig. 42.2 Somatotopic arrangement of tracts in the spinal cord: S, sacral; L, lumbar; T, thoracic; C, cervical. Reproduced with permission from Standring, S, *Gray's Anatomy*. © Elsevier, 2005.

3. The GP has arranged an MRI (Fig. 42.1). What is the radiological diagnosis (Fig. 42.3)?

There is a large mass with mixed signal intensity (A) extending from the left side of the spinal canal in the mid-thoracic region (T7) through the neural foramen (B) and into the chest cavity (C). The body and posterior elements of the T7 vertebra (D) are eroded by the mass. The spinal cord is displaced. These appearances are diagnostic of a large neurofibroma. This is a slow-growing benign tumour that grows along a nerve root and through the neural foramen. It typically expands on either side of the foramen, hence the term 'dumb-bell' neurofibroma.

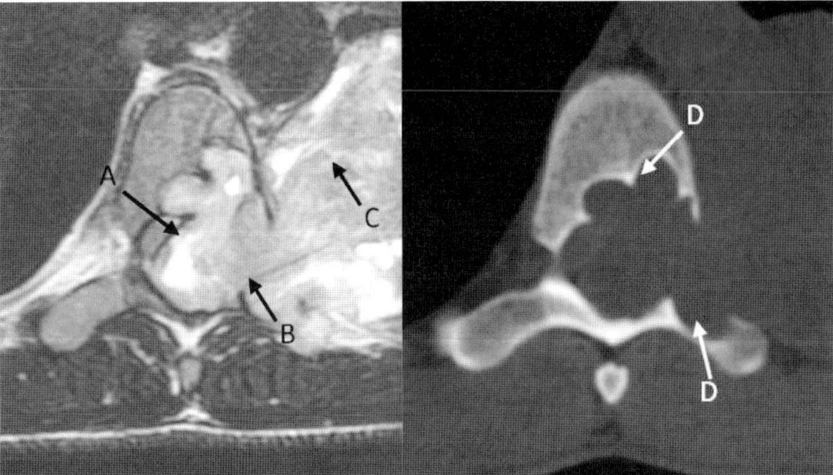

Fig. 42.3

4. The patient has numbness up to the umbilicus which corresponds to the T10 dermatome. Why is there a discrepancy between the level of the lesion (in this case T7) and the sensory level (at T10)?

It is common for the clinical 'sensory' level to be noted several (two or three) segments below the anatomical level of the pathology. The explanation for this is that the spinal cord is shorter than the spinal canal, and in the lower thoracic spinal canal this equates to two to three spinal levels.

5. How should the patient be counselled? If surgery is to be offered, how should it be done?

The patient has progressive spinal cord compression and will become paralysed if untreated. Surgery carries the rare risk of exacerbation of his neurological deficit.

If he chooses to go ahead with surgery, he should be given dexamethasone for a few days beforehand to reduce vasogenic oedema.

Surgery should aim to find the (hopefully well preserved) tissue plane deep to the tumour so that it can be removed completely from the spinal cord. There is a risk of the surgery resulting in instability and hence requiring supplementation with pedicle screws. The other consideration is that the larger part of the tumour is within the chest cavity; input from the cardiothoracic surgeons should be sought.

Further reading

Asazuma T, Toyama Y, Maruiwa H, Fujimura Y, Hirabayashi K (2004). Surgical strategy for cervical dumbbell tumors based on a three-dimensional classification. *Spine (Phila Pa 1976)*; **29**: E10–14.

Conti P, Pansini G, Mouchaty H, Capuano C, Conti R (2004). Spinal neurinomas: retrospective analysis and long-term outcome of 179 consecutively operated cases and review of the literature. *Surg Neurol*; **61**: 34–43.

Eden K (1941). The dumb-bell tumours of the spine. *Br J Surg*; **28**: 549–70.

Husband DJ, Grant KA, Romaniuk CS (2001). MRI in the diagnosis and treatment of malignant spinal cord compression. *Br J Radiol*; **74**: 15–23.

Jamieson DRS, Teasdale E, Willison HJ (1996). Lesson of the week. False localising signs in the spinal cord. *BMJ*; **312**: 243.

False localizing signs

This refers to neurological signs that are produced by lesions situated at locations other than those that would be expected for such a sign. Perhaps the best known false localizing sign is the sixth nerve palsy that occurs with raised intracranial pressure. Fifth and seventh nerve dysfunction has also been noted to occur with raised intracranial pressure. The presumed mechanism is stretching of the cranial nerves due to downward displacement of the brainstem by a supratentorial mass lesion. The Kernohan–Woltman notch phenomenon is also considered to be a false localizing sign and occurs when a supratentorial lesion causes ipsilateral uncal herniation and ipsilateral pupillary dilation in conjunction with an ipsilateral hemiparesis due to compression of the contralateral midbrain from displacement of the free edge of the tentorium. This is 'falsely localizing' as one would expect a supratentorial lesion to cause contralateral (rather than ipsilateral) hemiparesis (Fig. 42.4).

(continued)

False localizing signs *(continued)*

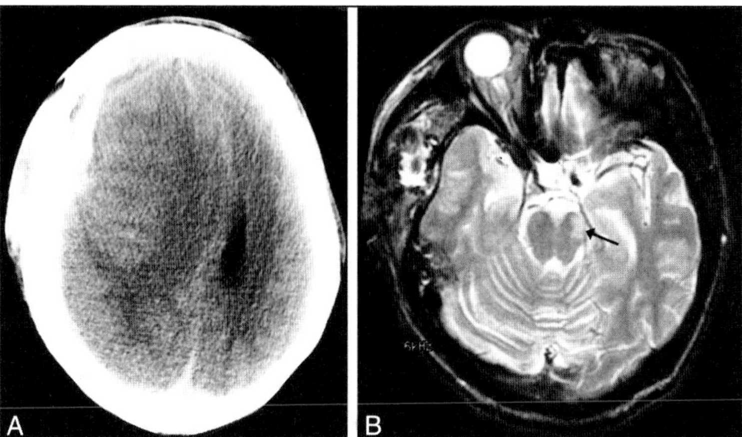

Fig. 42.4 Kernohan's notch phenomenon: a right subdural haematoma causing mass effect and compression of the left cerebral peduncle against the tentorium, causing right hemiplegia. (A) CT scan showing an acute right-sided subdural hematoma with midline shift. (B) T_2-weighted axial MRI demonstrating a hyperintense region in the contralateral left cerebral peduncle (arrow) giving rise to ipsilateral hemiparesis. Reproduced from *Neurology* **12**, December 2000; **55**(11): 1751. © Lippencott, Williams & Wilkins, 2000.

Types of spinal cord lesions

Spinal cord pathology can usually be reliably localized before imaging with a thorough clinical assessment. The most important anatomical concepts are as follows.

- **The structure of the grey and white matter of the spinal cord** The grey matter forms the central part of the spinal cord where synapses form between descending upper motor neurons and the lower motor neurons, and between the sensory afferents and their corresponding ascending tracts. The grey matter is more sensitive to acute and chronic compression and injury than the white matter surrounding it which forms the tracts taking information to and from the levels below. This is the anatomical basis of central cord syndrome.
- **Decussation of the pathways** The (ascending) spinothalamic tracts carry pain and temperature sensory information but the synapses between the first-order sensory afferents and the ascending neurons are on the contralateral side of the cord at the level of the sensory afferent. The (ascending) dorsal columns (cuneate and gracile fasciculae) carry vibration, proprioception, and light touch information, and do not cross at this level; they ascend and cross in the sensory decussation of the medulla. The (descending) corticospinal or pyramidal tracts decussate at the pyramidal decussation in the medulla and hence descend on the side of

(continued)

Types of spinal cord lesions *(continued)*

the cord at which they will synapse and exit. This is the basis of Brown–Séquard syndrome.

- **Lamellation of the spinal cord** Like the rest of the CNS, the white matter tracts around the edge of the cord are arranged somatotopically. There is preservation of spatial information by the organization of the white matter tracts. The outermost layers of the white matter subserve the anatomically most caudal areas, such that sacral sensation is conveyed by the outermost fibres of the whole cord. For example, at C5 the innermost white matter tracts are those supplying C5, the next innermost supply C6, and so forth. This forms the basis of the suspended or ascending sensory level. Pressure on the cord affects the outermost fibres (sacral and low lumbar) first, and as the pressure increases it affects the fibres towards the centre of the cord and the grey matter. Therefore the symptoms ascend to the level of the pathology, above which they cannot rise.

The key clinical features of pathology affecting the spinal cord and roots, which can be elicited by both history and examination, are as follows.

- **Pain** Axial pain (midline) can be used with accuracy to determine the level of pathology affecting the structures that offer mechanical stability to the spinal column. Expect pain, and sometimes tenderness to percussion, in cases of tumours infiltrating bone and epidural infections, particularly discitis. Pain is obviously a key feature of trauma but in this case the history will make the diagnosis. Radicular pain localizes pathology compressing a nerve root, either laterally above the conus medullaris (i.e. cervical or thoracic spine) or both laterally and centrally in the lumbar spine. Radicular arm pain follows a stereotyped dermatome to give the level involved. Radicular pain from the thoracic spine typically radiates around one or other side of the chest wall and is often misdiagnosed as musculoskeletal chest pain, indigestion, or angina.
- **Sensory disturbance** This may be incomplete or complete. In a single dermatome it reflects root compression and is usually preceded by a history of pain that gives way to numbness (occasionally over a short period). Sensory disturbance due to spinal cord compression may be symmetric (suggesting a central spinal canal pathology) or asymmetric (most commonly caused by a unilateral large disc prolapse in the cervical spine). The level of the sensory disturbance is not always the same as the level of the pathology causing it. Pathology such as a tumour pressing on the cord will affect the outermost fibres of the cord first; according to the lamellation of the cord, this will be the most caudal sensory fibres. Therefore an extradural tumour causing slowly progressive cord compression at T5 will initially cause numbness of the perineum (S2, S3, S4) followed by the calf and sole of the foot (S1), the anterior shin (L5), and so forth. The sensory loss will ascend and stop at the level of the pathology, where it will progress in severity. This is the suspended sensory level. In theory this also applies to motor deficits, but in practice these are harder to elicit clinically

(continued)

Types of spinal cord lesions *(continued)*

because of the inability to examine intercostal muscles individually and the natural differential strengths of the lower limb muscle groups.

- **Weakness** This is found in a pattern of upper or lower motor neuron weakness, or a combination of the two. Upper motor neuron weakness results in a loss of corticospinal control of the muscle group and increased tone and brisk monosynaptic (tendon) reflexes. Strength is affected later in the course of the illness and, given that upper motor neuron weakness due to spinal pathology is seen far more commonly in the legs than in the arms, the ability to walk is usually preserved. However, the loss of corticospinal control results in a spastic stiff gait which, combined with loss of proprioceptive feedback, may result in a tendency to fall. In contrast, lower motor neuron weakness due to compression of either the root or damage to the grey matter of the spinal cord at the level of the affected nerve root results in a loss of the monosynaptic reflex and loss of muscle tone, combined with severe weakness and loss of function.

Therefore the most common spinal cord syndromes are as follows.

- **Central cord syndrome** The patient is usually elderly with a relatively minor flexion–extension injury to the cervical spine on a background of degenerative disease (which maybe occult). The pathology is an acute compressive lesion to the cervical spinal cord which on MRI shows an expanded swollen spinal cord with signal change and often evidence of fresh haemorrhage (i.e. a contusion). Owing to the increased sensitivity to such injuries of the grey matter compared with the white matter of the spinal cord, the grey matter is affected more at the level of the injury. There is a resulting lower motor neuron weakness affecting the territory of the injury (most common at C5/6) with a flaccid weakness with absent reflexes of the arms and hands. The white matter tracts are typically also affected, but less so, and the lower limb power, although usually affected, is often better preserved than the upper limb power. There is often preservation of continence.
- **Brown–Séquard syndrome** (also known as Brown–Séquard hemiplegia) A lesion affecting one side of the cord produces ipsilateral pyramidal distribution weakness, ipsilateral loss of vibration, proprioception, and fine touch, and contralateral loss of pain and temperature sensation below the level of the lesion.

Case 43

A 12-year-old girl is admitted by the paediatricians. She was previously healthy but recently she was noticed to be running less and tending to walk more slowly or limp at times. She began to complain of neck pain and has started to use her hands more slowly and deliberately. Her GP was concerned about Guillain-Barré syndrome and sent her to the local emergency department.

Questions

1. What features of the history are important and what is the differential diagnosis?
2. An MRI scan is done (Fig. 43.1). Describe the labelled abnormality. What is the diagnosis?

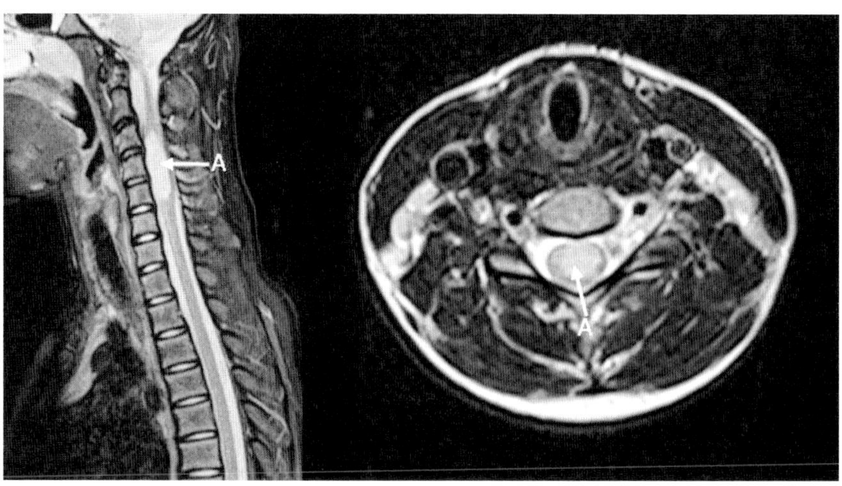

Fig. 43.1

Answers

1. What features of the history are important and what is the differential diagnosis?

The combination of neck pain with motor deficits in the upper and lower limbs that have evolved over a period of time points to an insidious pathological process affecting the cervical spinal cord. The neck pain is very important as it is classically associated with extradural pathology. In older people this would be degenerative or metastatic disease or trauma. Degnerative disease such as a disc prolapse is almost impossible in a 12-year-old and secondary deposits are very rare in a child with no previous history of malignancy. An abscess should be considered including tuberculosis (TB) depending on the social circumstances. Primary extradural tumours are also a possibility. Intradural pathology can cause neck pain, particularly if there is a disease process stretching the dura. This includes acute inflammatory processes such as Guillain–Barré syndrome and transverse myelitis as well as intradural tumours. It would be vital to enquire about any sensory loss or sphincter disturbance, as if present their pattern will provide further clues about the location of the lesion (see 'Spinal cord tumours and their associated symptoms', p. 307).

2. An MRI scan is done (Fig. 43.1). Describe the labelled abnormality. What is the diagnosis?

The sagittal T_2 image shows a hyperintense circumscribed mass in the spinal cord from C3 to C5 (A). The axial view demonstrates that the lesion (A), appearing hyperintense with normal cord around it which appears as a rim of hypointensity, is located within the spinal cord. This is an intramedullary tumour expanding the cord and there is a little dilation of the central canal of the cord below it.

Questions

3. What types of intramedullary tumours are there?
4. What is the initial management for this patient?
5. What is the role of surgery for intradural intramedullary tumours?

3. What types of intramedullary tumour are there?

The most common types are gliomas. Grade III gliomas (anaplastic astrocytomas) rather than glioblastoma are seen in the spinal cord. The other relatively common tumour (in children) is an ependymoma. These have a range of subtypes from benign (myxopapillary subtype) to more malignant (grade III). Other rare primary CNS tumours can also occur, as well as intramedullary metastases.

4. What is the initial management for this patient?

The initial management is dexamethasone to reduce any associated oedema and full neuro-axis MRI for staging.

5. What is the role of surgery for intradural intramedullary tumours?

The aims of surgery in the treatment of primary intramedullary tumours of the spinal cord should be considered in the following terms.

1. To biopsy tissue where there is diagnostic uncertainty and the result will influence the patient's management, such as the decision to proceed with radiotherapy or chemotherapy.
2. To debulk or excise the tumour where there is a realistic chance of so doing without unacceptable neurological deficit and with good prognosis.
3. To manage associated problems (e.g. syringomyelia) or to drain tumour cysts.

Selecting patients correctly for debulking or excision surgery versus conservative management is important. Where the tumour is well circumscribed (as with many ependymomas), surgery can potentially be curative and more aggressive strategies are justified. Similarly, for malignant tumours (grades III and IV), where the neurological deficit is profound and progressive, aggressive surgery, including cordectomy for patients with complete or near-complete paraplegia, is well described with the occasional long-term survivor reported. However, those patients with partial slowly progressive deficits presenting earlier in the course of their illness merit a more cautious approach.

In this case, the tumour is well circumscribed radiologically and surgery should aim for debulking or excision. However, the risks of major deficit are high. Surgery could be performed using continuous electrophysiological monitoring, typically motor and somatosensory evoked potentials (MEPs and SSEPs), to alert the surgeon to potential intraoperative damage.

This child underwent debulking of the tumour after MRI showed no other sites of tumour. MEPs were used and showed severe slowing at one point during dissection of the anterior part of the tumour. She woke up with severe weakness of her hands, but this improved over 6 days and she was able to feed herself and mobilize independently by day 8. Her bowel and bladder function remained intact. Histology showed a grade III ependymoma and she underwent adjuvant chemoradiotherapy.

Spinal cord tumours and their associated symptoms

Spinal tumours can be classified as extradural, intradural–extramedullary and intradural–intramedullary. The distiction is not always apparent on a sagittal MRI image but can be seen on coronal and axial views (Fig.43.2). Extradural tumours typically cause pain and signs of progressive external cord compression. Posteriorly sited tumours will affect the dorsal columns first, whereas laterally sited tumours will cause pain and affect the spinothalamic and corticospinal tracts. Spincter disturbance usually occurs at a later stage. Intradural–extramedullary tumours also present with pain at the spinal level but also radicular pain, and progress to signs of cord compression. Intradural–intramedullary tumours do not cause pain as often, and when pain does occur it can be poorly localized. It has the propensity to affect the spinal cord tracts from 'inside out'—sphincter disturbance may be an early feature and dissociated sensory deficits can occur.

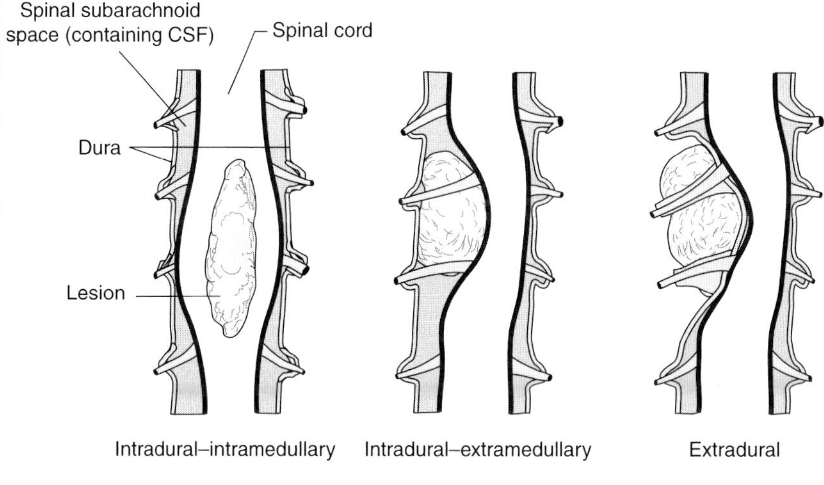

Fig. 43.2 Location of spinal tumours.

Case 44

A 67-year-old woman presents to the emergency department with increasing back pain for 2 months, preventing her from sleeping and driving. Her legs have been feeling slightly numb for 4 days, and for the past 2 days she has been confined to the ground floor of her house. This morning she fell and was unable to get up. She underwent a lobectomy and radiotherapy for small-cell lung cancer last year. She last saw her oncologist 3 months ago and is under clinical surveillance.

Questions

1. What features in a back pain history point to a more sinister cause?
2. The patient has reduced power at grade 3/5 in both lower limbs. Her lower limb reflexes are slightly brisk with plantars downgoing. There is a sensory level below the umbilicus. Anal tone is slightly reduced and a bladder scan shows a residual volume of 100mL. Her arms are normal.
   (a) How should the above neurological findings be interpreted?
   (b) Are there any investigations that may be of value in the emergency department?
3. X-rays are performed (Fig. 44.1). What do they show?

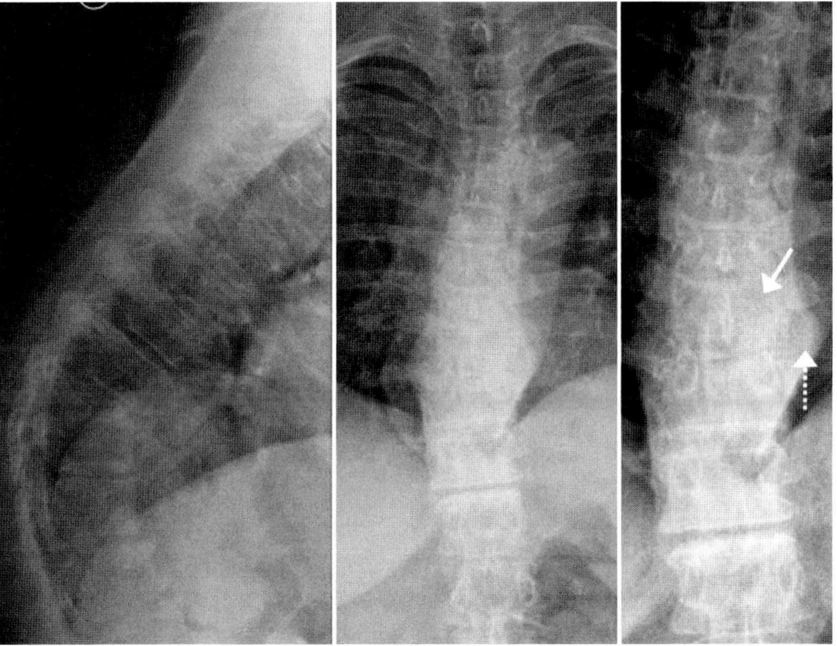

Fig. 44.1

Answers

1. What features in a back pain history point to a more sinister cause?

There are a number of 'red flags' that increase the likelihood of a sinister cause for the back pain (Table 44.1).

2. The patient has reduced power at grade 3/5 in both lower limbs. Her lower limb reflexes are slightly brisk with plantars downgoing. There is a sensory level below the umbilicus. Anal tone is slightly reduced and a bladder scan shows a residual volume of 100mL. Her arms are normal.

(a) How should the above neurological findings be interpreted?

The picture is mixed. There are certainly features consistent with spinal cord compression, but the reflexes and anal tone findings are slightly ambiguous and could be normal. Downgoing plantars are not typically associated with cord compression. Often a telephone referral does not paint a clear neurological picture, but if features consistent with cord compression are reported the patient should be managed as such until the diagnosis is excluded.

(b) Are there any investigations that may be of value in the emergency department?

If plain X-rays of the spine show bony destruction, an urgent MRI scan is required. Even if the X-rays are normal but there is clinical suspicion of cord compression, an MRI will still be indicated. The X-rays are not indicated for back pain *per se* but because of red flag symptoms. Other appropriate immediate investigations in view of the history of cancer are a chest X-ray and blood tests including serum calcium.

Table 44.1 Red flag symptoms in a back pain history

Red flag	Possible underlying cause of back pain
Neurological deficit (including sphincter disturbance)	Spinal cord compression due to any traumatic or mass lesion
Pain at rest or at night	Malignancy, inflammatory disorders
Localized spinal tenderness	Malignancy, spinal injury
History of malignancy	Malignancy
History of trauma	Spinal injury
Weight loss	Malignancy, infection
Fever	Infection, malignancy
Systemic Illness	Related to systemic illness
Steroid use	Osteoporotic fracture

3. X-rays are performed (Fig. 44.1). What do they show?

There is collapse and kyphotic angulation of a lower thoracic vertebrae (T9). The AP X-rays show a paraspinal mass (dotted arrow), and on re-windowing and closer viewing the adjacent pedicle of T9 is not clearly seen (solid arrow), a classic finding in metastatic bony disease.

An MRI (Fig. 44.2) shows tumour destroying the T9 body, extending posteriorly along the T9 pedicles and causing severe spinal cord compression.

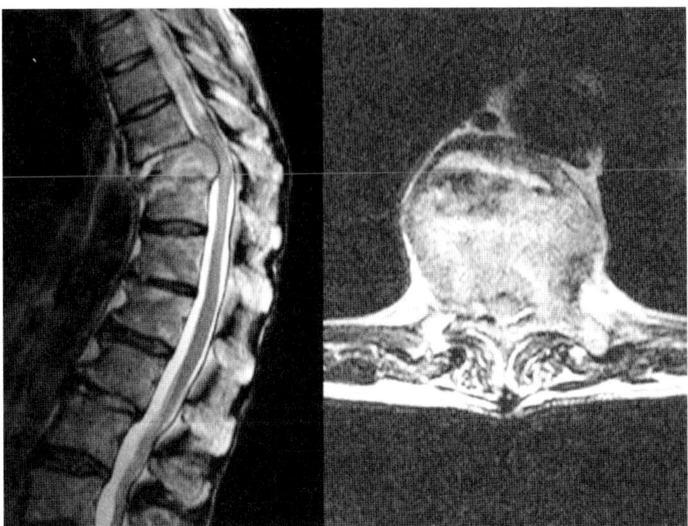

Fig. 44.2

Questions

4. Are there any evidence-based guidelines for the management of malignant spinal cord compression?
5. What are the management options in this case? What are the risks and benefits of each?
6. Are any other investigations appropriate to inform the decision-making?

Answers

4. Are there any evidence-based guidelines for the management of malignant spinal cord compression?

In the UK, NICE has produced a guideline on the management of malignant spinal cord compression. In terms of definitive management, each patient should receive individualized treatment after discussion between oncologists and specialist spinal surgeons.

5. What are the management options in this case? What are the risks and benefits of each?

This patient needs urgent treatment to prevent a complete cord lesion. The management options are radiotherapy or surgery. She should be commenced on dexamethasone. Radiotherapy avoids surgery with its attendant risks of haemorrhage, infection, and worsening the deficit, but it takes several days before it has an effect. During this time the deficit may worsen. Surgery has the advantage of providing immediate decompression but there are risks, as described above. She has anterior collapse and therefore a simple posterior decompression alone will leave the vertebral column unstable. Hence she may require stabilization, usually with pedicle screws and possibly an anterior cage. Instrumentation increases the operative time, blood loss, and complication risk.

6. Are any other investigations appropriate to inform the decision making?

She should have her cancer restaged with a CT scan, and a discussion with her oncologist about her prognosis and the desired management. CT scanning can also assess bony anatomy at the levels above and below (important if these bones are used for pedicle screw stabilization).

Her CT showed no definite evidence of disease elsewhere, but did raise suspicion of the bone density of the T8 vertebral body. She underwent surgery to decompress and stabilize the spine from T7 and T8 to T10. Afterwards she noticed improvement in her leg power immediately and walked by day 4 postoperatively. She received adjuvant radiotherapy after 6 weeks, and she was well and ambulant a year later.

Further reading

Abrahm JL, Banffy MB, Harris MB (2008). Spinal cord compression in patients with advanced metastatic cancer: 'All I care about is walking and living my life'. *JAMA*; **299**: 937–46.

British Association of Surgical Oncology (1999). British Association of Surgical Oncology Guidelines. The management of metastatic bone disease in the United Kingdom. The Breast Specialty Group of the British Association of Surgical Oncology. *Eur J Surg Oncol*; **25**: 3–23.

George R, Jeba J, Ramkumar G, Chacko AG, Leng M, Tharyan P (2008). Interventions for the treatment of metastatic extradural spinal cord compression in adults. *Cochrane Database Syst Rev*; **4**: CD006716.

Ibrahim A, Crockard A, Antonietti P, *et al.* (2007). Does spinal surgery improve the quality of life for those with extradural (spinal) osseous metastases? An international multicenter prospective observational study of 223 patients. *J Neurosurg Spine*; **8**: 271–8.

NICE (2011). *Metastatic Cord Compression. NICE Guideline CG75.* Available online at: http://www.nice.org.uk/CG075 (accessed 13 March 2011).

Patchell RA, Tibbs PA, Regine WF, *et al.* (2005). Direct decompressive surgical resection in the treatment of spinal cord compression caused by metastatic cancer: a randomised trial. *Lancet*; **366**: 643–8.

Case 45

A 32-year-old man consults his GP with a history of headaches for 3 months, with no vomiting or nausea. They are intermittent and not associated with diurnal variation. His friends have asked him to speak more clearly on occasion, and he has felt that his speech is less fluent. However, he has no imbalance and he has been playing tennis.

Questions

1. What is the differential diagnosis?
2. A CT scan (Fig. 45.1: pre-contrast, left; post-contrast, right) is done. Comment on the findings.
3. Coronal T_1, pre- and post-contrast, and axial T_2 MRI sequences are done (Fig. 45.2). What do they show? What treatment would you offer and what is the critical management concern?

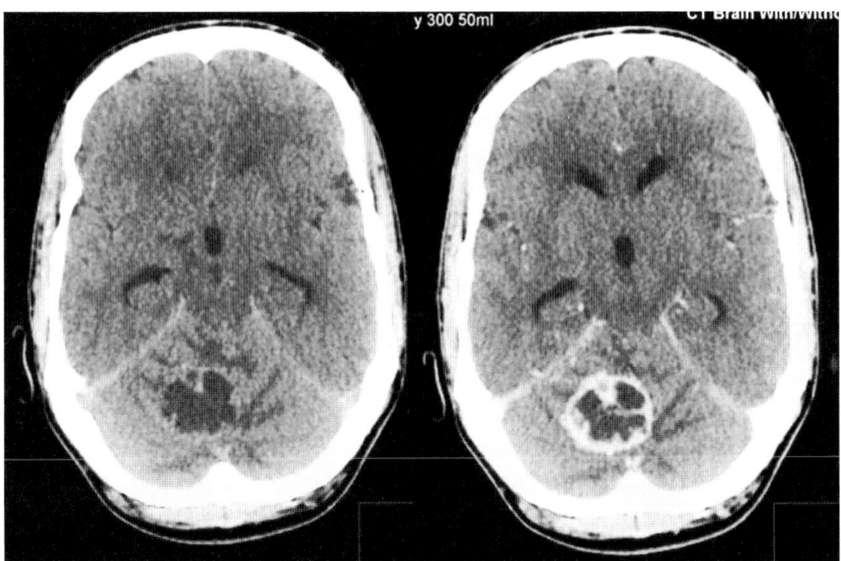

Fig. 45.1

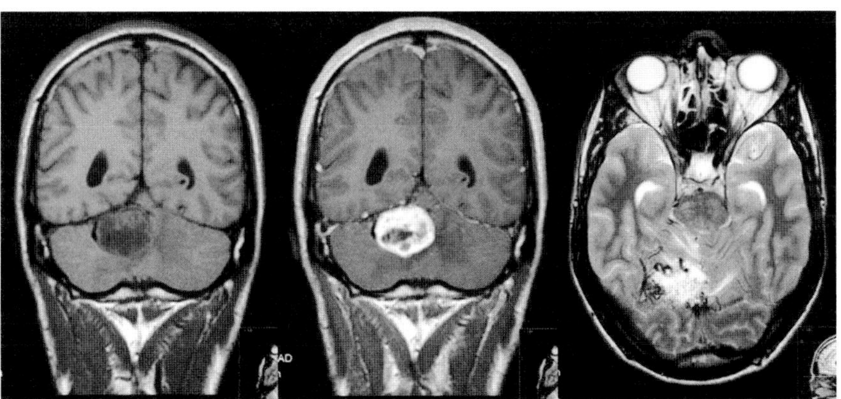

Fig. 45.2

Answers

1. What is the differential diagnosis?

Headaches and changes in speech coordination raise the possibility of a cerebellar mass with hydrocephalus. It would be unusual for a supratentorial mass to produce raised intracranial pressure with headaches and focal deficit in relation to mild speech disturbance (which in this case is more suggestive of dysarthria than dysphasia). The slow and minimally progressive nature of the symptoms suggests a benign lesion.

2. A CT scan (Fig. 45.1: pre-contrast, left; post-contrast, right) is done. Comment on the findings.

There is an obvious enhancing mass, which has an isodense capsule and hypodense contents, to the right of the midline in the cerebellum. There is mild surrounding oedema. The third ventricle is oval rather than slit-like and the temporal horns of the lateral ventricles are clearly visible, indicating hydrocephalus.

The most common enhancing tumour type within the cerebellum is metastatic disease. However, the patient's age and the duration make this unlikely. Primary posterior fossa tumours in adults are commonly haemangioblastomas, ependymomas, or pilocytic astrocytomas.

3. Coronal T_1, pre- and post-contrast, and axial T_2 MRI sequences are done (Fig. 45.2). What do they show? What treatment would you offer and what is the critical management concern?

The coronal T_1 pre- and post-contrast and axial T_2 images confirm a well-circumscribed avidly enhancing mass . The axial T_2 image through the upper part of the mass shows a number of surrounding black flow voids indicating blood vessels. Enlarged surrounding vessels are a typical feature of cerebellar haemangioblastoma, and the diagnosis should be questioned if they are not seen around a lesion of this size. There is no merit in conservative management for this patient as his symptoms will inevitably progress.

Haemangioblastomas are benign (WHO grade I) and therefore may be cured by complete surgical excision. Although usually sporadic, they do occur as part of von Hippel–Lindau disease, one of the neurocutaneous syndromes,where they may be multiple. They commonly occur as a cystic mass with a non-enhancing wall and a solid enhancing nodule; removal of the nodule alone is the surgical treatment. Solid haemangioblastomas, such as this one, are less common and enhance throughout. The tumour is highly vascular and an attempt should be made to remove it in one piece (en bloc).

Catheter angiography is useful, as knowledge of the blood supply may aid surgery, and embolization of the feeding vessels, where possible, can reduce vascularity, as shown for the patient in Fig. 45.3. The pre- and post-embolization lateral angiograms show an impressive reduction in tumour 'blush' from high vascular flow

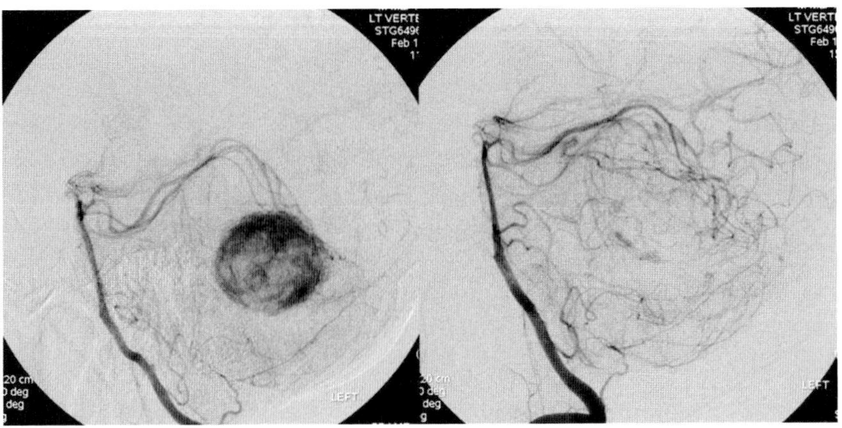

Fig. 45.3

through the superior cerebellar artery. His surgery was uneventful, with en bloc removal and minimal blood loss. He made a full recovery and was discharged on day 5 postoperatively.

Further reading

Eskridge JM, McAuliffe W, Harris B, Kim DK, Scott J, Winn HR (1996). Preoperative endovascular embolization of craniospinal hemangioblastomas. *Am J Neuroradiol*; **17**: 525–31.

Rachinger J, Buslei R, Prell J, Strauss C (2009). Solid haemangioblastomas of the CNS: a review of 17 consecutive cases. *Neurosurg Rev*; **32**: 37–47.

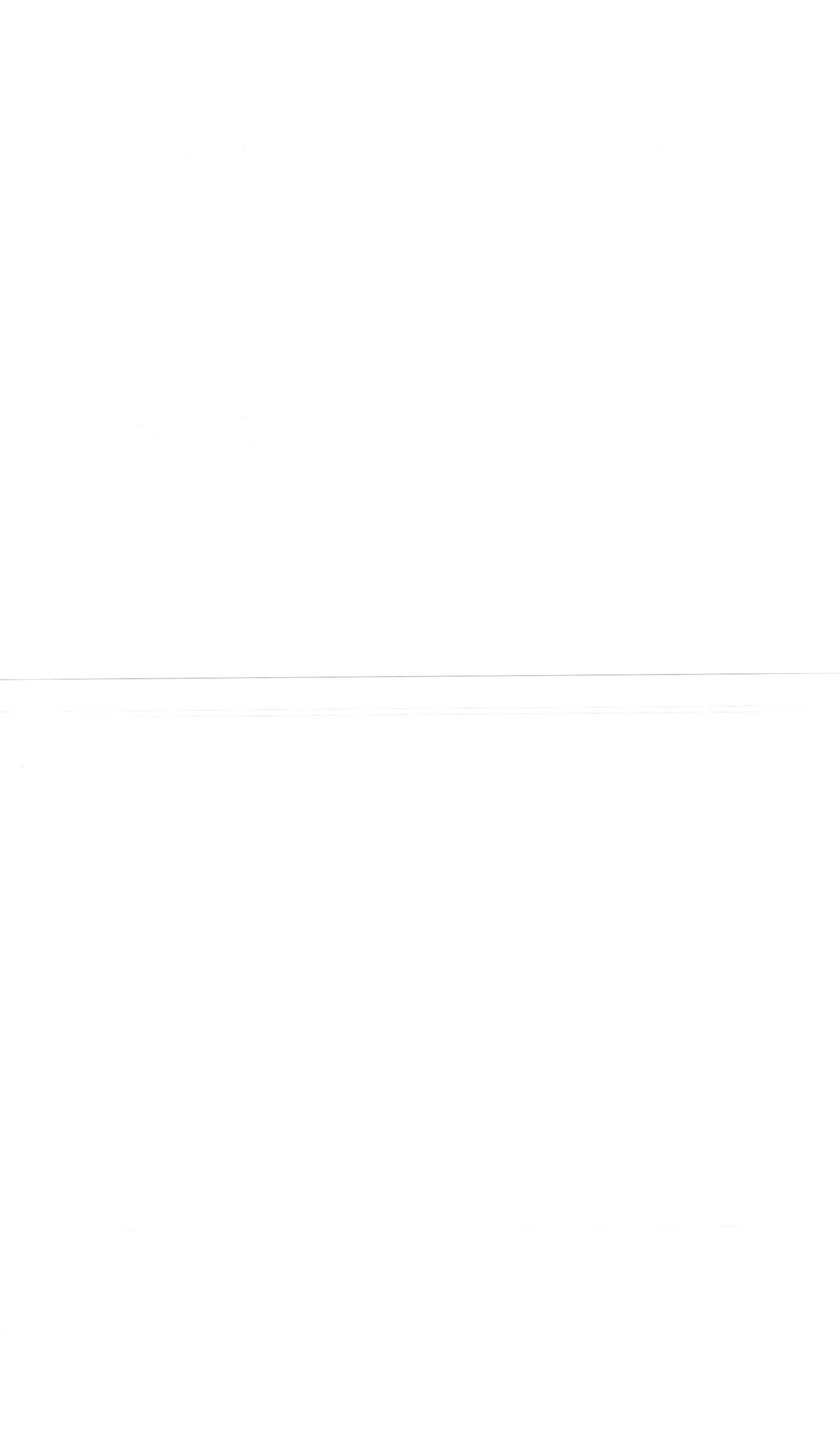

Section 5

Spinal neurosurgery

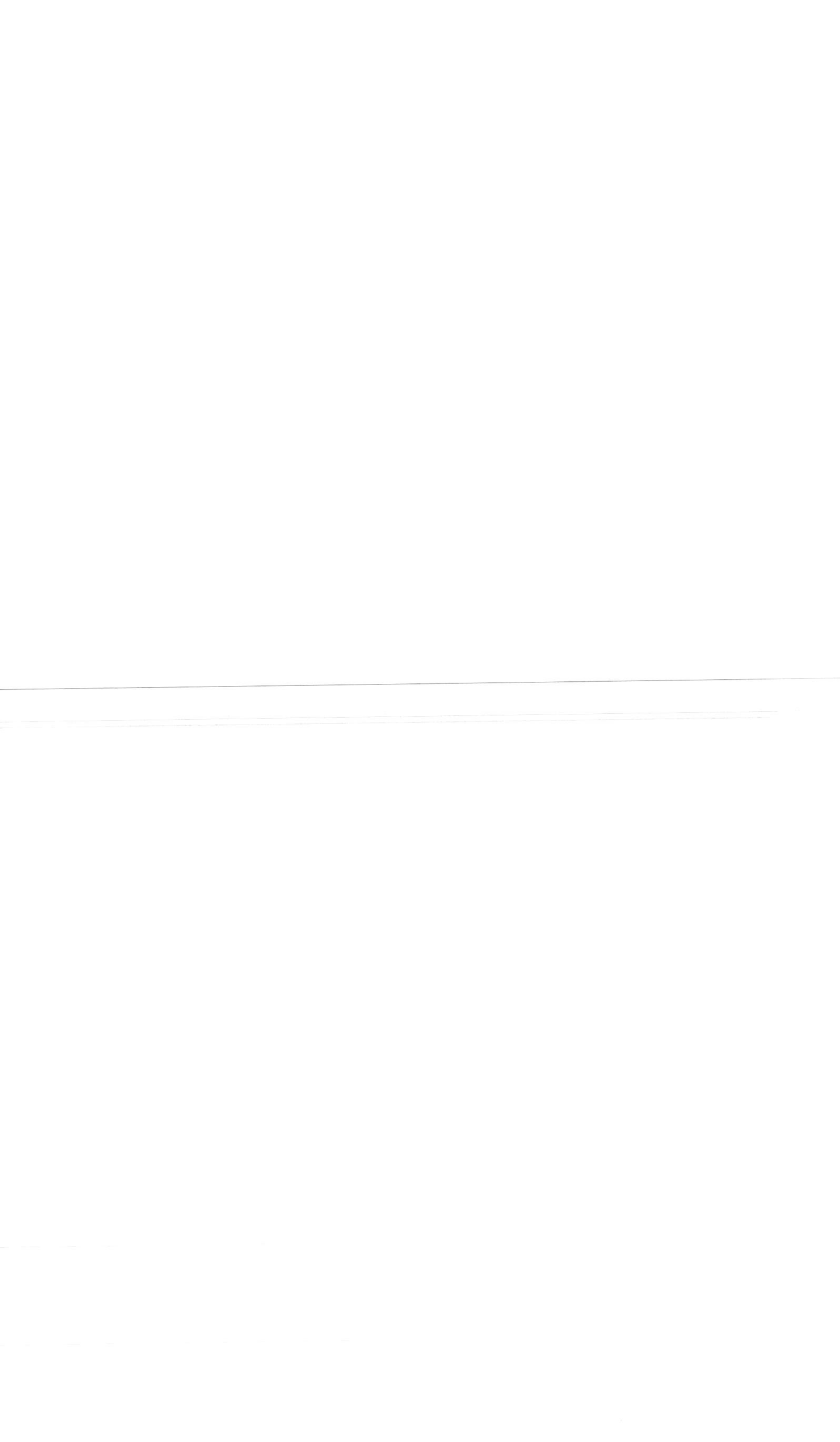

Case 46

A 37-year-old man, normally active and otherwise healthy, develops a sudden pain in his back and an 'electric shock' down his left leg. Over 5 weeks the back pain resolves but he is left with intermittent severe pain in the left leg which radiates down his calf into the sole of the foot and little toe. His right leg has been unaffected and he has normal sphincter function.

Questions

1. What is the likely diagnosis? Is there a differential diagnosis?
2. The patient walks with a mildly antalgic gait. What other signs would you look for on examination?
3. He tells you that he underwent an MRI scan last week and has brought it with him (Fig. 46.1) What is the diagnosis and how would you manage him at this stage?
4. What surgery would you offer and what risks would you discuss with him?

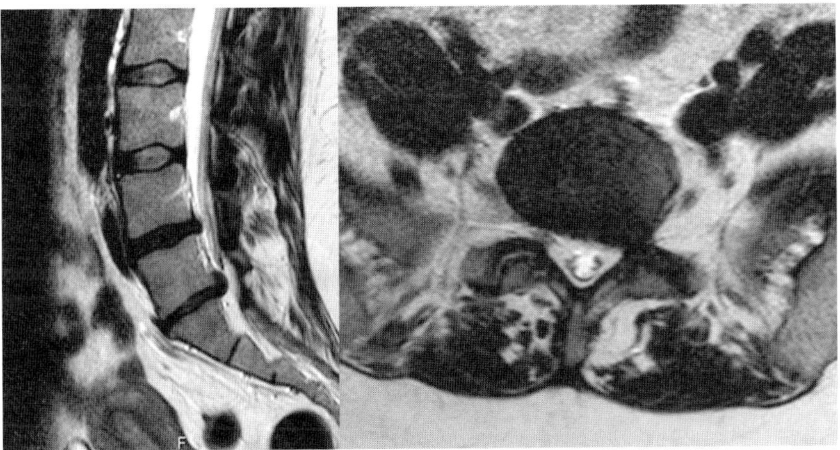

Fig. 46.1

Answers

1. What is the likely diagnosis? Is there a differential diagnosis?

The history is classical for a prolapsed L5/S1 intervertebral disc and left S1 dermatomal sciatica (see 'Nerve roots affected by a prolapsed disc', p. 328).

Hip and knee pathology can both mimic sciatica, especially in older people. Many patients will have back pain, and there may be dual pathology. Recent exacerbation of back pain with sciatica suggests the two are linked. Rarely, acute leg pain can be a presentation of vascular events such as limb ischaemia. Calf pain may be a symptom of DVT which should be considered in a patient with severe immobility due to back pain.

2. The patient walks with a mildly antalgic gait. What other signs would you look for on examination?

The most common finding will be a restriction of passive straight leg raise. He may have sensory change in the left S1 dermatome and an absent or diminished ankle jerk. In more severe cases there is S1 numbness and weakness of ankle plantarflexion.

He has restricted straight leg raise at 40°. Apart from mild sensory loss and a weak ankle jerk, he is intact.

3. He tells you that he underwent an MRI scan last week and has brought it with him (Fig. 46.1). What is the diagnosis and how would you manage him at this stage?

There are two degenerate discs at L4/5 (A) and L5/S1 (B). The L5/S1 bulges posteriorly a little more than the L4/5, and the axial slices confirm a left posterolateral

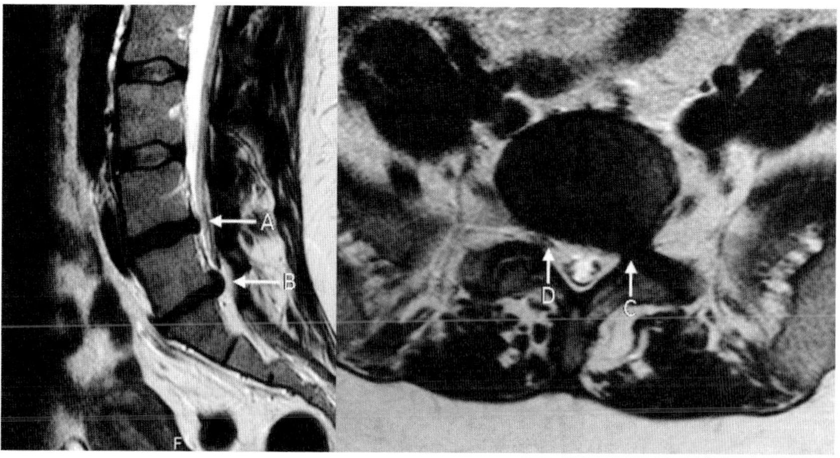

Fig. 46.2

disc prolapse compressing the left S1 nerve root in the lateral recess (C) and the normal right nerve root (D). Note that the left S1 root is not visible separate from the disc. The right S1 root is clearly shown surrounded by fat in the lateral recess.

Most disc prolapses will settle with conservative management. Therefore patients should be managed conservatively with rest and analgesia in the first instance. If there is neurological deficit there is a stronger case for early surgery, especially if the deficit is a foot drop which is a disabling problem. The point at which surgery is considered for sciatica depends on the degree of pain, and how much it impacts on the patient's quality of life. Six weeks is a reasonable period to allow for spontaneous resolution, but waiting longer will continue to confer better likelihood of resolution.

4. What surgery would you offer and what risks would you discuss with him?

As leg pain is his main complaint he should be offered a lumbar discectomy for the L5/S1 fragment. Discectomy for leg pain with typical symptoms and clinical–radiological correlation has a high chance (≥90%) of relieving his leg pain. There may be a secondary improvement in his back pain as a result of the increased mobility afforded by relief from the sciatica.

The risks of a lumbar discectomy should be small. He should be informed of the general risks of haemorrhage and infection. There is a very small risk of infective discitis, which results in progressive back pain and, rarely, sepsis some weeks following surgery, and would require a prolonged course of antibiotics. The risk of very serious neurological complication (i.e. cauda equina syndrome) from such an operation should be extremely small, although it should be discussed during the consent process. Similarly, the risk of S1 weakness should be mentioned as a rare occurrence. Early recurrence in the first few weeks following surgery can be treated by repeat surgery, usually with a good result.

Further reading

Jegede KA, Ndu A, Grauer JN (2010). Contemporary management of symptomatic lumbar disc herniations. *Orthop Clin North Am*; **41**: 217–24.

Moliterno JA, Knopman J, Parikh K, *et al.* (2010). Results and risk factors for recurrence following single-level tubular lumbar microdiscectomy. *J Neurosurg Spine*; **12**: 680–6.

Pearson AM, Blood EA, Frymoyer JW, *et al.* (2008). SPORT lumbar intervertebral disk herniation and back pain: does treatment, location, or morphology matter? *Spine (Phila Pa 1976)*; **33**: 428–35.

van der Windt DA, Simons E, Riphagen II, *et al.* (2010). Physical examination for lumbar radiculopathy due to disc herniation in patients with low-back pain, *Cochrane Database Syst Rev*; **2**: CD007431.

Weinstein JN, Tosteson TD, Lurie JD, *et al.* (2006). Surgical vs non-operative treatment for lumbar disk herniation: the Spine Patient Outcomes Research Trial (SPORT): a randomized trial. *JAMA*; **296**: 2441–50.

Case 47

A 38-year-old woman presents to the emergency department with 2 weeks of back pain radiating down her left leg. On the previous day, she noticed difficulty passing urine and partial numbness of her buttocks.

Questions

1. What is the diagnosis?
2. What are the important questions to ask?
3. On examination there was some weakness of plantarflexion and hip extension on the left. The left ankle reflex was absent. Pinprick sensation was preserved throughout the lower limbs but sensation was absent in the perineum. However, when more pressure was applied to the pin, the patient reported that she could feel the sharp pin in the perineum. The rest of the examination was normal.
   (a) Identify the level of the pathology
   (b) Are the clinical findings consistent with the suspected diagnosis?
4. What investigations are required? What would you do if the patient was claustrophobic and unable to tolerate an MRI scan?
5. The patient undergoes an MRI scan of the lumbar spine (Fig. 47.1). Describe the findings on the scan.
6. What is the management, and on what time scale?
7. The patient is reviewed the following morning when she complains of recurrent left leg pain. How should her symptoms be managed?

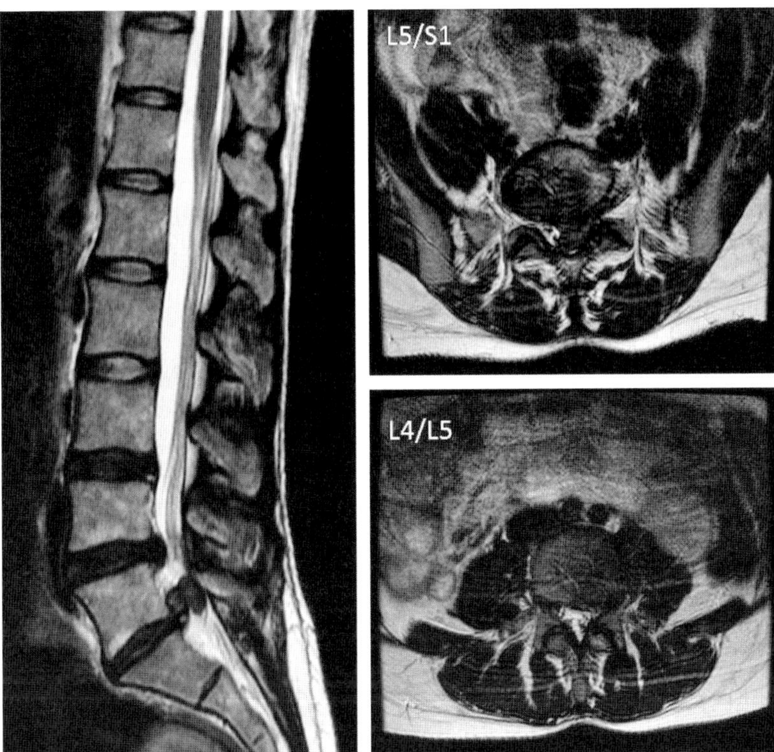

Fig. 47.1

Answers

1. What is the diagnosis?

Cauda equina syndrome until proven otherwise. This is a clinical syndrome resulting from compression of the cauda equina. It presents with a variable combination of leg pain (classically bilateral), anaesthesia in the sacral distribution, and urinary retention with overflow incontinence. In this case, the most likely cause of cauda equina compression is a prolapsed lumbar intervertebral disc. Other lesions, including tumours, abscesses, and trauma, can also cause cauda equina syndrome.

2. What are the important questions to ask?

The exact nature of the urinary symptoms must be determined because it helps to distinguish cauda equina syndrome from urinary retention due to back pain, urinary tract infection, or pre-existing bladder problems (see 'Disorders of micturition in neurosurgery', p. 342). The timing of onset of symptoms is also critical because it influences the timing of surgery. The completeness of the symptoms is strongly correlated with the recovery potential, with patients with incomplete cauda equina syndrome having a better prognosis.

3. On examination there was some weakness of plantarflexion and hip extension on the left. The left ankle reflex was absent. Pinprick sensation was preserved throughout the lower limbs but was absent in the perineum. However, when more pressure was applied to the pin, the patient reported that she could feel the sharp pin in the perineum. The rest of the examination was normal.

(a) Identify the level of the pathology

The left ankle reflex is affected, suggesting involvement of the S1 nerve root. Ankle plantarflexion and hip extension also have contributions from S1. Therefore the level of compression is likely to be at L5/S1 (see 'Nerve roots affected by a prolapsed disc', p. 328 and Table 52.3, p. 352).

(b) Are the clinical findings consistent with the suspected diagnosis?

Examining perineal sensation can be challenging if the patient's response is inconsistent. As a general rule, if perineal pinprick sensation is less than reported elsewhere when the same pressure is applied, it should be assumed that there is impairment. If a sharp sensation is elicited when the pin is pressed harder, impairment is not excluded. If a sharp sensation is not elicited at all, impairment is confirmed. Therefore these findings are consistent with cauda equina compression.

4. What investigations are required? What would you do if the patient was claustrophobic and unable to tolerate an MRI scan?

If the clinical diagnosis is suspected, an MRI scan of the lumbar spine is required immediately. Claustrophobic patients may tolerate the MRI scanner with sedation. If not, the options include a CT myelogram or a MRI under general anaesthetic.

5. The patient undergoes an MRI scan of the lumbar spine (Fig. 47.1). Describe the findings on the scan (Fig. 47.2).

On the sagittal view there is a large disc prolapse at L5/S1 filling the width of the canal (1). The axial view at this level shows that the disc is laterally sited to the left (2). Note that the thecal sac (surrounded by a small amount of CSF which appears white on this T_2 image) is displaced to the right (3). There is a smaller left-sided disc protrusion at the level above, where the canal is more capacious (see L4/L5 image above).

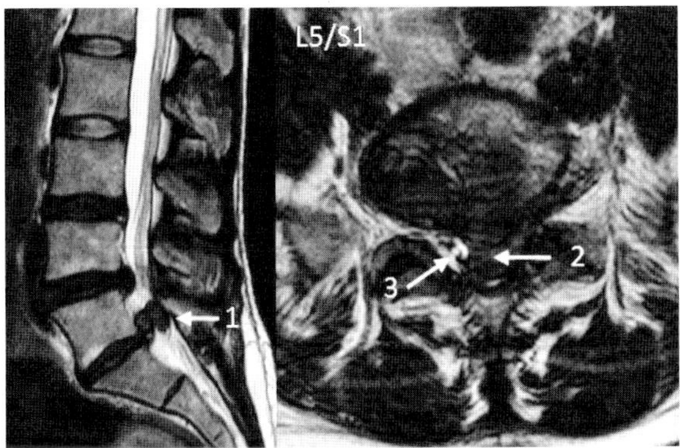

Fig. 47.2

6. What is the management, and on what time scale?

This patient presents within 24 hours of onset of urinary symptoms, so surgery should be performed immediately. The operation is a discectomy, involving a midline posterior approach, laminectomy, and removal of the prolapsed segment of disc. This patient was operated on overnight and reported an improvement in leg pain and some recovery of perineal sensation postoperatively.

7. The patient is reviewed the following morning when she complains of recurrent left leg pain. How should her symptoms be managed?

The symptoms have deteriorated following lumbar decompression. The differential diagnosis includes residual disc or postoperative haematoma causing neural compression, infection, and post-surgical oedema affecting the nerve roots. An MRI scan is required to exclude persistent neural compression. However, this showed normal postoperative appearances and the patient was managed with analgesia and discharged several days later.

Further reading

Cohen MS, Wall EJ, Kerber CW, Abitbol J-J, Garfin SR (1991). The anatomy of the cauda equina on CT scans and MRI. *J Bone Joint Surg Br*; **3**: 381–4.

Crocker M, Jones T, Rich P, Bell BA, Papadopoulos MC (2010). The clinical value of early postoperative MRI after lumbar spine surgery. *Br J Neurosurg*; **24**: 46–50.

Findlay G (2008). Meta-analysis and the timing of cauda equina surgery. *Br J Neurosurg*; **22**: 137–8

McCarthy MJ, Aylott CE, Grevitt MP, Hegarty J (2007). Cauda equina syndrome. Factors affecting long-term functional and sphincteric outcome. *Spine*; **32**: 207–16.

Advice box

Compression of the cauda equina does not always produce the complete triad of leg pain, urinary disturbance, and saddle anaesthesia. The diagnosis should always be suspected in any patient who has sensory changes in the sacral dermatomes S2, S3, or S4, even if it is only subjective or unilateral. There should be a low threshold for emergency scanning under these circumstances.

Nerve roots affected by a prolapsed disc

The nerve roots as they exit the spinal canal through the intervertebral foramina are situated just above the level of the numbered disc. A unilateral lumbar disc prolapse therefore tends to compress the traversing nerve roots, whereas a far lateral disc prolapse will tend to compress the exiting nerve root at that level. (Fig. 47.3.)

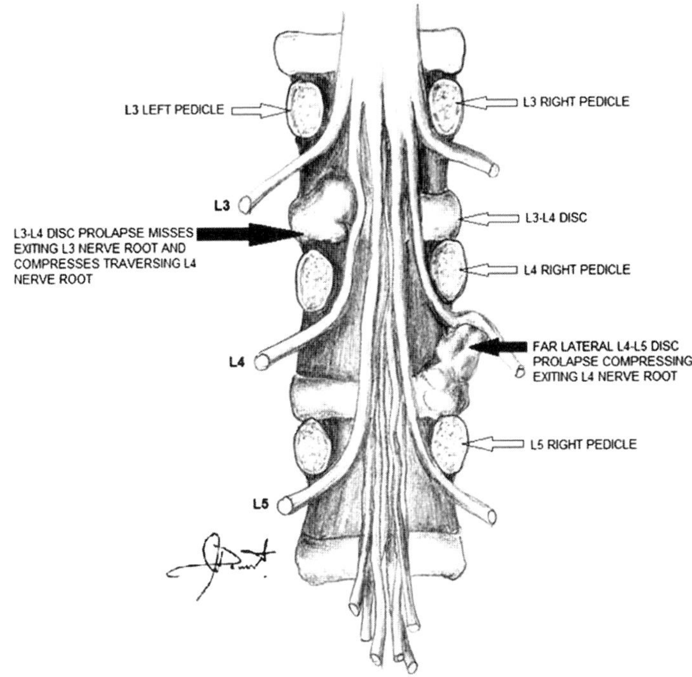

Fig. 47.3 Nerve roots affected by a prolapsed disc. Reproduced with permission from Juergen Kraemer, *Intervertebral Disk Diseases: Causes, Diagnosis, Treatment and Prophylaxis*. © Thieme, 2008.

Case 48

A 43-year-old woman has a 1-year history of right arm pain felt around the elbow and radiating into the thumb and index finger. It has settled a little but she has a continuous tingling feeling in the same region. There is no history of neck pain or trauma.

Questions

1. What is the differential diagnosis, and what features of the history or examination are key?
2. On closer assessment she confirms that the thumb and index finger, rather than the thumb and the lateral two and a half fingers, are affected. Spurling's sign is positive and you arrange an MRI. The T_2 sagittal images of the midline and to the right of the midline and the axial image of the C5/6 disc are shown in Fig. 48.1. Comment on the findings.
3. What are the options?
4. What are the surgical options?
5. What are the pros and cons of each?

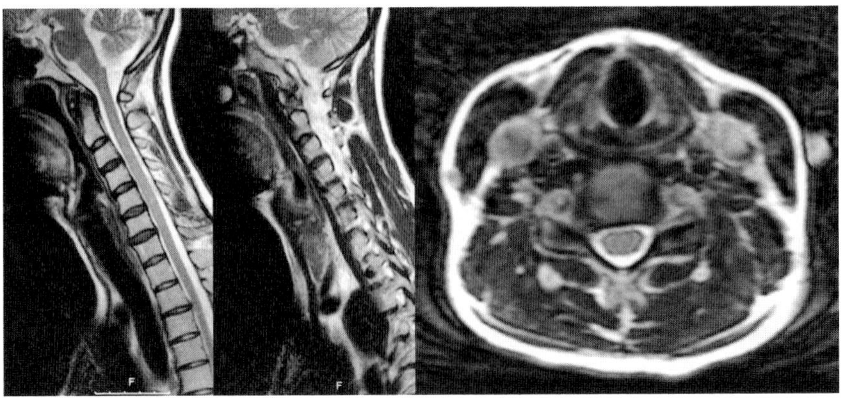

Fig. 48.1

Answers

1. What is the differential diagnosis, and what features of the history or examination are key?

The differential diagnosis is of neurological or musculoskeletal pain. The tingling in recent months suggests the symptoms to be more neurological in origin. The two most likely diagnoses are carpal tunnel syndrome, which may radiate proximally beyond the wrist to the elbow or the shoulder, and radiculopathy, classically C6 if the thumb and index finger are involved. Musculoskeletal causes of forearm pain should be considered and include lateral epicondylitis (tennis elbow) and tenosynovitis. These should be distinguished from neurological pain by point tenderness at the site of the inflammation exacerbated by passive movement of the associated tendons. Carpal tunnel syndrome classically responds to Tinel's test of tapping the median nerve in the carpal tunnel to provoke the symptoms, and Phalen's test of flexing the wrist in pronation for a short period to reproduce the symptoms. Cervical radicular pain can be reproduced by asking the patient to look up and turn their head to the contralateral side (Spurling's sign) to reduce the calibre of the affected nerve root exit foramen and reproduce symptoms.

2. On closer assessment she confirms that the thumb and index finger, rather than the thumb and the lateral two and a half fingers, are affected. Spurling's sign is positive and you arrange an MRI. The T_2 sagittal images of the midline and to the right of the midline and the axial image of the C5/6 disc are shown in Fig. 48.1. Comment on the findings.

There is loss of the normal cervical lordosis. This is very common in patients with acute and chronic cervical spine pathology. The discs appear healthy on the midline T_2 image and there is no loss of disc height or osteophyte formation of note. However, the sagittal image to the right of the midline shows some loss of CSF signal adjacent to the disc at the C5/6 level. The axial scans of the C5/6 level show the left C6 nerve root with CSF surrounding it, but there is narrowing of the foramen around the right C6 root due to lateral disc or osteophyte.

3. What are the options?

She does not have a progressive deficit and surgery should be offered if her pain is intractable or intolerable. A radiologically guided nerve root infiltration with steroids may be offered for temporary relief, or she could continue with appropriate oral analgesia.

4. What are the surgical options?

The aim of surgery should be to decompress the C6 nerve root in the C5/6 neural foramen. Therefore the options are an anterior cervical discectomy (ACD) or foraminotomy (a posterior approach to de-roof the right C6 neural foramen).

5. What are the pros and cons of each?

An ACD will remove the primary pathology (disc prolapse) and has higher success rates in alleviating the brachalgia (95%). Foraminotomy has slightly lower success rates (80%). However, an ACD has more significant potential morbidity from complications such as recurrent laryngeal nerve palsy and oesophageal, carotid injury, and neck wound haematoma.

ACD is preferred where there is a greater compressive component from anteriorly, where the nerve root may be 'bowstringed' over the disc/osteophyte and therefore still under tension if a posterior foraminotomy were performed.

The MRI shown in Fig. 48.2 is of a 55-year-old woman with a short history of neck pain, right shoulder and upper arm pain, and subsequent right arm weakness. There is a large C4/5 disc prolapse with probable compression of the C5 root and the lateral spinal cord at this level. This would be innappropriate for a foraminotomy as the neural compression is very marked and is exclusively from the front. She underwent an ACD and fusion with a cage and made a rapid and uneventful recovery.

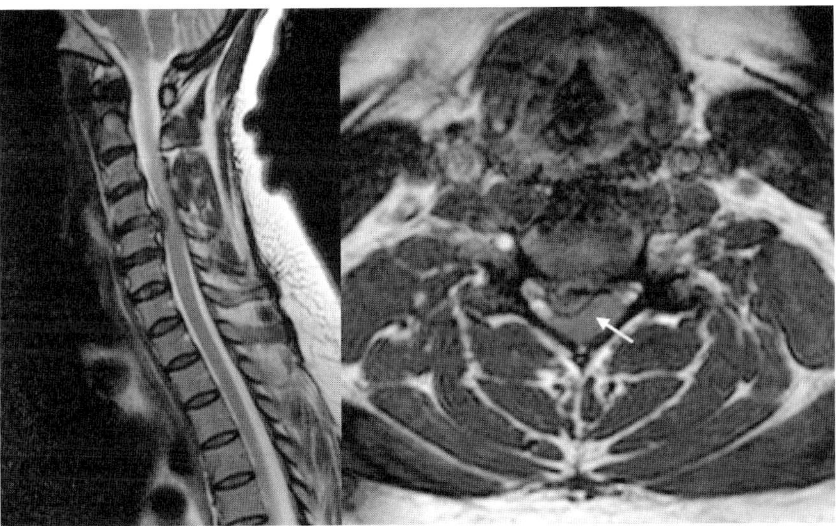

Fig. 48.2

Further reading

Heary RF, Ryken TC, Matz PG, *et al.* (2009). Joint Section on Disorders of the Spine and Peripheral Nerves of the American Association of Neurological Surgeons and Congress of Neurological Surgeons. Cervical laminoforaminotomy for the treatment of cervical degenerative radiculopathy. *J Neurosurg Spine*; **11**: 198–202.

Matz PG, Holly LT, Groff MW, *et al.* (2009). Joint Section on Disorders of the Spine and Peripheral Nerves of the American Association of Neurological Surgeons and Congress of Neurological Surgeons. Indications for anterior cervical decompression for the treatment of cervical degenerative radiculopathy. *J Neurosurg Spine*; **11**: 174–82.

Case 49

A 55-year-old woman has experienced left arm and neck pain for 18 months. Her usual pain radiates from the shoulder through the elbow into the thumb and index finger. However, a recent severe exacerbation involved the whole hand and lasted for 2 months. During that time she underwent an MRI and was referred for a surgical opinion.

On examination she describes slight sensory change in her left index finger but has no deficit in terms of power or deep tendon reflexes.

Questions

1. What is the differential diagnosis of her pain? Are there any provocative tests that might help in assessment?
2. The patient's MRI is shown in Fig. 49.1 (sagittal T_2, to the left of the midline, and axial T_2 through the C5/6 and the C6/7 discs). What are the findings and how do they fit with the history? What are the management options?

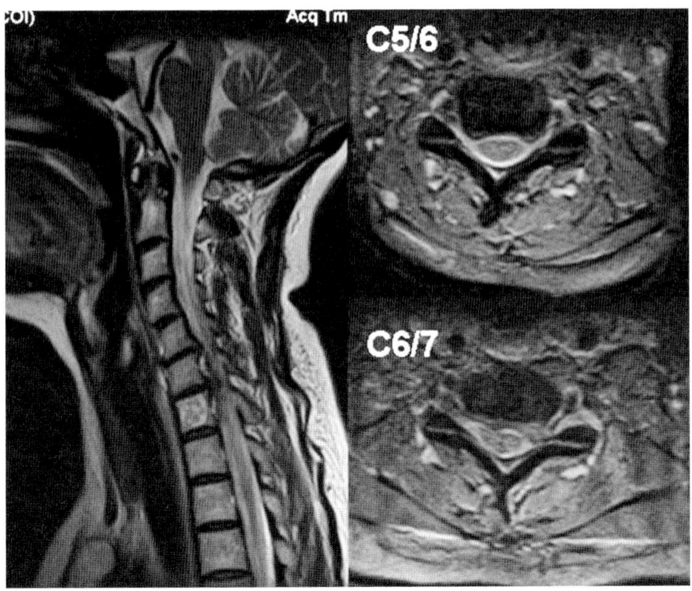

Fig. 49.1

Answers

1. What is the differential diagnosis of her pain? Are there any provocative tests that might help in assessment?

The differential diagnosis of lateral forearm pain includes a number of common conditions.

- Cervical radiculopathy: nerve root irritation in the exiting foramen of the spinal canal. This is usually due to a disc bulge or facet joint arthropathy and osteophyte formation. It may be reproduced by asking the patient to look up and to the side of the pain (Spurling's sign).
- Lateral epicondylitis (tennis elbow): inflammation of the common extensor origin at the head of the radius. Pressure over this area during passive supination/pronation is painful.
- Carpal tunnel syndrome: median nerve compression at the wrist. This typically involves the radial two and a half fingers and the thumb, but may often have forearm pain and easily be confused with C6 radiculopathy. Forced flexion of the wrist in pronation may reproduce the symptoms (Phalen's test) as may tapping on the volar surface of the wrist in mild extension (Tinel's test).

2. The patient's MRI is shown in Fig. 49.1 (sagittal T_2, to the left of the midline, and axial T_2 through the C5/6 and the C6/7 discs. What are the findings and how do they fit with the history? What are the management options?

There are two degenerate discs at C5/6 and C6/7 with posterior bulges on the sagittal images. On the axial images there is bilateral foraminal stenosis at C5/6, which is worse on the left, due to a low-signal bulge posterolaterally from the C5/6 disc. The C6/7 image also shows a posterolateral bulge, although it is higher signal than the level above. This suggests a higher water content and therefore may be a more recent disc prolapse than the radiologically less impressive protrusion above.

This is in keeping with her symptoms. She has a chronic (and hence fairly stable) entrapment of the left C6 root at C5/6, in keeping with the distribution of her chronic pain. Her recent exacerbation involving the whole hand was due to an acute disc prolapse at C6/7 which has settled down as most acute disc prolapses do.

Surgery for degenerative disease should be directed at the present symptoms rather than previous symptoms that have resolved, or to prevent future disease. The C6/7 level is asymptomatic currently and should be left alone. The bony stenosis at C5/6, as the cause of the ongoing symptoms, can be treated if the patient considers the risks acceptable. Nerve root decompression of the left C6 root in the C5/6 foramen will carry a high (>90%) chance of improving her pain if the correct level has been identified preoperatively. If uncertainty remains over the culprit level there are three options which might help this patient.

- Repeating the MRI as the symptoms have changed: if the C6/7 disc prolapse has improved radiologically the diagnosis is firm.

- Electrophysiology: EMG studies may show chronic C6 changes, but they are also likely to show C7 changes for some time after a period of compression and hence they may not move her diagnosis forward at all.
- CT-guided nerve root infiltration of steroid and local anaesthetic to the left C6 root in the C5/6 foramen. If this results in significant improvement (although temporary) in her pain syndrome, it is reasonable to hope for a qualitatively similar, but long-lasting, improvement as a result of decompressive surgery.

If surgical decompression is agreed on, there are two options: anterior cervical discectomy or posterior cervical foraminotomy.

Further reading

Kaiser MG (2006). Multilevel cervical spondylosis. *Neurosurg Clin N Am*; **17**: 263–75.

Rao RD, Currier BL, Albert TJ, *et al.* (2007). Degenerative cervical spondylosis: clinical syndromes, pathogenesis, and management *J Bone Joint Surg Am*; **89**: 1360–78.

Case 50

A 72-year-old man is referred by his GP. He is normally healthy with a 6-month progressive deterioration in mobility. He reports that his legs are strong and have normal sensation, but when he walks they feel heavy and become numb. He slows down after walking 300m and has to sit before continuing. He has no sphincter disturbance and no back pain.

Questions

1. What other features of the history are important?
2. What would you look for on examination?
3. There are no signs of vascular disease and the patient undergoes an MRI scan (Fig. 50.1). A sagittal T_2 and two axial T_2 scans are shown at the L4/5 level and the L3/4 level for comparison. What are the findings?
4. What are the treatment options? Are there any risks to consider?

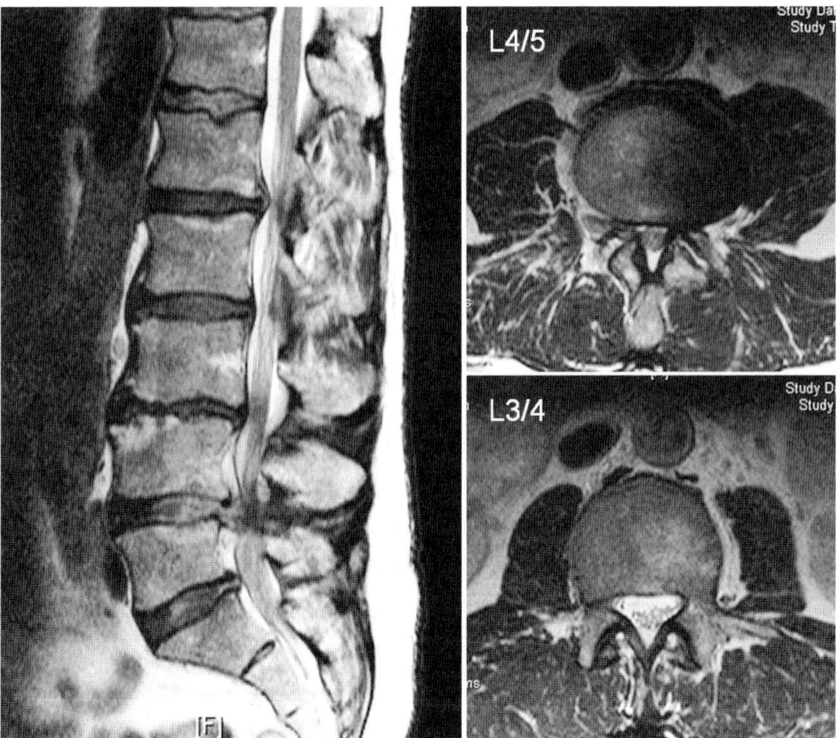

Fig. 50.1

Answers

1. What other features of the history are important?

The differential diagnosis is vascular or spinal claudication. Vascular claudication is exercise dependent, whereas spinal claudication is worse when lumbar lordosis is exaggerated by standing upright, causing buckling of the hypertrophic ligamentum flavum and nerve root compression. These aspects sometimes fit the history: vascular claudicants will still have symptoms when riding a bicycle, whereas spinal claudicants will not. Patients with lumbar stenosis may report being able to walk for longer if leaning forward for support (e.g. pushing a lawnmower or shopping trolley). They may also find walking uphill easier than walking downhill because of the difference in posture.

2. What would you look for on examination?

There are frequently no positive findings on physical examination in patients with spinal claudication. There may be dull lower limb reflexes, but these are usually intact. Peripheral foot pulses should be checked to rule out peripheral vascular disease.

3. There are no signs of vascular disease and the patient undergoes an MRI scan (Fig. 50.1). A sagittal T_2 and two axial T_2 scans are shown at the L4/5 level and the L3/4 level for comparison. What are the findings?

There is evidence of marked degenerative disease of the lumbar spine. There is narrowing of the spinal canal at the L4/5 level. On the axial scans the central part of the canal is patent but there is marked facet joint hypertrophy and hypertrophy of the ligamentum flavum, causing stenosis of the lateral recesses of the spinal canal.

4. What are the treatment options? Are there any risks to consider?

Symptoms usually worsen slowly in a predictable manner and surgery should be offered electively when the patient's symptoms become intolerable and oral analgesia is no longer sufficient. Surgery typically involves a laminectomy with undercutting of the hypertrophic facet joints, also known as lumbar decompression. The posterior midline elements are removed (spinous process, laminae, and underlying ligamentum flavum) and the anteromedial part of the facet joints that contacts the theca and compresses the nerve roots is removed to improve the dimensions of the spinal canal. Severe monoradiculopathy in a patient with spinal stenosis may be managed with analgesia and nerve root injections.

The risks of surgery include those of general anaesthesia for patients who are often elderly. Haemorrhage and infection are uncommon. The risk of dural tear is higher than in lumbar disc surgery as the canal is narrowed and the dura may be stuck to degenerate ligament. The risks of nerve root injury are also higher, although still small. The risks of iatrogenic cauda equina syndrome are very low, but would be severely disabling if it occurred.

An alternative option in patients whose symptoms are better in lumbar flexion is the surgical insertion of an interspinous spacer. These act at individual levels of the spine to wedge one or two segments of the lumbar spine in forward flexion, thus preventing extension and buckling of the hypertrophic ligamentum flavum responsible for stenotic symptoms. Efficacy can be limited and hence the procedure (which can be performed under local anaesthetic) is often reserved for medically unwell patients or those unwilling to accept the risks of laminectomy.

The preoperative MRI of a patient undergoing an X-stop interspinous implant insertion is shown in Fig. 50.2. This patient had a relatively capacious spinal canal when supine in the MRI scanner; the axial scans confirmed this but there was marked flaval hypertrophy, accounting for his very marked postural stenotic symptoms. Therefore he underwent X-stop placement at L4/5 (right) which resulted in improvement in his symptoms. They recurred after 5 months and he underwent laminectomy with lasting resolution of his leg pain.

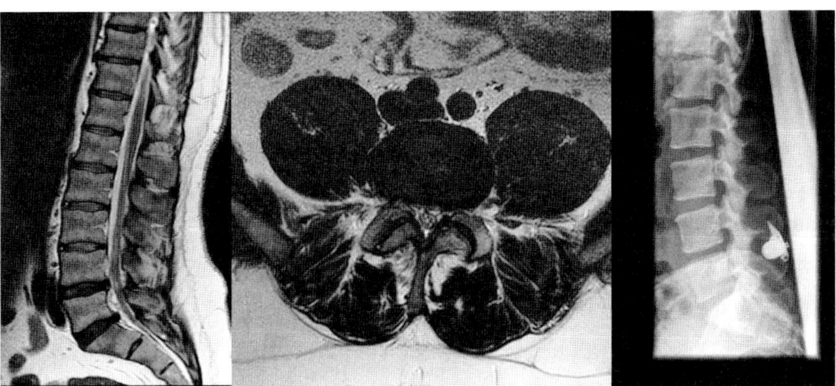

Fig. 50.2

Further reading

Barbagallo GM, Olindo G, Corbino L, Albanese V (2009). Analysis of complications in patients treated with the X-Stop Interspinous Process Decompression System: proposal for a novel anatomic scoring system for patient selection and review of the literature. *Neurosurgery*; **65**: 111–19.

Burnett MG, Stein SC, Bartels RH (2010). Cost-effectiveness of current treatment strategies for lumbar spinal stenosis: nonsurgical care, laminectomy, and X-STOP. *J Neurosurg Spine*; **13**: 39–46.

Orbai AM, Meyerhoff JO (2010). The effectiveness of tricyclic antidepressants on lumbar spinal stenosis. *Bull NYU Hosp Jt Dis*; **68**: 22–4.

Siebert E, Prüss H, Klingebiel R, Failli V, Einhäupl KM, Schwab JM (2009). Lumbar spinal stenosis: syndrome, diagnostics and treatment. *Nat Rev Neurol*; **5**: 392–403.

Disorders of micturition in neurosurgery

Continence is maintained by the balance of activity between the internal and external urethral sphincters and the detrusor muscle. Interruption to the nerve supply to these structures can affect continence. The innervation of the bladder consists of the following:

- Efferent
  - Sympathetics (T9–T12): relaxes detrusor, contracts internal sphincter, allows bladder filling
  - Parasympathetic (S2–S4): contracts detrusor, relaxes internal sphincter, empties bladder
  - Somatic (S2–S4; pudendal nerve): voluntary control of external urethral sphincter
- Afferent
  - Runs with all three fibres above
- Central
  - Fibres from the cerebral cortex, basal ganglia, and pontine micturition centre travel down the spinal cord in the medial and lateral reticulospinal tracts.

Normal micturition is initiated when the bladder wall is stretched. Activation of the visceral afferent pathways results in reflex contraction of the detrusor muscle (parasympathetic, promoting micturition) and the urge to void, mediated by afferent connections to higher centres. Continence is maintained by activation of the sacral somatic nerves (which activates the external urethral sphincter) and lumbar sympathetics (leading to contraction of the internal urethral sphincter and relaxation of detrusor).

Lesions in the spinal cord and above

A lesion in the spinal cord can interfere with the central control of micturition by interrupting the micturition pathway running from the pontine micturition centre to the sacral segments of the cord. This may result in detrusor instability, which results from disinhibition of the detrusor muscle and leads to urgency of micturition, urge incontinence, and low residual volume, or detrusor-sphincter dyssynergia, which results from involuntary detrusor contraction without relaxation of the external urethral sphincter and leads to urinary urgency with incomplete emptying of the bladder. Detrusor-sphincter dyssynergia is most often seen with spinal cord lesions, whereas detrusor hyper-reflexia can be seen in both spinal cord and cortical or basal ganglia pathology including cerebrovascular disease, normal pressure hydrocephalus, and frontal lobe tumours.

(continued)

Disorders of micturition in neurosurgery *(continued)*

Cauda equina syndrome

Classically there is painless urinary retention and overflow incontinence due to interruption of the parasympathetic and somatic pathways to the bladder. Absent bladder sensation (ask if the patient can feel a distended bladder, or the tug on a catheter) suggests impaired sacral outflow. Intact sensation does not exclude impaired sacral outflow as bladder afferents also travel with the sympathetic nerves. A bladder ultrasound may help in this situation. A full bladder with incontinence is consistent with cauda equina syndrome, whereas an empty bladder is not. However, various types of bladder dysfunction have been noted to occur in cauda equina syndrome, and there should be a low threshold for performing an MRI scan of the lumbar spine when the diagnosis is suspected. Note that acute back pain by itself can also cause urinary retention.

Case 51

A 55-year-old woman is referred by her GP with acute severe lumbar pain which had started 6 weeks previously whilst walking a friend's dog when it lurched suddenly. Her symptoms were settling but there had been an exacerbation a week prior to this consultation, and she feels that she is as bad as she was initially. She has an antalgic gait and sits awkwardly, is not overweight, and localizes the pain to her lower lumbar area.

Questions

1. What are 'red flag' symptoms?
2. She is keen to have an MRI scan. What do you advise?

Answers

1. What are 'red flag' symptoms?

'Red flag' symptoms are a set of symptoms that should alert the clinician to possible serious pathology underlying back pain. They must always be asked about in a back pain history (see Case 44 for a list of red flag symptoms). She has no red flag symptoms but is very anxious about her prognosis. She has undergone a lumbar spine X-ray which is normal.

2. She is keen to have an MRI scan. What do you advise?

The most recent NICE guidance (2009) recognizes that non-specific low back pain (i.e. without red flag symptoms) is not evaluated well with X-rays. MRI scanning is most unlikely to result in a change in her management, which should be non-surgical in the expectation that her symptoms will improve.

Questions

3. You advise her that an MRI is not appropriate. What will you suggest instead?
4. She returns 2 weeks later with an MRI scan that her GP arranged (Fig. 51.1). What does it show and what are the options for her management? She specifically asks about spinal fusion.

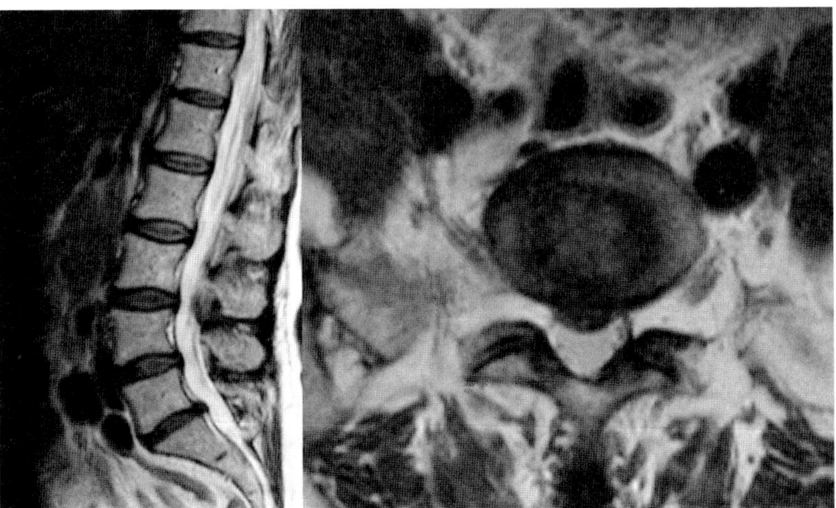

Fig. 51.1

Answers

3. You advise her that an MRI is not appropriate. What will you suggest instead?

She should be advised that she will get better with time and conservative treatment. There is good evidence to support exercise as a treatment for non-specific low back pain. She should take regular analgesia and be able to engage in structured exercise offered through physiotherapy. Non-weight-bearing exercise, particularly swimming or 'core stability' exercises including Pilates and yoga, may also be of value.

4. She returns 2 weeks later with an MRI scan that her GP arranged (Fig. 51.1). What does it show and what are the options for her management? She specifically asks about spinal fusion.

The MRI shows slight loss of height of the L5/S1 disc with a suggestion of a posterior disc prolapse. This is confirmed on the axial images through L5/S1 which shows a central disc herniation without neural compression (Fig. 51.2, arrow).

The options for her management should not change in view of this finding. The prolapsed disc is likely to settle with conservative treatment. A lumbar discectomy would carry a much lower chance of improving her back pain than the chance of improving leg pain in association with a disc prolapse.

Spinal fusion as a treatment for low back pain has variable degrees of evidence to support it. The largest trial of surgery versus structured therapy found a minimal difference between the two groups. Therefore fusion for unselected patients is of minimal benefit. Well-selected patients may benefit from fusion surgery for persistent 'discogenic back pain' and this may require a discogram (radiologically guided injection of contrast into the L5/S1 disc to try to reproduce the back pain). Lumbar disc replacement has been used as an alternative to fusion to treat low back pain. Currently, it is also supported by an equivocal evidence base, but clinical trials are ongoing.

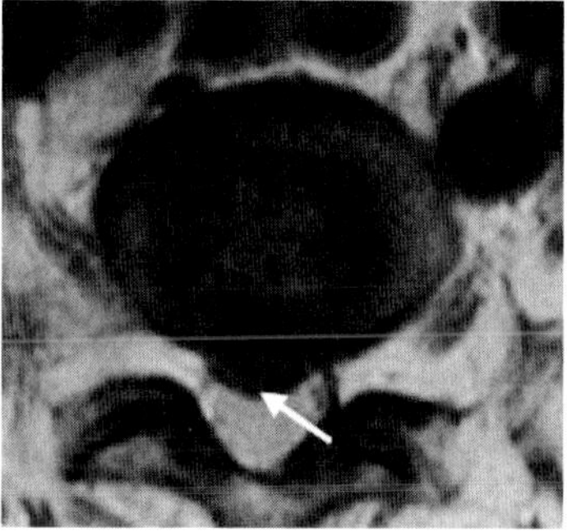

Fig. 51.2

Further reading

Fairbank J, Frost H, Wilson-MacDonald J, Yu LM, Barker K, Collins R (2005). Spine Stabilisation Trial Group. Randomised controlled trial to compare surgical stabilisation of the lumbar spine with an intensive rehabilitation programme for patients with chronic low back pain: the MRC spine stabilisation trial. *BMJ*; **330**: 1233.

Maher CG (2004). Effective physical treatment for chronic low back pain. *Orthop Clin North Am*; **35**: 57–64.

Mirza SK, Deyo RA (2007). Systematic review of randomized trials comparing lumbar fusion surgery to nonoperative care for treatment of chronic back pain. *Spine (Phila Pa 1976)*; **32**: 816–23.

NICE (2009). Low back pain. NICE Guideline CG88. Available online at: http://www.nice.org.uk/CG088 (accessed 13 March 2011).

van den Eerenbeemt KD, Ostelo RW, van Royen BJ, Peul WC, van Tulder MW (2010). Total disc replacement surgery for symptomatic degenerative lumbar disc disease: a systematic review of the literature. *Eur Spine J*; **19**: 1262–80.

Case 52

A 77-year-old woman is referred to the outpatient clinic with back pain for 3 years and recent pain radiating from her back through her hips into her legs and feet. The pain is intermittent and occurs when she walks or stands. Within 5 minutes of walking she will be unable to continue because of pain. She does not have any bowel or bladder disturbance. Her past medical history includes hypertension and osteoporosis. An MRI scan of the lumbar spine is performed.

Questions

1. The MRI is shown in Fig. 52.1. What does it show, and does it explain the symptoms?
2. Describe the Meyerding and Wiltse–Newman–MacNab classifications. How would this patient's disease be classified?
3. What is the management of this condition?

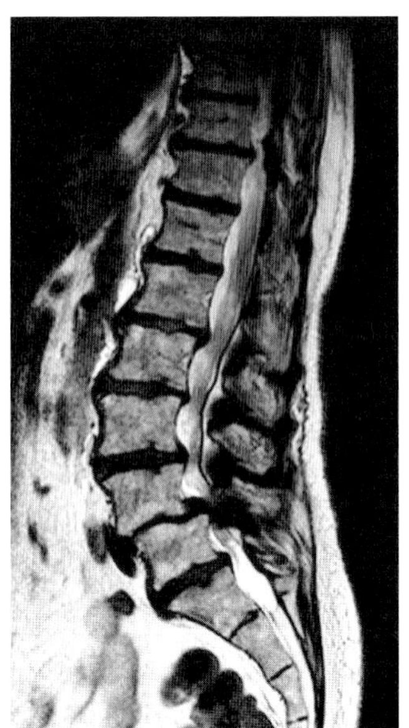

Fig. 52.1

Answers

1. The MRI is shown in Fig. 52.1. What does it show, and does it explain the symptoms?

There is spondylolisthesis: anterior displacement of L4 on the L5 vertebra. The L4/5 disc has lost height and protrudes posteriorly, and there is marked thickening of the ligamentum flavum at this level. Patients often present with back pain and neurogenic claudication from compression of the exiting nerve roots. Therefore symptoms are worse on walking or standing and are relieved by leaning forward, which increases the diameter of the spinal canal. A slip at the L4/5 level commonly affects the L5 nerve roots, which is consistent with this patient's symptoms (see 'Nerve roots affected by a prolapsed disc', p. 328). The resting neurological examination is

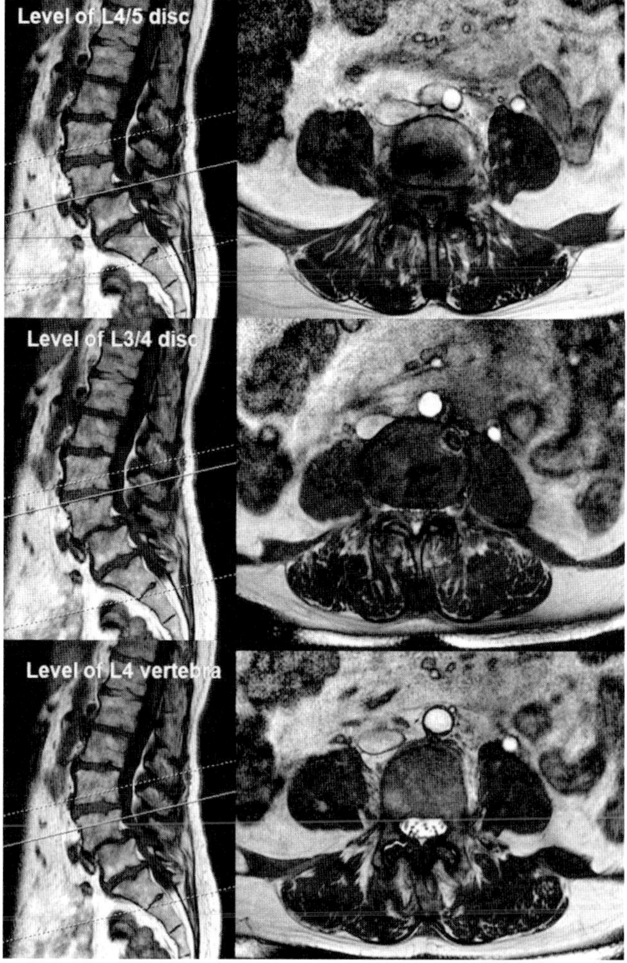

Fig. 52.2

often normal. Significant compression of the thecal sac may cause compression of the cauda equina. The axial view at the level of the slip (Fig. 52.2) shows obliteration of the spinal canal at this level, although the patient does not have symptoms of cauda equina syndrome. For comparison, an axial view at the disc space above (L3/4) and also at the level of the L4 vertebra is also shown, and demonstrates progressively more capacious space in the spinal canal (indicated by the white CSF).

2. Describe the Meyerding and Wiltse–Newman–MacNab classifications. How would this patient's disease be classified?

The Meyerding classification (Table 52.1) describes the amount of displacement at the level of the spondylolisthesis. The Wiltse–Newman–MacNab classification (Table 52.2) is an aetiological classification.

This patient's spondylolisthesis would be classified as a Meyerding grade 1, Wiltse–Newman–MacNab grade 3.

3. What is the management of this condition?

Management of spondylolisthesis is considered in operative or non-operative terms and depends on both the grade of spondylolisthesis and symptoms. Non-operative management consists of analgesia, muscle relaxants, and graded exercise. Surgery may be considered for persistent symptoms lasting over at least several weeks. The aims of surgery are to relieve pain and neurological deficit, and to prevent progression of the deformity. The approaches include posterior decompression alone or decompression with fusion/instrumentation. This patient underwent laminectomies at L3, L4, and L5 and pedicle screw stabilization with screw and rod fixation at L4/5, and experienced good improvement in her symptoms. The postoperative X-rays are shown in Fig. 52.3.

Table 52.1 Meyerding classification

Grade 1	Up to 25% displacement over vertebra below
Grade 2	Up to 50% displacement over vertebra below
Grade 3	Up to 75% displacement over vertebra below
Grade 4	Up to 100% displacement over vertebra below

Table 52.2 Wiltse–Newman–MacNab classification

Type 1	Dysplastic (congenital)
Type 2	Isthmic (pars articularis fracture)
Type 3	Degenerative
Type 4	Traumatic
Type 5	Pathological

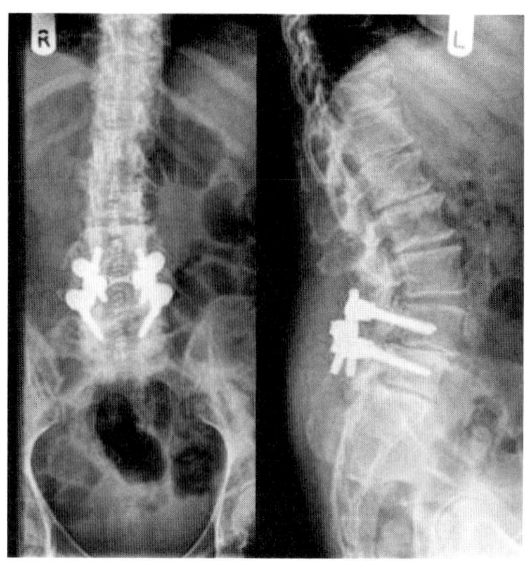

Fig. 52.3

Table 52.3 Myotomes for neurological examination

Movement	Nerve root	Muscle	Nerve
Upper limb			
Shoulder abduction	C5, C6	Deltoid	Axillary nerve
Elbow flexion (supinated)	C5, C6	Biceps	Musculocutaneous nerve
Elbow flexion (half pronated)	C5, C6	Brachioradialis	Radial
Elbow extension	C6, C7, C8	Triceps	Radial
Wrist flexion	C7		
Wrist extension	C7	Long extensors	Radial
Finger flexion	C8	Flexor digitorum profundus (FDP)	Median (FDP 1–3) Ulnar (FDP 3 & 4)
Finger abduction	T1	Abductor digiti minimi	Ulnar
Lower limb			
Hip flexion	L1, L2	Iliopsoas	Femoral
Knee extension	L3, L4	Quadriceps	Femoral
Dorsiflexion	L4	Tibialis anterior	Deep peroneal nerve

(continued)

Table 52.3 *(continued)* Myotomes for neurological examination

Movement	Nerve root	Muscle	Nerve
Big toe extension	L5	Extensor hallucis longus (EHL)	Deep peroneal nerve
Plantar flexion	S1, S2	Gastrocnemius, soleus	Tibial nerve
Knee flexion	L5, S1, S2	Hamstrings	Sciatic nerve
Hip extension	L5, S1, S2	Gluteus maximus	Inferior gluteal nerve
Hip adduction	L2, L3	Adductors	Obturator nerve
Inversion	L4, L5	Tibialis posterior	Tibial nerve
Eversion	L5, S1	Peroneus longus and brevis	Superficial peroneal nerve*

* Eversion will be weak in common peroneal nerve palsy, *but* other L5 innervated muscle groups will be strong (EHL, inversion). In L5 lesion, all L5 associated movements will be weak including ankle eversion.

Section 6

Paediatric neurosurgery and hydrocephalus

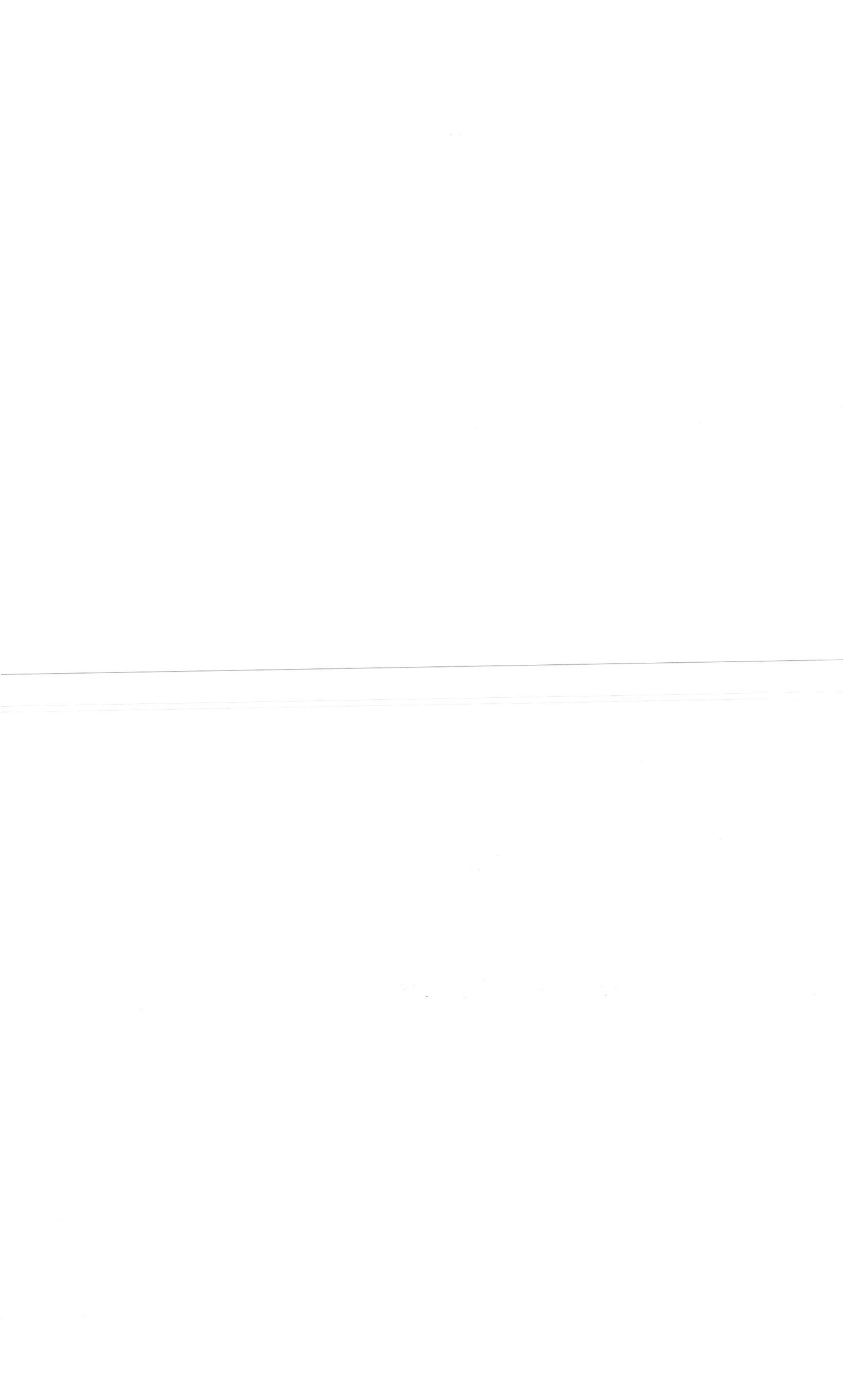

Case 53

A 72-year-old man was referred by the neurologists with a 2-year history of progressive difficulty with mobility. He was previously very active and enjoyed long walks outdoors, but these have been curtailed recently because of a number of falls. On even ground he finds he has slowed and on uneven ground he frequently trips. His wife has become somewhat frustrated with his deterioration. In addition he is reported by his family as being 'less sharp' than he used to be and he is no longer able to complete crosswords. They also say he has become forgetful at times. His GP referred him to a neurologist where an MRI scan of the brain was performed (Fig. 53.1) and he has been referred for a neurosurgical opinion.

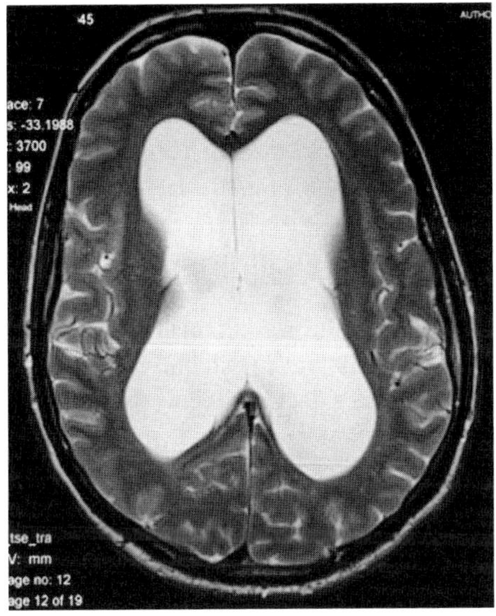

Fig. 53.1

Questions

1. What does the MRI show, and what is the differential diagnosis? Are there any other features of the history that are relevant?
2. How would you proceed?
3. If shunting is indicated, what kind of shunt would you place, and why?

Answers

1. What does the MRI show, and what is the differential diagnosis? Are there any other features of the history that are relevant?

The MRI scan shows marked ventricular enlargement. There is no signal change around the ventricles: therefore this is a chronic process of ventricular enlargement. The lower slices of the scan should be reviewed to ensure there is no mass lesion or other reason for the hydrocephalus (there is not) (see 'CSF circulation and hydrocephalus', p. 360).

The differential diagnosis clinically includes spinal disease to explain the gait disturbance, although this would not account for the memory disturbance. In the light of the imaging, the diagnosis is either cerebral atrophy and a chronic progressive dementia, or chronic hydrocephalus of unknown aetiology, so-called normal-pressure hydrocephalus (NPH). Ventricular dilation without raised CSF pressure remains a poorly understood phenomenon. Current explanations suggest a failure of CSF absorption, either at the level of the arachnoid granulations or due to poor CSF flow through the subarachnoid space. Laplace's law states that the wall tension of a hollow object such as a balloon, or in this case the ventricles, is inversely related to the size of the object. Therefore the larger ventricles are less able to resist small increases in CSF pressure, perhaps even those occurring under normal physiological conditions.

Normal-pressure hydrocephalus was originally described by Hakim. The classical symptoms are known as Hakim's triad and consist of dementia, ataxia, and incontinence. The incontinence does not follow the pattern of spinal cord lesions (painless retention and overflow); rather, it is the apparently normal passage of urine in response to a full bladder, but without the patient being aware or particularly concerned by it. It is best thought of as part of the cognitive decline rather than a separate entity. In elderly patients it may be confused with urgency or gait problems preventing them getting to the toilet in time.

2. How would you proceed?

The principal differential diagnosis (assuming cervical myelopathy is clinically or radiologically eliminated) is a degenerative neurological condition causing dementia, which is essentially not treatable. It is difficult to distinguish patients with true NPH who may benefit from CSF diversion from those with dementia and cerebral atrophy causing dilation of the ventricles which expand to fill the space left by the shrinking brain (hydrocephalus *ex vacuo*). There is an argument to be made for offering CSF diversion (i.e. VP shunting) to all such patients on the grounds that it is the only option available to make the patient any better. However, there are reasons not to shunt all such patients; these include both the intraoperative risk and the risks associated with shunting in patients with very large ventricles, such as intracerebral and subdural haematomas. In addition, shunting a patient who subsequently fails to improve will inevitably raise concerns over blockage of the shunt, either postoperatively or in the future when their condition progresses, and may result in multiple shunt explorations.

Therefore it is desirable to offer the patient and their family some evidence to support the diagnosis. Measurement of CSF pressure by ICP monitoring or LP can occasionally be helpful if there are B-waves (an ICP pressure >20mm Hg for >5 minutes). However, the baseline pressure is usually normal and an absence of B-waves does not exclude the diagnosis. A valuable alternative is to perform therapeutic CSF drainage, temporarily mimicking the actions of a shunt, during which time the patient can be assessed for improvement. This is optimally done with a formal physiotherapy and psychological assessment as a baseline, followed by CSF drainage either by LP to drain around 40mL CSF or by insertion of a lumbar drain to continuously drain CSF for 24–48 hours. During the post-drainage period the patient should be monitored for improvement, preferably by full physiotherapy and psychological reassessment. An objective improvement strengthens the mandate for shunting; no improvement allows the surgical team to be more circumspect about the diagnosis.

This man's timed 10m walk improved from 29 to 24 seconds following LP. His Mental State Examination was 25/30 before and improved to 28/30 after. Therefore he proceeded with VP shunt insertion.

3. If shunting is indicated, what kind of shunt would you place, and why?

One of the greatest concerns in shunting any patient with very large ventricles is that overdrainage of CSF may produce subdural collections and haematomas. This is often a concern with normal pressure hydrocephalus.

The CSF pressure in a patient with a VP shunt is regulated by the valve. High-pressure valves only open when the CSF pressure is high; low-pressure valves open when the CSF pressure is high or normal, and only close at low pressure. Patients with NPH will ultimately need CSF to be drained at low pressure; however, doing so immediately with a shunt carries a high risk of subdural haematoma. The accepted solution, although it has yet to be supported by good evidence, is to place a variable-pressure valve in the shunt. This can be adjusted externally using a magnetic programmer through the skin, without the need to operate on the shunt or anaesthetize the patient. The usual practice is to place the shunt at a higher setting of the valve, and then to lower the pressure setting of the valve sequentially over the next few weeks. The theory is to allow the brain to expand gradually, rather than collapsing it quickly and encouraging subdural collections. A variety of programmable shunt valves are available commercially. However, they can be reset by very strong magnetic fields, and patients should have their shunt setting confirmed before and after any MRI scans they undergo.

This patient underwent placement of a right occipital VP shunt with a programmable valve. The pressure setting was lowered on day 3 postoperatively prior to discharge, at 3 months, and finally at 6 months in clinic. He and his family reported a gradual improvement in his walking and his cognitive decline stabilized, although it did not improve.

Further reading

Ringel F, Schramm J, Meyer B (2005). Comparison of programmable shunt valves vs standard valves for communicating hydrocephalus of adults: a retrospective analysis of 407 patients. *Surg Neurol*; **63**: 36–41.

Shprecher D, Schwalb J, Kurlan R (2008). Normal pressure hydrocephalus: diagnosis and treatment. *Curr Neurol Neurosci Rep*; **8**: 371–6.

Wallenstein MB, McKhann GM 2nd (2010). Salomón Hakim and the discovery of normal-pressure hydrocephalus. *Neurosurgery*; **67**: 155–9.

CSF circulation and hydrocephalus

Cotungo is credited for the discovery of cerebrospinal fluid and Dandy for the experimental verification of its circulation. The ventricular system consists of the two paired lateral ventricles, which communicate with the third ventricle through the foramina of Monro, from which CSF passes via the aqueduct of Sylvius to the fourth ventricle. The fourth ventricle communicates with the cranial and spinal subarachonid space via the foramen of Magendie and the paired foramina of Luschka (Fig. 53.2). Most (70%) of the CSF is secreted by choroid plexus but some is derived from capillary ultrafiltrate and metabolic water production. Secretion of CSF is an energy-dependent process requiring the Na^+/K^+-ATP (sodium–potassium adenosine triphosphate) pump with sodium being secreted into the subarachnoid space and water following it. The rate of CSF production is approximately 450mL/day and the total volume is around 150mL with one-sixth (25mL) in the ventricular system (the remainder is in the spinal canal and the subarachnoid space). The choroid plexus consists of a single layer of cuboidal epithelial cells surrounding blood capillaries. It is found in the floor, body, and roof of the temporal horns of the lateral ventricles, the roof of the third ventricle, and within the fourth ventricle. CSF is absorbed from arachnoid granulations in the superior sagittal sinus. These operate as a pressure-dependent valve, transmitting CSF when the ICP is higher than the venous pressure. Some CSF is also absorbed by veins. The rate of CSF absorption largely regulates CSF pressure as production remains relatively constant. CSF production is decreased by carbonic anhydrase inhibitors (acetazolamide) and noradrenaline and increased by CO_2 and volatile anaesthetics. It is also controlled by the raphe nuclei.

Hydrocephalus results from an imbalance between production and absorption of CSF, resulting in increased CSF volume and pressure. It must be distinguished from ventriculomegaly (i.e. dilated ventricles with low or normal CSF pressure) which occurs in cerebral atrophy and NPH, amongst other conditions. Acute hydrocephalus may be characterized by an area of periventricular 'lucency' which refers to an area of low density on a CT scan, typically at the tips of the frontal horns of the lateral ventricles. This represents CSF egress into the adjacent white matter and indicates high intraventricular pressure. Acute hydrocephalus is a

(continued)

CSF circulation and hydrocephalus *(continued)*

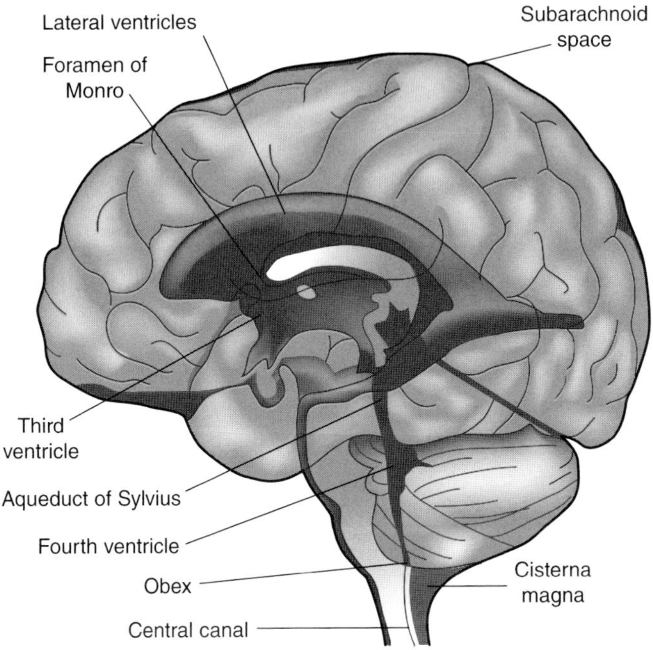

Fig. 53.2 The ventricular system. Reproduced from Samandouras G, (2010). *The Neurosurgeon's Handbook*. © Oxford University Press.

neurosurgical emergency which, if left untreated, can rapidly lead to brain herniation and death. Infants can tolerate an increase in CSF volume more than adults because of the non-union of cranial sutures. Therefore the head enlarges, and macrocephaly is a common presentation of hydrocephalus in infants. Hydrocephalus can be classified as obstructive or communicating; the former results from obstruction of CSF flow within the ventricular system and the latter from obstruction at the arachnoid villi. In obstructive hydrocephalus the ventricles proximal to the obstruction will be dilated, whereas those distal will be relatively small.

Case 54

A 6-week-old baby boy was referred by the paediatricians. A health visitor alerted the GP as the child's head circumference was raised on two successive measurements and she was concerned. The child was born by a normal vaginal delivery. The pregnancy was uneventful; the mother had already had two older children with no medical problems. Both the 12- and 20-week ultrasound scans were normal. Since birth the baby had been feeding well and not crying unduly. He has not had other symptoms such as fevers or unusual patterns of vomiting.

Questions

1. How should a baby be examined neurologically?
2. What is the differential diagnosis of an enlarged head in a baby? What additional findings would you look for on examination?
3. The baby undergoes a CT scan (Fig. 54.1). What is the diagnosis? Does the sagittal reformat of the scan (Fig. 54.2) make the diagnosis any clearer?
4. What are the treatment options? What would you have done if the diagnosis of hydrocephalus had been made antenatally?

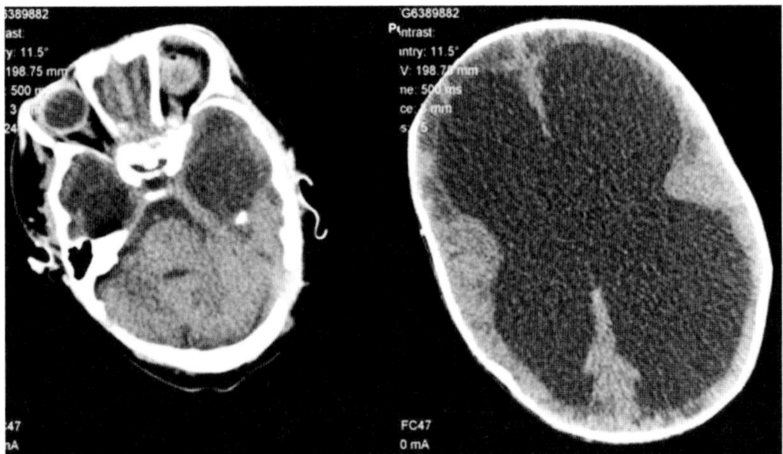

Fig. 54.1

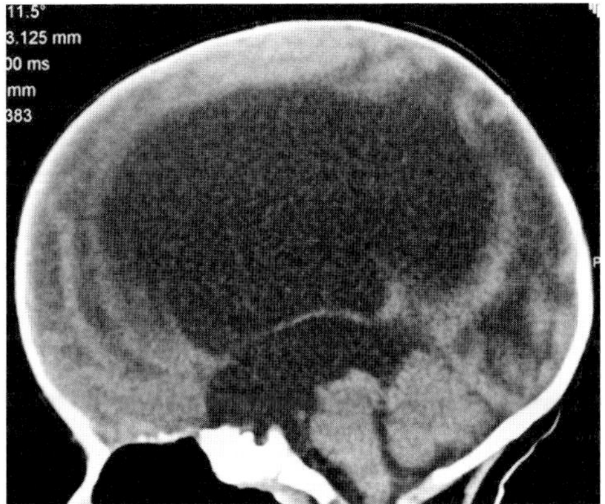

Fig. 54.2

Answers

1. How should a baby be examined neurologically?

The general conscious state should be noted by observing whether the baby is alert and interacting normally, miserable, or drowsy. The pupils and gaze should be assessed; impaired upward gaze (sunsetting) may signal raised intracranial pressure. The fontanelle should be palpated; a bulging fontanelle is consistent with a high ICP, and a sunken one is not. The head circumference should be measured, and the tone and movements of the limbs noted, as should the observation chart (temperature, pulse, blood pressure).

On examination the baby was alert. The anterior fontanelle was tense and bulging. His head circumference was 44.2cm (well above the 95th centile). It was 38cm at birth (around the 90th centile).

2. What is the differential diagnosis of an enlarged head in a baby? What additional findings would you look for on examination?

Macrocephaly is not always pathological. Some children have a large head with normal-sized ventricles and no underlying cause. This is often familial. Pathological enlargement of the head is most commonly due to hydrocephalus, either obstructive (e.g. tumour, aqueduct stenosis) or communicating (e.g. perinatal haemorrhage, meningitis). Macrocephaly without hydrocephalus is less common and may be due to a large space-occupying lesion—occasionally an astrocytoma or large tumour, a large arachnoid cyst, or a chronic subdural haematoma. Increased volume of brain tissue may enlarge the head as seen in a number of the neurocutaneous syndromes, most commonly neurofibromatosis. Venous hypertension due to a large arteriovenous malformation may cause macrocephaly. In addition, there are a number of metabolic causes including the endocrinopathies of hypoparathyroidism and adrenal insufficiency.

Only a few of these are capable of causing the head circumference to cross the centiles quite as spectacularly as in this child. In this case hydrocephalus is the most likely diagnosis. The associated features of raised CSF pressure, apart from the bulging fontanelle, are distended scalp veins. If the child is fixating normally (which begins around 6 weeks post gestation) it may be possible to elicit a loss of upgaze—the inability to look above the horizontal plane (Parinaud's syndrome). This is strongly suggestive of ventricular dilation causing stretching of the tectal plate.

3. The baby undergoes a CT scan (Fig. 54.1). What is the diagnosis? Does the sagittal reformat of the scan (Fig. 54.2) make the diagnosis any clearer?

There is massive dilation of the lateral ventricles. However, the fourth ventricle is small. Therefore this is a non-communicating hydrocephalus with an obstruction either in the third ventricle or between the third and fourth ventricles. Obstruction in the third ventricle would most commonly be a tumour. Obstruction between the third and fourth ventricles could again be a tumour in the pineal region or aqueduct stenosis.

The reformatted CT clearly shows the enlarged third and the small fourth ventricle. The pineal region is seen clearly and appears normal. The cerebral aqueduct is not seen clearly at all, and therefore the diagnosis is aqueduct stenosis.

4. What are the treatment options? What would you have done if the diagnosis of hydrocephalus had been made antenatally?

The child needs CSF diversion on a fairly urgent basis (within a few days). If there is any doubt about the underlying cause of the hydrocephalus, an MRI might be performed which would give a better appreciation of the anatomy of the cerebral aqueduct but is unlikely to change the management.

The two forms of permanent CSF diversion are a VP shunt or endoscopic third ventriculostomy (ETV). Shunting is the default option for both communicating and non-communicating hydrocephalus as it allows CSF to be absorbed outside the CNS. ETV requires functioning CSF absorption pathways and a patent subarachnoid space as it creates a direct pathway from the third ventricle to the basal cisterns and subarachnoid space; however, it is only likely to be successful in patients with non-communicating hydrocephalus. Where possible, ETV is considered superior to shunting as it allows physiological CSF absorption and problems of siphoning causing overdrainage are avoided. The risk of acute blockage is lower with a third ventriculostomy than with a shunt.

Aqueduct stenosis is the form of non-communicating hydrocephalus most amenable to ETV as CSF composition is entirely normal (unlike post-haemorrhagic or post-meningitic hydrocephalus) and the bar to CSF absorption is anatomical, which is bypassed by the creation of the hole (stoma) in the floor of the third ventricle. As such, success rates are high (>90%) in adults with aqueduct stenosis. However, success rates are far lower in babies for reasons that may include underdevelopment of the subarachnoid space because of a lack of CSF pressure during gestational CNS development. Some neurosurgeons would place a shunt with the plan that if and when the shunt first blocks, the child should undergo an ETV to try to make them shunt-independent.

This boy was treated with a VP shunt using a low-pressure valve. He was discharged with a sunken fontanelle and stable head circumference. Over the next 3 months his head circumference returned to the 90th centile where it remained. After 3 years his shunt had not blocked and therefore he has not undergone ETV.

Fetal anomaly scanning at 20 weeks gestation incorporates detailed assessment of development of the brain and spine, as well as the ventricular system. Abnormalities found may point to an increased risk of a certain condition, such as trisomy 21 (Down's syndrome) or may be diagnostic, as in the case of spina bifida and hydrocephalus.

It is very hard to come to terms with neurological disability of a child. The parents will need careful counselling. Most structural abnormalities of the fetal brain can be further imaged with MRI which should be performed in a specialist centre. Fig. 54.3 shows an MRI scan of a twin pregnancy with the uppermost baby showing marked ventricular dilation. The findings should be interpreted and discussed with the parents by a paediatric neurologist or neurosurgeon. The mode of delivery of the baby requires consideration, informed by further ultrasound scans later in the pregnancy which will document the degree of ventricular dilation. Knowledge of hydrocephalus is limited in the general population, and the parents should be advised of the probable need for surgical treatment at some point in the first few weeks of life. Regardless of aetiology, endoscopic ventriculostomy has a low success rate in neonates and therefore the hydrocephalus will require a shunt.

Parents may also wish to consider termination of the pregnancy. If so, they will want to know about the risk to future pregnancies of the same condition. This is dependent on the aetiology of the hydrocephalus, but as this may be hard to establish, particularly after a termination, advising the parents will be difficult in this area. Nearly all cases of congenital hydrocephalus that can be detected antenatally are sporadic and, whilst it is usual to test the mother for various conditions, including infections, that may have been implicated, these effects are unlikely to be realized a second time. The aetiology of the hydrocephalus and hence the neurological prognosis for the baby may be informed by either amniocentesis or chorionic villous sampling.

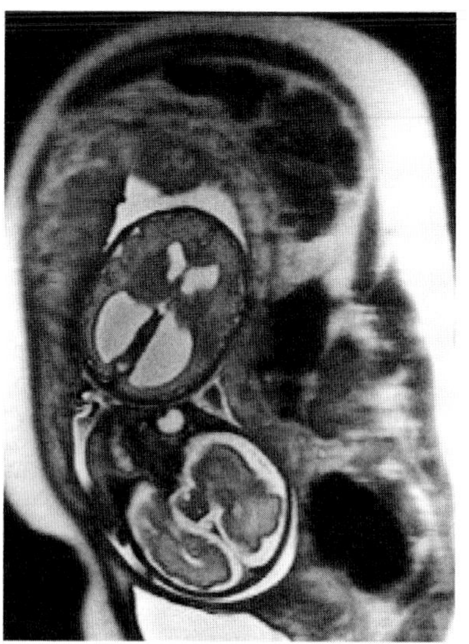

Fig. 54.3

Further reading

Kadrian D, van Gelder J, Florida D, *et al.* (2005). Long-term reliability of endoscopic third ventriculostomy. *Neurosurgery*; **56**: 1271–8.

Kulkarni AV, Drake JM, Kestle JR, *et al.* (2010). Predicting who will benefit from endoscopic third ventriculostomy compared with shunt insertion in childhood hydrocephalus using the ETV Success Score. *J Neurosurg Pediatr*; **6**: 310–15.

Lingman G (2005). Management of pregnancy and labour in cases diagnosed with major fetal malformation. *Curr Opin Obstet Gynecol*; **17**: 143–6.

Ogiwara H, Dipatri AJ Jr, Alden TD, Bowman RM, Tomita T (2010). Endoscopic third ventriculostomy for obstructive hydrocephalus in children younger than 6 months of age. *Childs Nerv Syst*; **26**: 343–7.

Peruzzi P, Corbitt RJ, Raffel C (2010). Magnetic resonance imaging versus ultrasonography for the in utero evaluation of central nervous system anomalies. *J Neurosurg Pediatr*; **6**: 40–5.

Case 55

A 32-year-old woman is referred to the outpatient clinic. She is 36 weeks pregnant with a baby who has been diagnosed with spina bifida. A myelomeningocoele is present at L4/5. There is an associated Chiari malformation and hydrocephalus.

Questions

1. How should this patient be counselled? Why do Chiari malformations and hydrocephalus occur with myelomeningocoeles? What other abnormalities are associated with this condition?
2. The baby is delivered by Caesarean section. It was noted to have a small head but the anterior fontanelle was normal. There was good tone in the limbs, and the arms, hips, and knees were moving. Fig. 55.1 shows the myelomeningocoele. How should the baby be nursed and what should be done with the defect pending surgery?
3. The myelomeningocoele is closed the day after birth. What postoperative precautions are necessary?
4. The mother asks what the risks are for her subsequent pregnancies to be affected. How would you reply?
5. Two years later, the infant is referred to the outpatient clinic with increasing unsteadiness. What is the differential diagnosis?

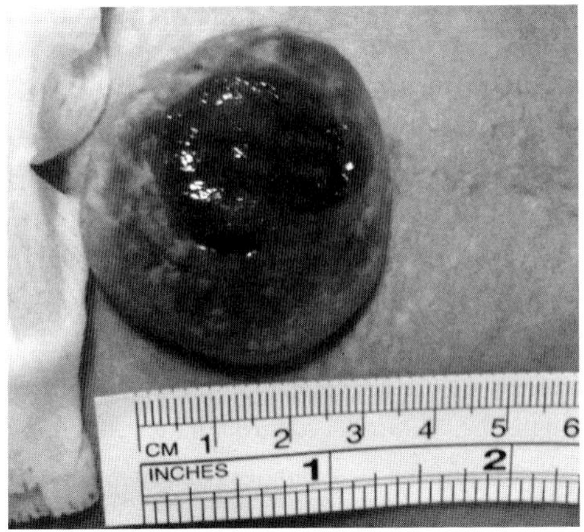

Fig. 55.1

Answers

1. How should this patient be counselled? Why does the Chiari malformation and hydrocephalus occur with myelomeningocoele? What other abnormalities are associated with this condition?

The mother should be aware of the implications of the diagnosis and the perinatal issues, and the immediate and longer-term consequences for the child should be reviewed. The issues include the following.

- The method of birth—a Caesarean section may reduce the risk of infection (and therefore meningitis) being introduced through the defect during a vaginal delivery.
- The uncertain nature of the neurological deficit, which could potentially be severe.
- The need for early surgery (usually within 48 hours of birth) to close the defect, the aim of which is to prevent meningitis and preserve neural function. It will not reverse the deficits that the baby already has.
- Complications of the operation, including wound breakdown, CSF leak, meningitis, and dermoid inclusion tumours.
- The need to monitor the progression of hydrocephalus in the postnatal period and the potential need for CSF diversion (most commonly a VP shunt).
- The potential for neurological, orthopaedic, and cognitive problems later in life due to tethered cord, hydrocephalus, and shunt problems. In addition, the Chiari malformation may lead to brainstem compression and syringomyelia.
- The availability of a multidisciplinary service to provide a complete package of care for the physical and social development of the child.

The myelomeningocoele results from a failure of the neural tube to close in the third week of embryonic life. This results in defective formation of the cranial vesicles, leading to a small posterior fossa. The fetal cerebellum and brainstem grow into a diminished space, causing their downward displacement through the foramen magnum. Hydrocephalus arises as a direct consequence of this because of obstruction of CSF outflow from the posterior fossa. Myelomeningocoeles are associated with numerous other developmental abnormalities including abnormal gyri, agenesis of the corpus callosum, cerebellar dysplasia, and abnormal anatomy of the ventricular system and brainstem.

2. The baby is delivered by Caesarean section. It was noted to have a small head but the anterior fontanelle was normal. There was good tone in the limbs, and the arms, hips, and knees were moving. Fig. 55.1 shows the myelomeningocoele. How should the baby be nursed and what should be done with the defect pending surgery?

The baby should be nursed on its front or side. A sterile moist dressing should be used to keep the defect covered.

3. The myelomeningocoele is closed the day after birth. What postoperative precautions are necessary?

The wound must be inspected to check the integrity of the closure and for signs of CSF leak. The development of hydrocephalus must be monitored by serial head circumference measurements or cranial ultrasound. This baby had progressive hydrocephalus and underwent a VP shunt.

4. The mother asks what the risks are for her subsequent pregnancies to be affected. How would you reply?

There is a genetic component to the disease, with an approximately 10% risk of an offspring having the condition if either parent or a sibling is affected. The use of folic acid in the prenatal and antenatal period has been shown to reduce the incidence of spina bifida.

5. Two years later, the infant is referred to the outpatient clinic with increasing unsteadiness. What is the differential diagnosis?

The possibilities include shunt malfunction, tethered cord, Chiari malformation, hydromyelia, and syringomyelia. In practice, shunt dysfunction is probably the most common cause of neurological deterioration in this population. This should be evaluated, following which full craniospinal imaging is required to exclude the other differential diagnoses.

Further reading

Stapleton S (2004). Spinal dysraphism. In: Moore AJ, Newell DW (eds), *Neurosurgery*. London: Springer.

Case 56

A 20-year-old woman is referred by the orthopaedic surgeons. She has been complaining of rather indistinct bilateral leg pains, a little worse on the right side. These have been present for about 2 years and have been tolerable, but more recently she has found that the right lower leg pain has subsided and she has had some difficulty, particularly with the right foot, when walking and running. Her medical history is relevant only for removal of a fatty lump from her lower back as a child, which was performed abroad. Since childhood she has never developed proper bladder control and voids using intermittent self-catheterization.

Examination finds absent ankle jerks bilaterally. The right foot is arched more than the left and there is some contracture of the calf, holding it in slight plantarflexion.

Questions

1. What is the differential diagnosis?
2. An MRI is done (sagittal and axial T_2) (Fig. 56.1). What is shown (A–C)? What is the likely cause of her symptoms? What would you advise her?

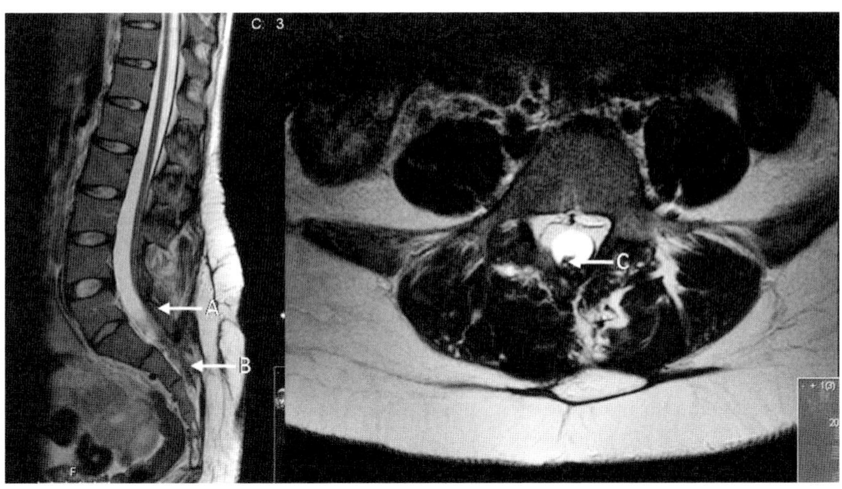

Fig. 56.1

Answers

1. What is the differential diagnosis?

The bilateral leg pain may be caused by a number of pathologies including peripheral neuropathy, sciatica, and hip or knee disease. However, the pes cavus suggests a slow denervation of the muscles maintaining the foot arch. The urinary symptoms are very important and would be likely to have been investigated in the past.

The combination of symptoms suggests a lesion affecting the cauda equina which has been present for many years (hence the failure to develop normal bladder control) with recent progression. The fatty lump she may know little about is a clue to a likely underlying spinal dysraphism.

Spinal dysraphism is a spectrum of conditions. Some are very severe, such as the open myelomeningocoele seen antenatally, requiring closure after birth, with a high incidence of associated severe neurological deficits. At the other end of the scale are truly occult spina bifida defects which are asymptomatic throughout life and only detected incidentally on imaging or clinical examination. The underlying problem is a failure of formation of the posterior aspects of the neural arch. These structures are the spinal cord, arachnoid, dura, fat, bone, and skin. In open myleomeningoceole, there is neural tissue on view with CSF leaking from it at birth. The milder versions are typically covered with skin, may have a hairy patch or dimple in association, and have defects of the bone underneath. A lipoma may be present under the skin and running down and mixed in with the nerve roots.

2. An MRI is done (sagittal and axial T_2) (Fig. 56.1). What is shown (A–C)? What is the likely cause of her symptoms? What would you advise her?

The vertebral bodies and discs are normal and well aligned, and the spinal canal is of normal calibre. However, the spinal cord does not end normally at L1/2; rather, it continues and its termination is indistinct but related to an area with overlying scar and a defect in the lumbar fascia (A). The bony elements do not form normally and there is a suggestion that the spinal subarachnoid space communicates with the subcutaneuous fat opposite the S2 segment (B). The axial image confirms the low-lying spinal cord lying dorsally in the thecal sac and related to the soft tissues overlying it (C). There is agenesis of the laminae bilaterally here and the facet joints are also abnormal.

This is a spinal dysraphic defect with a low-lying cord. In combination with the clinical features of progressive leg symptoms the diagnosis is of spinal cord tethering, with the cord being stretched by its attachment to the subcutaneous lipoma.

The progressive nature of her symptoms makes conservative management unattractive and likely to be associated with worsening disability. The rule for spinal cord disease is typically that lost function, specifically spincter control, sensation, or motor function, will not be recovered with surgery which only prevents deterioration. Once a definite progression of symptoms is established, surgery should be considered strongly.

Surgery will aim to free the low-lying cord and cauda equina from the intradural component of the lipoma and associated thickened arachnoid. It risks damaging the nerve roots and the cord as there will be no normal anatomy at the site of the dysraphic defect. It will necessarily involve a laminectomy and durotomy at least one level above the site of presumed tethering to identify normal dura and then open it to free the neural structures, progressing caudally through the defect. The filum terminale, which attaches the conus medullaris to the sacral hiatus, is also usually identified and divided in such an operation. Cord-tethering syndromes are more common in children as the cord and spine grow at a differential rate, unmasking the tethering. Therefore such an operation is likely to be more familiar to a clinician with an interest in paediatric neurosurgery.

Further reading

Bowman RM, Mohan A, Ito J, Seibly JM, McLone DG (2009). Tethered cord release: a long-term study in 114 patients. *J Neurosurg Pediatr*; **3**: 181–7.

Stetler WR Jr, Park P, Sullivan S (2010). Pathophysiology of adult tethered cord syndrome: review of the literature. *Neurosurg Focus*; **29**: E2.

Case 57

A 20-year-old woman has been seen by the neurologists. She has a 3-week history of severe headaches and progressive visual failure, and originally saw an optician who suggested that she needed to be seen in hospital. She has an approximately symmetrical loss of visual acuity, not correctable by glasses, which is now 6/24 bilaterally. In addition, she describes the edges of her vision closing in and feels that she is 'looking down a tunnel'. She has no diplopia, no vomiting, no seizures, and no focal neurological symptoms or signs. Fundoscopy shows gross papilloedema bilaterally.

Questions

1. What is the cause of her visual failure? An MRI has been done (sagittal T_1, axial T_2, and AP venogram) (Fig. 57.1). What are the key findings?
2. How would you proceed?

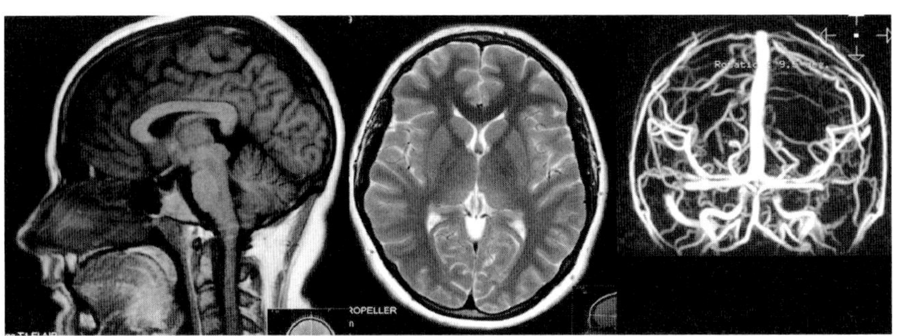

Fig. 57.1

Answers

1. What is the cause of her visual failure? An MRI has been done (sagittal T_1, axial T_2, and AP venogram) (Fig. 57.1). What are the key findings?

She has raised intracranial pressure. The pattern of visual failure, with the field restriction she describes and the loss of acuity due to the swelling of the optic nerve, is typical of raised pressure. She may have an enlarged blind spot bilaterally. The lack of focal neurological deficit suggests that the raised pressure is due to either hydrocephalus or a mass lesion large enough to cause raised ICP but otherwise remaining undetected. Such a lesion would have to be located in non-eloquent brain, typically the right frontal or temporal lobe.

If hydrocephalus is the cause, she may have a small benign obstructive lesion, such as a colloid cyst or meningioma, in the third ventricle. A fourth ventricular tumour is a possibility but there is usually a history of imbalance or other cerebellar dysfunction. Hydrocephalus due to aqueduct stenosis usually presents in childhood but may occasionally become evident in adulthood for reasons that are often unclear. Other causes of hydrocephalus, such as haemorrhage or meningitis, usually have symptoms of the underlying disease early in their course. The final possibilities are benign intracranial hypertension (BIH) or a major venous sinus thrombosis such as a sagittal sinus occlusion.

The key findings supportive of BIH are normal-sized ventricles and cortical CSF spaces, best seen on the T_2 sequences. The sagittal image shows low signal intensity within the pituitary fossa, consistent with CSF replacing pituitary tissue—the 'empty sella'. The venogram shows defects in both transverse sinuses laterally approaching the transverse–sigmoid junction, but they are not thought to be thrombosed. These are all key features of BIH.

BIH, also known as idiopathic intracranial hypertension (IIH) or pseudo-tumour cerebri, more commonly affects women more commonly than men and is associated with obesity. The term 'benign' has fallen out of favour, as it may result in severe and even complete visual failure. The aetiology remains unknown and debated, but CSF diversion is still considered a definitive treatment.

2. How would you proceed?

The rate of her visual deterioration is of crucial importance in deciding her management. Most patients are managed medically by a combination of neurology and ophthalmology services to whom they present prior to neurosurgical consultation. Her assessment should include (if it has not already taken place) a detailed ophthalmological examination including perimetry tests. In addition she should have an LP to measure the opening pressure, for CSF analysis, and to remove enough CSF therapeutically to lower the pressure by half. The opening pressure for a patient with BIH may be higher than 40cmH_2O. Draining enough to lower it below 20cm H_2O will relieve headaches where they are present and also stabilize the visual failure.

Medical management is usually preferred for patients with BIH. Acetazolamide is usually given to reduce CSF production and may be sufficient for some months or years but many patients will become refractory to acetazolamide and require shunting.

Because the ventricles are small, or at best of normal size, there is often a preference to divert CSF with a lumbar–peritoneal shunt. This also avoids the risk of cranial surgery. However, lumbar–peritoneal shunts have a greater tendency to block or displace, and a number of patients subsequently require a ventricular shunt.

This patient's visual failure had progressed despite maximal therapy with acetazolamide and LPs every other day. Accordingly, she underwent placement of a VP shunt which resulted in sustained improvement of her headaches immediately. Her visual acuity improved to 6/9 bilaterally at 6 months postoperatively.

In recent years there has been great interest in the venous sinus stenoses seen on venography, which have been postulated to be the primary causative factor in BIH. As a consequence some centres have used endovascular techniques to stent the venous sinuses to improve venous drainage, with the expectation that this will improve CSF pressure. Small series have reported good outcomes using this technique. The counter-argument is that the raised intracranial pressure causes venous obstruction, and this is supported by venograms done shortly after therapeutic LPs showing resolution of the previously seen stenosis after reduction in CSF pressure.

Three weeks after shunt placement she attends the ward urgently. She has had recurrent headaches for the last 36 hours with the same features as the headaches she had preoperatively, although she has no visual failure as yet. She has also noticed an uncomfortable tense lump at the site of the abdominal wound where the distal end of the shunt was inserted. She has not been febrile or vomiting.

On examination the cranial end of the shunt is well healed and not tender. The abdominal wound is also well healed, but there is a tense firm limp underneath it which is tender. There is no guarding or peritonism.

Questions

3. What is the differential diagnosis?
4. X-rays of the shunt are taken (Fig. 57.2). What do they show?
5. How should she be managed?

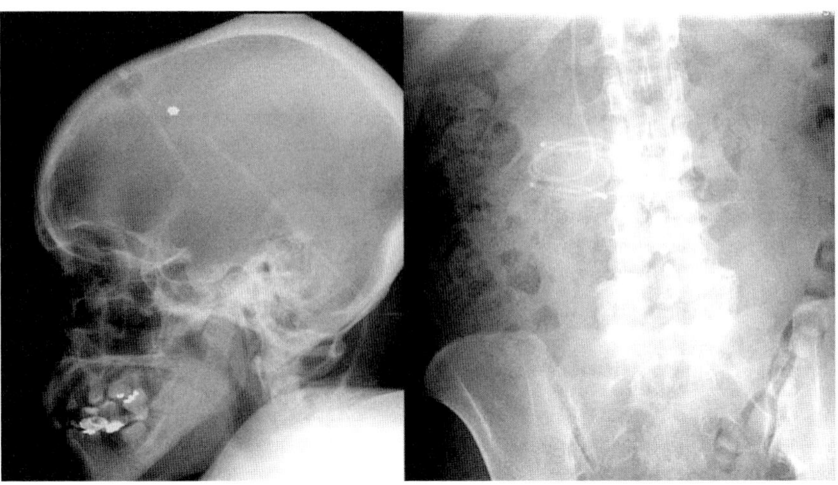

Fig. 57.2

Answers

3. What is the differential diagnosis?

The recurrence of symptoms suggests that the shunt is not working. Given the small size of her ventricles, it is possible that they have collapsed around the shunt and blocked it. However, the tender abdominal lump suggests a local abdominal problem causing the shunt to fail. This might be peritoneal scarring from previous surgery, but the most likely cause is that the shunt has become pulled out of the peritoneum and CSF is now collecting subcutaneously at high pressure causing local tenderness and raised CSF pressure.

4. X-rays of the shunt are taken (Fig. 57.2). What do they show?

The cranial tubing is unremarkable. However, at the abdominal end the shunt tubing is coiled up in a small area in the right upper quadrant. This suggests that it has pulled out of the peritoneum and CSF is failing to be absorbed at a low enough pressure to keep her headaches at bay. A lateral X-ray would confirm this but is not necessary given the clinical likelihood. This is a more common problem in obese patients because of technical difficulties with the abdominal component of the shunt surgery.

5. How should she be managed?

The bottom end of the shunt should be explored and re-implanted in the peritoneal cavity. It may be sutured carefully to the rectus sheath to reduce the chance of recurrence. Careful closure of the peritoneum and rectus sheath may also prevent herniation of the abdominal contents, including the shunt tubing. Assistance of a general surgeon with a laparoscope may make this component of the surgery easier.

Further reading

Bussière M, Falero R, Nicolle D, Proulx A, Patel V, Pelz D (2010). Unilateral transverse sinus stenting of patients with idiopathic intracranial hypertension. *Am J Neuroradiol*; **31**: 645–50.

Cozzens JW, Chandler JP (1997). Increased risk of distal ventriculoperitoneal shunt obstruction associated with slit valves or distal slits in the peritoneal catheter. *J Neurosurg*; **87**: 682–6.

De Simone R, Ranieri A, Bonavita V (2010). Advancement in idiopathic intracranial hypertension pathogenesis: focus on sinus venous stenosis. *Neurol Sci*; **31** (Suppl 1): S33–9.

Digre KB (1999). Idiopathic intracranial hypertension. *Curr Treat Options Neurol*; **1**: 74–81.

Lee SW, Gates P, Morris P, Whan A, Riddington L (2009). Idiopathic intracranial hypertension; immediate resolution of venous sinus 'obstruction' after reducing cerebrospinal fluid pressure to $<10cmH_2O$. *J Clin Neurosci*; **16**: 1690–2.

Wang VY, Barbaro NM, Lawton MT, *et al.* (2007). Complications of lumboperitoneal shunts. *Neurosurgery*; **60**: 1045–8.

Case 58

A 33-year-old man who had a ventriculoperitoneal shunt in infancy for congenital hydrocephalus, which has never been revised, presented to the emergency department with increasing headaches, nausea, and vomiting.

Questions

1. What are the important questions to ask in the history?
2. How can a potentially blocked shunt be assessed at the bedside?
3. List two radiological investigations that can be performed to check for a blocked shunt
4. How should this patient be investigated?
5. The results of the investigations for this patient are as follows:
   - fundoscopy—patient did not tolerate procedure
   - shunt valve—does not refill on compression
   - shunt series X-rays—no abnormalities found
   - serum inflammatory markers—normal
   - CT brain is shown in Fig. 58.1.

   What will you do next?

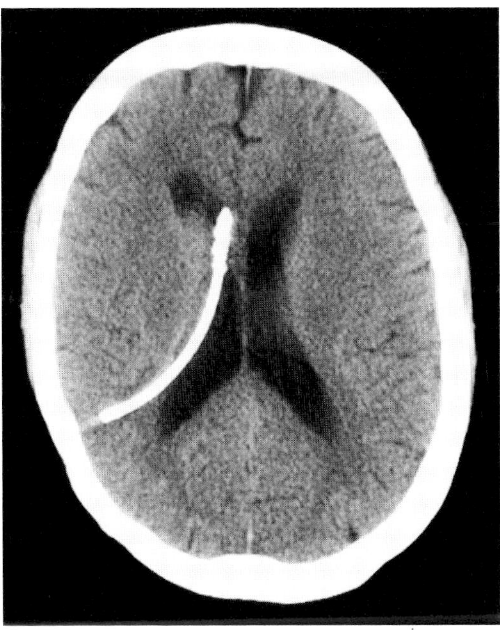

Fig. 58.1

Answers

1. What are the important questions to ask in the history?

In any patient presenting with a shunt-related problem, the essential questions to ask are as follows.

- About the shunt:
  - location of the distal end of the shunt (peritoneum, pleura, superior vena cava)
  - type of shunt (pressure setting, programmable or not)
  - the diagnosis requiring the shunt
  - when the shunt was first inserted
  - date and nature of subsequent revisions (which part of the shunt was revised, whether it was removed, etc.).
- About the symptoms:
  - associated with raised ICP (blocked shunt)—headaches, nausea, vomiting, visual disturbance
  - associated with infection—pyrexia, altered mental state
  - associated with problems at the distal end of the shunt (e.g. abdominal pain).

Patients and their relatives are often very aware of the presenting symptoms when the shunt has blocked in the past, and it is always worthwhile paying attention to these symptoms when assessing the patient.

2. How can a potentially blocked shunt be assessed at the bedside?

Several bedside tests can reveal information about whether the shunt is functioning adequately.

- **Papilloedema** indicates raised intracranial pressure and is therefore consistent with a blocked shunt. It does not indicate which part of the shunt is blocked.
- **Pressing on the reservoir** may indicate whether the proximal (ventricular catheter) end is working. Press the valve and release: if the valve refills, the ventricular catheter is patent; if it depresses and does not fill, blockage of the ventricular catheter is a possibility, although a low ICP may also be possible. Even if the valve fills, a blocked shunt is not excluded as the shunt tubing distal to the valve may still be blocked. This is generally an unreliable technique, especially in older shunts, as one may be pressing on a ventricular access reservoir or the valve may have become incompetent.
- **Tapping the shunt** is a commonly performed test which involves passing a narrow (usually 25G) needle into the reservoir of the shunt valve. A manometer and syringe may be connected to it. There are various results from such a test:
  - CSF easily aspirated at high pressure—suggests distal blockage.

- CSF easily aspirated at low pressure—shunt may be working, does not exclude blockage.
- CSF difficult to aspirate—suggests proximal blockage.

3. List two radiological investigations that can be performed to check for a blocked shunt

- X-ray shunt series enables the shunt tubing to be examined for breakages or disconnections.
- CT brain will enable the size of the ventricles to be assessed. Ventriculomegaly (especially if there is an increase in size of the ventricles compared with a previous CT scan performed when the patient did not have a blocked shunt) is consistent with a blocked shunt. Some patients can have 'stiff ventricles' that do not dilate when under pressure and so a normal CT scan does not exclude a shunt blockage. Ultimately the decision to explore a shunt for potential blockage depends on careful assessment of the patient's symptoms.

4. How should this patient be investigated?

The patient clinically has a blocked shunt. The fundi should be examined for papilloedema. The shunt valve can be examined to see if it refills after compression. The patient also requires a shunt series X-ray to identify problems with the shunt tubing, and a CT scan to assess the size of the ventricles. The serum inflammatory markers should also be checked as shunt infection can present with similar symptoms, and there may be both infection and blockage (the former leading to the latter). Tapping the shunt can be avoided as it carries the risk of introducing infection and the clinical suspicion of shunt infection is low.

5. The results of the investigations for this patient are as follows:

- fundoscopy—patient did not tolerate procedure
- shunt valve—does not refill on compression
- shunt series X-rays—no abnormalities found
- serum inflammatory markers—normal
- CT brain is shown in Fig. 58.1.

What will you do next?

The shunt catheter is positioned in the ventricle and the ventricles are not particularly dilated. An old CT when the shunt was known to be working was not available for comparison. Shunt infection is unlikely because the shunt was last operated on a very long time ago. The shunt valve is not filling, which is consistent with obstruction of the proximal (ventricular) catheter, but this finding in itself is not sufficient evidence for blockage. Confirmation could be sought by measuring the CSF pressure. This can be done by tapping the shunt valve with a needle and attaching a manometer, but this carries the risk of introducing infection into the shunt system. An LP carries less risk of introducing infection. In this patient an LP was considered safe and therefore was performed. It revealed an opening CSF pressure of >40cmH_2O. The patient proceeded to surgery, during which the proximal catheter was found to be blocked. This could not be removed as it had adhered to brain over many years. Therefore a new catheter was inserted with the old one still in place. The patient's symptoms resolved postoperatively.

A CT head should be performed after shunt revision so that a baseline scan (with a functioning shunt) is available for comparison if the patient presents with shunt-related problems in the future. The postoperative CT scan of this patient, in which both the old and the new catheter can be seen, is shown in Fig. 58.2.

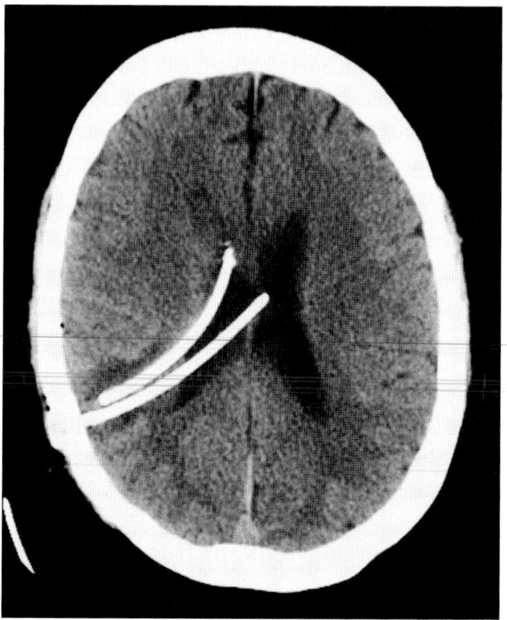

Fig. 58.2

Advice box

- Patients with a blocked shunt may have normal-sized ventricles on CT. The diagnosis of a blocked shunt must not be excluded on the basis of a CT scan showing normal-sized ventricles.
- The decision to explore a shunt is ultimately based on the patient's symptoms.
- A patient and his or her family are often the best source of information for how a shunt blockage has presented in the past for that particular patient.

Case 59

A district general hospital refers a 30-year-old woman who presented to the emergency department following three generalized tonic–clonic seizures. She has a VP shunt which was inserted following traumatic intracranial haemorrhage at 15 months of age. She has had numerous shunt revisions, the last of which was 3 months ago. For the past 2 days, her family noted that she was quiet and not her usual self, although she herself did not complain of any symptoms. On arrival at the local emergency department she was post-ictal and drowsy but responsive with a GCS of 12/15 (E3, V3, M6). During assessment she deteriorates to a GCS of 3/15 and is intubated. Her pupils are size 3, equal and reactive. Her CT scan is shown in Fig. 59.1.

Questions

1. Describe the appearances on the scan (Fig. 59.1). What would be your advice over the telephone?
2. A scan from a recent hospital admission (during which the shunt was revised) is shown in Fig. 59.2. Comment on the appearances and its relevance to the current presentation.
3. The patient arrives at your hospital intubated and ventilated. Where will you direct the patient and what will your immediate actions be?
4. At surgery, the shunt tubing is found to be patent throughout and the CSF pressure is low. A sample of CSF was sent to the microbiology laboratory intraoperatively, and the following results were obtained: red cell count, 167; white cell count, 1035 (92% polymorphs); Gram stain, Gram-negative rods. What is the management?

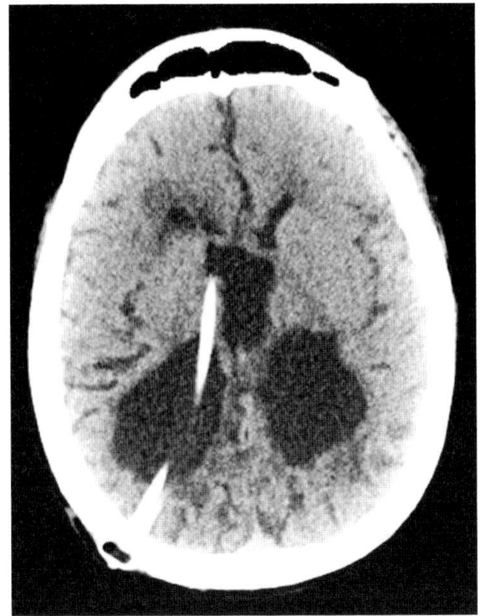

Fig. 59.1

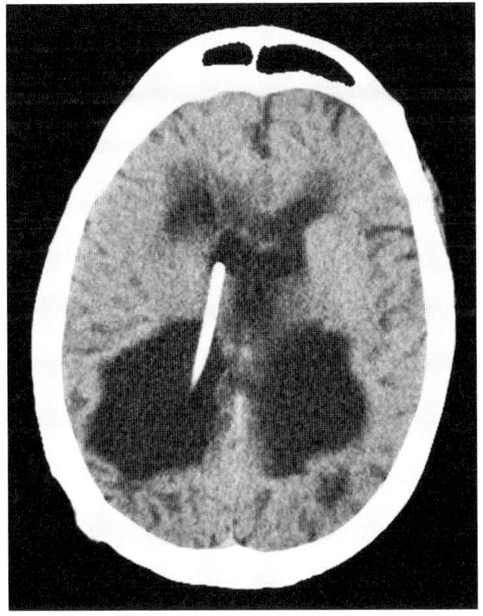

Fig. 59.2

Answers

1. Describe the appearances on the scan (Fig. 59.1). What would be your advice over the telephone?

The third ventricle and the occipital horns of the lateral ventricles are dilated. A ventricular catheter traverses the right lateral ventricle and lies in the third ventricle. Some low density, which may represent transependymal flow and raised intracranial pressure, is seen around the frontal horns.

Clinical deterioration, ventriculomegaly, and transependymal flow are consistent with a blocked shunt. This patient requires urgent transfer to the neurosurgical department for evaluation. The local clinicians may be asked to aspirate some fluid from the shunt or perform an LP if there is likely to be a delay in transfer. If available, previous imaging should be consulted to see if there has been any interval change in the size of the ventricles. Blood tests should be processed at the local hospital so that the patient can proceed directly to theatre on arrival with reference to those results.

2. A scan from a recent hospital admission (during which the shunt was revised) is shown in Fig. 59.2. Comment on the appearances and its relevance to the current presentation.

The ventricles are larger on the previous scan. A shunt catheter is seen with its tip in the right frontal horn of the lateral ventricle. There is more transependymal flow compared with the current scan. In other words, the current scan looks 'better' than the previous one. In this situation it is important to establish whether the old scan was performed before or after a shunt revision. In any case, a current scan that looks 'better' than a previous scan does not necessarily exclude shunt blockage because there may have been initial improvement followed by deterioration. A blocked shunt must always be suspected (regardless of radiological appearances) if there has been clinical deterioration.

Seizures or coma from a metabolic cause are also a possibility and should be considered, although priority should be given to exploring the shunt. Since a shunt revision operation has been performed only 3 weeks ago, infection needs to be excluded as shunt infections are more common in the postsurgical period, with their likelihood decreasing progressively with time since last revision.

3. The patient arrives at your hospital intubated and ventilated. Where will you direct the patient and what will your immediate actions be?

The patient should be transferred to the operating theatre immediately as an operation can rapidly and simultaneously address diagnosis (blocked shunt or infection) and management (revise shunt if blocked or remove shunt if infected). If the shunt is found to be patent and the CSF sterile, another cause for the neurological deterioration must be sought. The pupillary responses should be checked on a regular basis, in this case on the patient's arrival in the department and before surgery.

4. At surgery, the shunt tubing is found to be patent throughout and the CSF pressure is low. A sample of CSF was sent to the microbiology laboratory intraoperatively, and the following results were obtained: red cell count, 167; white cell count, 1035 (92% polymorphs); Gram stain, Gram negative rods. What is the management?

These findings are consistent with bacterial infection (see 'CSF analysis in the diagnosis of ventriculomeningitis', p. 393). The management for a shunt-associated infection is as follows.

- Remove the entire shunt system if feasible (if the patient is not fit for surgery, antibiotics may be used with the shunt left *in situ*, but this is associated with a worse outcome).
- Provide interim CSF drainage (e.g. with an external ventricular drain). This enables continuous drainage of CSF, CSF sampling to monitor the response of infection to antibiotic therapy, and administration of intrathecal antibiotics if necessary.
- Identify the source of infection.
- Commence intravenous antibiotics.
- Re-insert the shunt when the CSF is sterile.

Questions

5. List the routes by which internal ventricular catheters may become infected. What is the difference between meningitis and ventriculitis and which affects patients with infected shunts?
6. Are there any evidence based guidelines for the treatment of shunt-associated ventriculitis/meningitis?

Answers

5. List the routes by which internal ventricular catheters may become infected. What is the difference between meningitis and ventriculitis and which affects patients with infected shunts?

- Contamination of the shunt by the patient's skin flora at the time of insertion (most common)
- Breakage of the skin overlying the shunt
- Contamination of the distal end of the shunt (e.g. peritonitis for ventriculoperitoneal shunts)
- Haematogenous.

By definition, meningitis involves inflammation of the meninges, whereas ventriculitis involves inflammation of the ventricular ependyma. Patients with an infected shunt or external ventricular drainage device initially develop ventriculitis. They may or may not develop meningitis depending on the extent of residual communication between the ventricular system and the subarachnoid space.

6. Are there any evidence-based guidelines for the treatment of shunt-associated ventriculitis/meningitis?

Better outcomes are achieved by removing the shunt system rather than leaving it *in situ*. There are no evidence-based guidelines for the type and duration of antimicrobial therapy, although recommendations have been published. Intravenous antibiotics should generally be continued for 7–14 days and negative CSF cultures should be obtained throughout this period before the shunt is re-inserted. Intrathecal antibiotics may be considered in resistant cases or when the shunt apparatus cannot be removed.

Further reading

Connell T, Curtis T (2005). How to interpret a CSF—the art and the science. *Adv Exp Med Biol*; **568**: 199–216.

Straus SE, Thorpe KE, Holroyd-Leduk J. (2006). How do I perform a lumbar puncture and analyze the results to diagnose bacterial meningitis? *JAMA*; **296**: 2012–22.

Tunkel AR, Hartman BJ, Kaplan SL, *et al.* (2004). Practice guidelines for the management of bacterial meningitis. *Clin Infect Dis*; **39**: 1267–84.

van de Beek D, Drake JM, Tunkel AR (2010). Nosocomial bacterial meningitis. *N Engl J Med*; **362**: 146–54.

CSF analysis in the diagnosis of ventriculomeningitis

CSF analysis plays a vital part in the diagnosis of infection in neurosurgical patients. CSF can be obtained by LP, tapping a shunt reservoir or an external drainage device, or intraoperatively. CSF cell count, Gram stain, and culture are used to diagnose and monitor infection. Culturing an organism is the definitive test of infection but the results are not immediately available, whereas the cell count and Gram stain provide a rapid assessment.

The white cell count in normal CSF in adults and infants over 2 months of age should be <5 (slightly more in neonates due to the increased permeability of the blood–brain barrier). The presence of neutrophils is consistent with bacterial infection, whereas lymphocytes are elevated in viral infection. The Gram stain may identify the type of organism and aid selection of antibiotics, but the sensitivity of Gram staining for infection can be as low as 56%. Therefore a negative Gram stain does not exclude infection. The CSF may contain red blood cells if the CSF was obtained by a traumatic LP, there has been intracranial haemorrhage, or a surgical procedure has been performed. The presence of red blood cells in the CSF may elevate the white cell count in the absence of infection. The normal ratio of white blood cells to red blood cells in blood contaminated CSF is assumed to be one white cell to 500–750 red cells, to mirror the ratio in whole blood. The white cell count can be 'corrected' in the presence of red cells (e.g. if the white cell count is 30 but the red cell count is 25 000, the expected number of white cells is calculated as 25000/750 = 33. Therefore a white cell count of 30 is normal in this situation). These ratios are derived from (several) *in vitro* studies. Although these ratios are widely used in clinical practice to interpret blood-contaminated CSF in neurosurgical patients, the effectiveness of applying this method to the diagnosis of infection is unproven.

Case 60

A 6-month-old boy presents via the paediatricians with progressively enlarging head circumference. His head now measures 51.5cm, which makes it far above the 95th centile (5th to 95th centile range 41.5–46cm). There is no medical history of note; he was born by ventouse delivery at 38 weeks and is developmentally normal. Examination finds that there is a bulging fontanelle but no loss of upgaze, and the boy seems alert and normal apart from his head, which is clearly enlarged.

Questions

1. A CT scan is done (Fig. 60.1). Comment on the findings and the management options.
2. Would you have any concerns about shunting this boy over and above the usual concerns about VP shunt placement in a child?

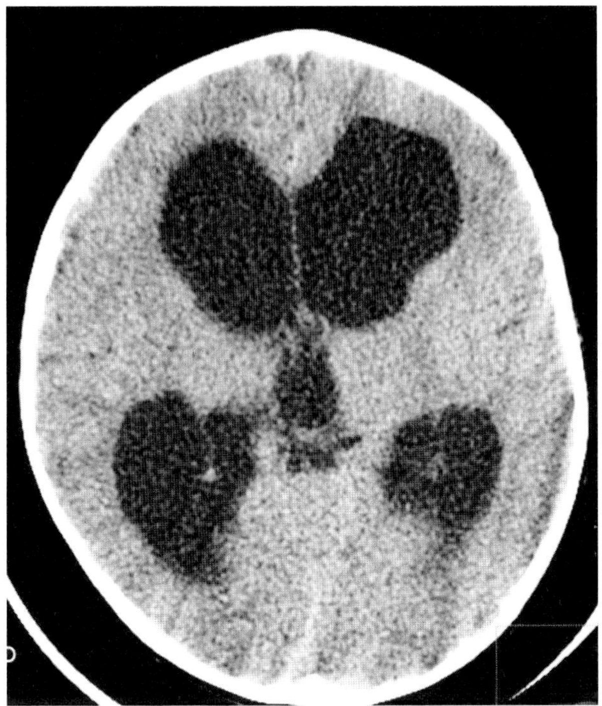

Fig. 60.1

Answers

1. A CT scan is done (Fig. 60.1). Comment on the findings and the management options.

The CT shows grossly dilated ventricles. The most likely cause is aqueduct stenosis or another congenital malformation. However, an MRI does not show aqueduct stenosis, and therefore the diagnosis is considered to be 'idiopathic' hydrocephalus.

The child requires treatment of the hydrocephalus to avoid developmental delay. Given his age (under 1 year) and the lack of obstruction to CSF circulation (e.g. tumour, aqueduct stenosis) as a cause of the hydrocephalus, treatment should be a ventriculoperitoneal shunt rather than endoscopic third ventriculostomy, which, athough preferable as a successful treatment for hydrocephalus, has lowest success rates in children under 1 year old and patients with communicating hydrocephalus.

2. Would you have any concerns about shunting this boy over and above the usual concerns about VP shunt placement in a child?

The degree of the ventricular dilation raises concern about draining CSF too rapidly. The skull will not collapse as it would in a neonate, and hence there is concern about the cortex falling away from the skull because of the loss of CSF volume. In this situation the child may be drowsy for some time post surgery or may develop subdural effusions. Strategies to minimize this include programmable (variable opening pressure) shunt valves or prolonged bed rest after shunt placement to prevent over-drainage due to siphoning effects of the shunt tubing.

A VP shunt is placed with a medium–low pressure (70mmH_2O) valve. The boy is discharged 2 days later, but is taken to his GP after 3 weeks with progressive irritability, fluctuating consciousness, and vomiting. His GP suspects that the shunt is blocked and refers him directly for a CT scan.

Question

3. What does the CT scan (Fig. 60.2) show and how would you treat the patient?

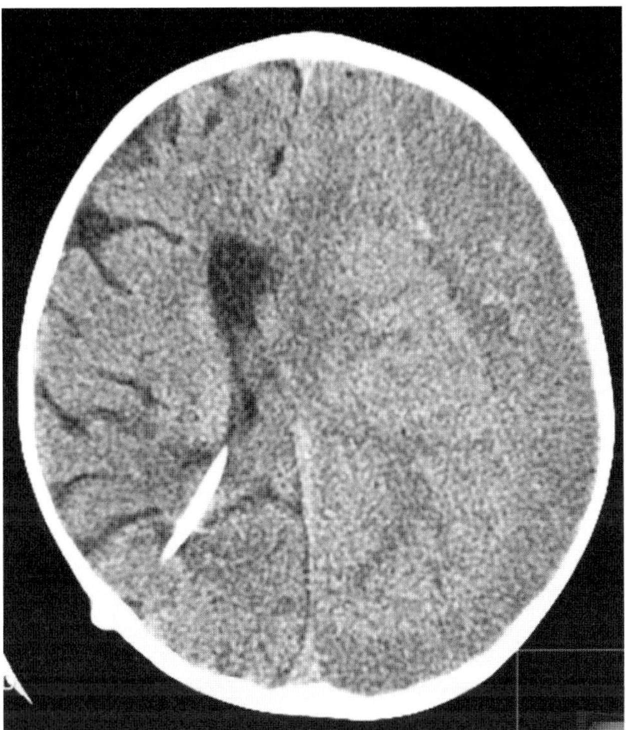

Fig. 60.2

Answer

3. What does the CT scan (Fig. 60.2) show and how would you treat the patient?

The CT does not suggest that the shunt is blocked as the ventricles are small. Rather, it suggests that the shunt is working too well; the ventricles are now far smaller and there is CSF overlying the cortex on the right side. However, there is a large slightly hypodense (compared with brain) collection overlying the left cerebral hemisphere with midline shift to the right due to a subdural haematoma. The shunt catheter is seen within the occipital horn of the right lateral ventricle.

The subdural haematoma has arisen because of the lower intracranial pressure and collapse of the brain due to over-drainage of ventricular CSF. Simply draining the subdural haematoma will invite it to recur. There must also be a change in the CSF drainage process. This will involve changing the function of the shunt. There are three options, in addition to draining the haematoma.

1. Tie off the shunt temporarily with a view to untying it after the subural haematoma has resolved clinically and radiologically.
2. Change the valve for one with a higher opening pressure.
3. Change the valve for one with variable opening pressure.

Option 3 is probably preferable for this boy. The brain can be encouraged to re-expand by a period of higher CSF pressure and after a few weeks, when another CT scan has confirmed that the subdural collection has gone, the shunt pressure can be turned down in small graduated steps. It is hoped that any recurrence of the subdural haematoma will be small enough to be managed non-operatively by cautious reprogramming of the valve.

Further reading

Aschoff A, Kremer P, Benesch C, Fruh K, Klank A, Kunze S (1995). Overdrainage and shunt technology. A critical comparison of programmable, hydrostatic and variable-resistance valves and flow-reducing devices. *Childs Nerv Syst*; **11**: 193–202.

Zemack G, Romner B (2000). Seven years of clinical experience with the programmable Codman Hakim valve: a retrospective study of 583 patients. *J Neurosurg*; **92**: 941–8.

Case 61

A 24-year-old female hairdresser is referred to the clinic. She has noticed a progressive change in sensation in both her hands, on the right a little more than the left, over the past 2 years. This has not been particularly intrusive and she has not noticed any functional impairment and is still working normally. However, about 2 months previously she burnt her thumb very badly on some curling tongs and did not notice until someone pointed it out, at which point she attended the emergency department. Severe loss of pain and temperature sensation was found and her GP subsequently arranged an MRI scan.

Questions

1. What do the patient's symptoms represent and what is the differential diagnosis?
2. She undergoes an MRI of her cervical spine (Fig. 61.1). What does it show? How would you investigate her further?
3. More scans are done (Fig. 61.2). What is the aetiology of her symptoms?
4. What are the treatment options? Which would you prefer in this case?
5. How would you counsel her about surgery? What risks should be mentioned?

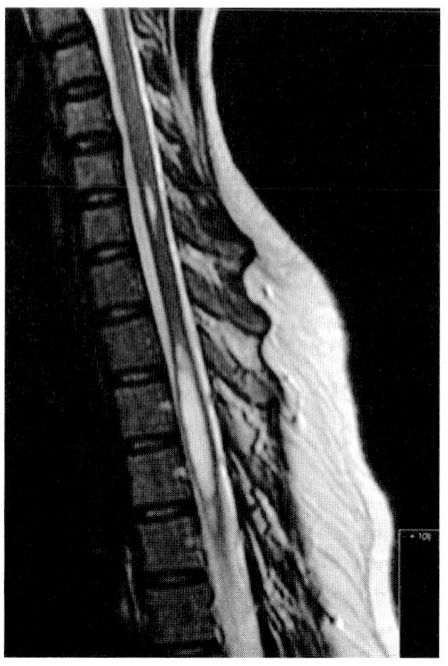

Fig. 61.1

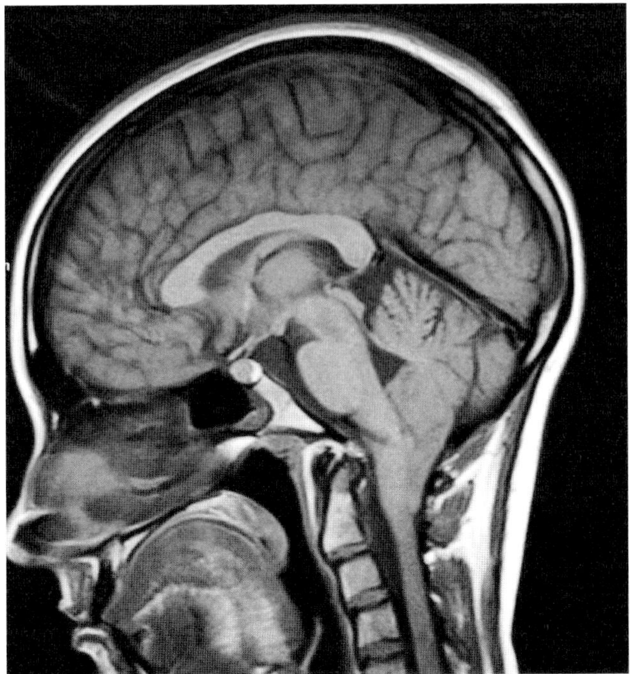

Fig. 61.2

Answers

1. What do the patient's symptoms represent and what is the differential diagnosis?

She has symptoms of loss of pain and temperature, but not fine touch or motor control. This is a form of dissociated sensory loss due to interruption of the spinothalamic tracts which decussate at the level of entry into the spinal cord before they ascend, and is strongly suggestive of a lesion within the spinal cord. The long history suggests either a very slow growing neoplasm or syringomyelia.

2. She undergoes an MRI of her cervical spine (Fig. 61.1). What does it show? How would you investigate her further?

The sagittal T_2 MRI shows at least two areas of high signal, compatible with fluid, in the spinal cord at the mid-cervical level and the cervicothoracic junction. This is syringomyelia.

She should have further MRI sequences. Syringomyelia can be idiopathic but is more commonly due to an associated abnormality. Pathologies presenting with syringomyelia include spinal cord tumours (which may be at a site remote from the syrinx itself), hydrocephalus, tethering of the spinal cord, and Chiari malformation. For these reasons she should have an MRI scan of the entire craniospinal axis, particularly the foramen magnum to look for Chiari malformation and post-contrast sequences to look for enhancing tumours.

3. More scans are done (Fig. 61.2). What is the aetiology of her symptoms?

There is a Chiari malformation. There is cerebellar tonsillar descent through the foramen magnum to the level of the body of C2. However, there is not a particularly vertical cerebellar tentorium or appreciable platybasia. Tonsillar descent in isolation is a feature of the Chiari I malformation, which usually presents in adulthood with cough headaches. Further anomalies of the skull base and in the posterior fossa are features of the Chiari II malformation, which is a more complex embryological problem, almost always in association with an open neural tube defect. It typically presents in childhood, either in association with spina bifida or hydrocephalus, or with brainstem compression and swallowing problems.

4. What are the treatment options? Which would you prefer in this case?

She is symptomatic due to the syrinx and there is an argument for treating the syrinx directly with a syringosubarachnoid shunt. However, routine practice should be to perform a foramen magnum decompression in the first instance to attempt to normalize CSF dynamics around the foramen magnum. Additionally, tonsillar resection may be performed to increase the space around the medulla and spinal cord in the foramen magnum. The hope is that improving CSF flow around the foramen magnum will help resolve the syringomyelia. If she develops clinically worsening syringomyelia despite an adequate foramen magnum decompression, a syringo-subarachnoid shunt may be required.

5. How would you counsel her about surgery? What risks should be mentioned?

She should be advised of the benign but progressive nature of syringomyelia. She should additionally be advised that her symptoms may not improve despite surgery, and therefore that surgery is to halt decline rather than reverse it. There are a number of risks to surgery. Despite surgery she may continue to decline and require a syringo-subarachnoid shunt. Some patients without hydrocephalus develop it following surgery and require VP shunting. Additionally, there are risks of posterior fossa surgery including persistent CSF leak and pseudomeningocoele, which is particularly common after this operation. She is also likely to feel very nauseated and dizzy following the surgery, although this will gradually settle.

She undergoes a foramen magnum decompression, C1 and C2 laminectomy, and tonsillar resection. She recovers from the surgery well and is discharged with headaches that are improving on day 5. However on day 10 she attends the emergency department with worsening severe headaches and associated vomiting and nausea. She has been unable to get out of bed with the headaches and has continuing neck stiffness. She has a CT scan (Fig. 61.3).

Question

6. What are the salient features? What is the diagnosis and management?

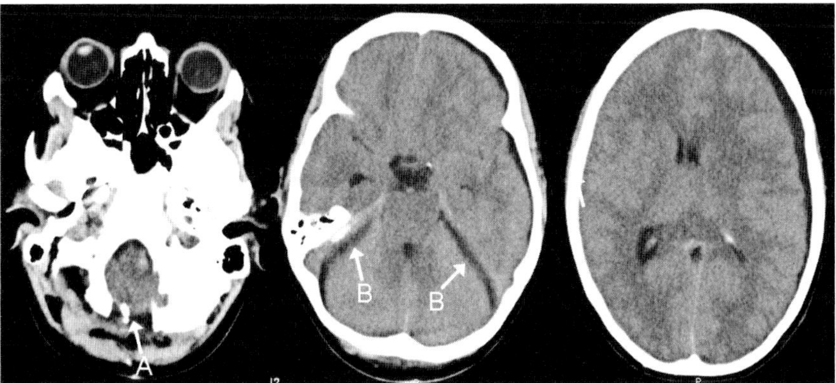

Fig. 61.3

Answer

6. What are the salient features? What is the diagnosis and management?

The foramen magnum decompression is evident (the bony defect created by the operation to decompress the foramen magnum is labelled A). However, there is crowding of the enlarged foramen magnum. There is a left-sided subdural collection which is also evident around the cerebellum and the tentorium (B). There is a little midline shift to the right.

There are two possible diagnoses. One is that there has been sufficient brain shift to cause shearing of a bridging vein and that this is a subdural haematoma (the most common cause of a subdural collection with midline shift). However, the collection is however very hypodense and is isodense with CSF, suggesting that it is a subdural effusion caused by low intracranial pressure and asymmetrical 'brain slump' rather than actively pressing the brain to one side. It would more commonly manifest as bilateral subdural effusions. This would be supported by the collection being around the tentorium as well. The likely aetiology is CSF leak into the area of the foramen magnum, which usually causes a pseudomeningocoele. The key feature of the history is the postural variation; if the headaches are worse when she sits up or stands they are more in keeping with low CSF pressure.

The management of subdural haematoma after cranial surgery is usually burr-hole drainage. However, drainage of subdural collections with low CSF pressure will result in increased brain slump, pneumocephalus, and worsening of the patient's neurological condition including drowsiness and even coma. Therefore this patient should be managed supportively with fluids, analgesia, and flat bed rest if the headaches continue. If she develops refractory subdural effusions a subdural–peritoneal shunt without a valve may be considered.

Further reading

Fernández AA, Guerrero AI, Martínez MI, *et al.* (2009). Malformations of the craniocervical junction (Chiari type I and syringomyelia: classification, diagnosis and treatment). *BMC Musculoskelet Disord*; **10** (Suppl 1): S1.

Hida K, Iwasaki Y (2001). Syringosubarachnoid shunt for syringomyelia associated with Chiari I malformation. *Neurosurg Focus*; **11**: E7.

Park YS, Kim DS, Shim KW, Kim JH, Choi JU (2009). Factors contributing improvement of syringomyelia and surgical outcome in type I Chiari malformation. *Childs Nerv Syst*; **25**: 453–9.

Prat R, Galeano I (2009). Pain improvement in patients with syringomyelia and Chiari I malformation treated with suboccipital decompression and tonsillar coagulation. *J Clin Neurosci*; **16**: 531–4.

Section 7

Miscellaneous

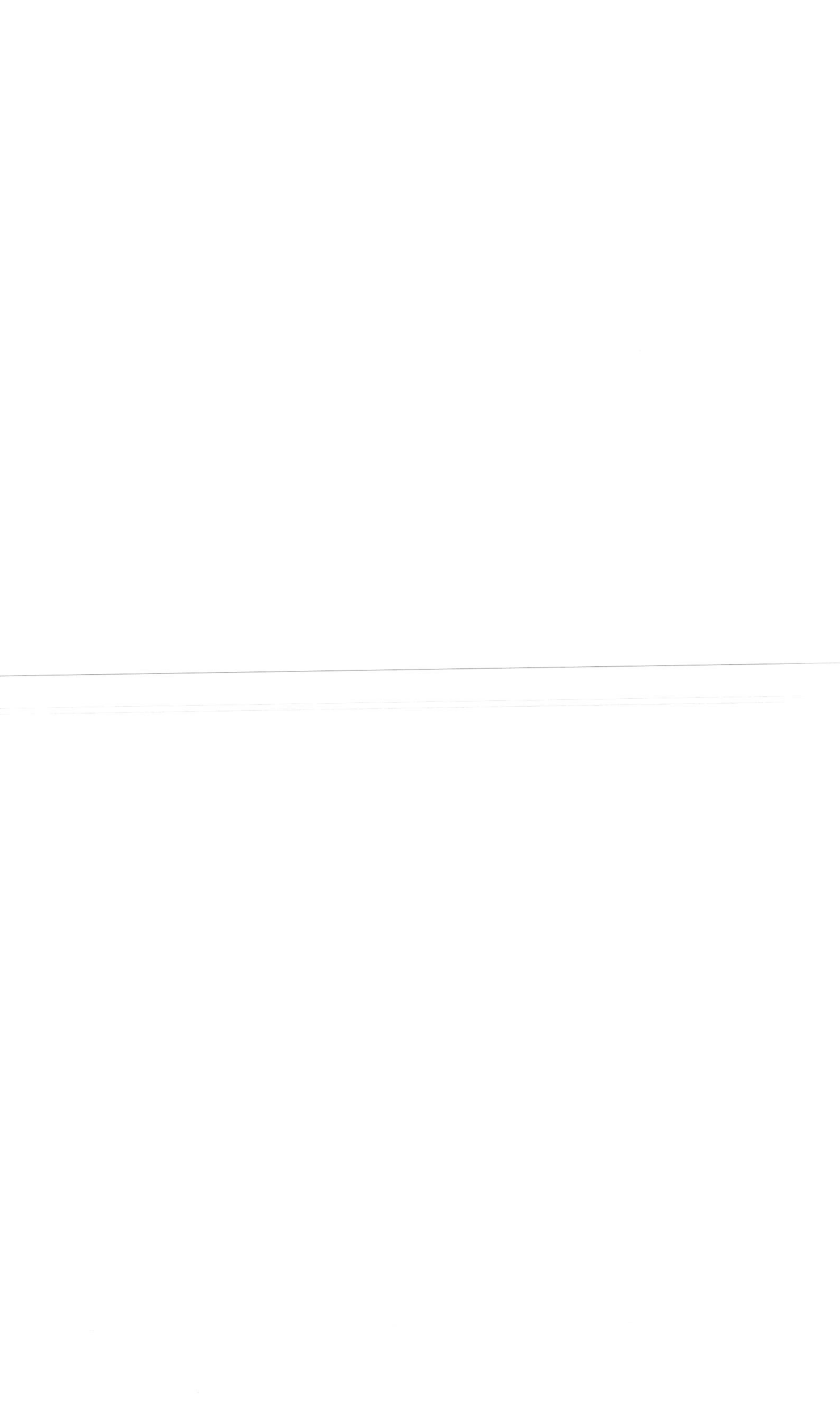

Case 62

A 60-year-old man was referred with a 3-year history of right-sided facial pain. The pain, which was described as 'stabbing', was in the cheek. It had been occasional but had now increased in frequency such that he was experiencing several episodes a day. The pain was triggered by anything that touched the face and when he ate or brushed his teeth. The severity was such that he could not eat or talk normally.

Questions

1. What is the diagnosis?
2. What investigations are required, and what are the other possible diagnoses to consider?
3. What are the management options?

Answers

1. What is the diagnosis?

The diagnosis is trigeminal neuralgia in the maxillary division. The pain of trigeminal neuralgia is characterized by recurrent severe pain, classically triggered by tactile stimulus and described as sharp or stabbing. The pain can last from seconds to minutes and is confined to a distribution of the trigeminal nerve, most commonly in the maxillary or mandibular divisions. Alternative diagnoses must be considered if pain occurs outside the area supplied by the trigeminal nerve.

2. What investigations are required, and what are the other possible diagnoses to consider?

A dental cause for the pain should be excluded. MRI may show a blood vessel impinging on the trigeminal nerve at the 'root entry zone' as it exits the brainstem. Other causes of trigeminal neuralgia include tumours, cysts, and vascular malformations, and for this reason an MRI is mandatory in the early stages of management. The gradient echo MRI shown in Fig. 62.1 demonstrates compression of the right trigeminal nerve (arrowhead) by a blood vessel (appearing as grey dots).

3. What are the management options?

The initial management is with carbamazepine. Surgery is considered for severe prolonged symptoms or if medication is not tolerated. Surgical options include percutaneous procedures, including radiofrequency thermocoagulation and glycerol rhizolysis of the trigeminal ganglion, gamma knife surgery, and microvascular decompression. Microvascular decompression provides the best long-term outcome although it carries the highest morbidity. Patients at high risk from general anaesthesia (although not necessarily the elderly) and those with relatively minor symptoms may opt for the less invasive approaches, whereas those with severe symptoms who are otherwise well may opt for microvascular decompression.

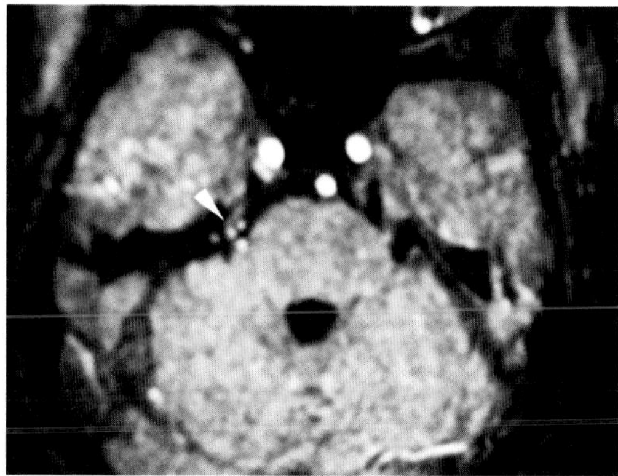

Fig. 62.1

This patient underwent microvascular decompression. A small artery arising from the basilar artery was found to be in contact with the trigeminal nerve. It was lifted off the nerve and a piece of Teflon gauze was placed in between. The patient made a good recovery and was pain free immediately after the operation.

Question

4. What other neurovascular compression syndromes are there?

Answer

4. What other neurovascular compression syndromes are there?

Compression of the facial nerve, vestibulocochlear nerve, and glossopharyngeal nerve lead to hemifacial spasm, pulsatile tinnitus, and glossopharyngeal neuralgia, respectively.

Further reading

Bennetto L, Patel NK, Fuller G (2007). Trigeminal neuralgia and its management. *BMJ*; **334**: 201–5.

Case 63

A 56-year-old man with a history of hypertension presented with a sudden-onset headache. On examination his GCS was 15/15 and his pupils were equal and reactive. He had a left hemiparesis of grade 4/5. A CT scan was performed, and is shown in Fig. 63.1.

Question

1. What does the CT scan show? How does it explain the patient's presentation?

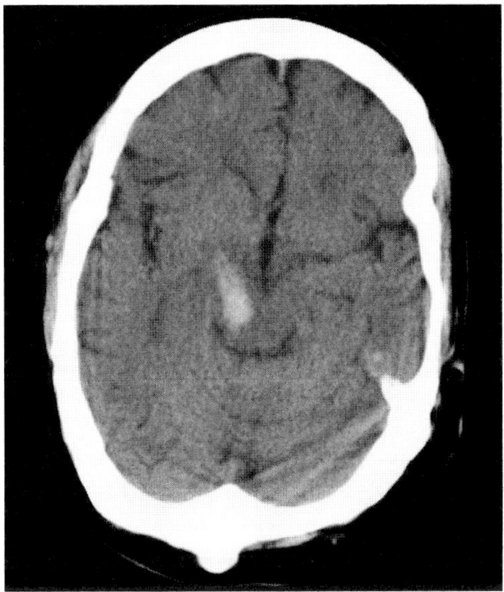

Fig. 63.1 Reproduced with permission from *Mov Disord* 2009 Aug 15; **24**(11): 1697–8.

Answer

1. What does the CT scan show? How does it explain the patient's presentation?

The scan shows a small focal haematoma in the area of the right midbrain. The hemiparesis has resulted from interruption of the corticospinal tract as it traverses the cerebral peduncle. At this level the fibres from the cortex have not crossed and the patient has a contralateral hemiparesis.

Questions

2. Four days later the patient begins to have involuntary twisting of the left arm, which was held in extension most of the time, and sudden flinging movements of the whole arm. What condition does the patient have, and lesions to which areas of the brain cause it?
3. Medical management has not been successful and the patient is referred for functional neurosurgery. What are the surgical options?
4. What is the mechanism of action of deep brain stimulation? What are the possible complications?

Answers

2. Four days later the patient begins to have involuntary twisting of the left arm, which was held in extension most of the time, and sudden flinging movements of the whole arm. What condition does the patient have, and lesions to which areas of the brain cause it?

The patient has dystonia and hemiballismus of the left arm. These movement disorders can occur with lesions to various structures including the thalamus, basal ganglia, deep white matter, and in some cases the cerebral cortex. Hemiballismus was traditionally considered to be pathognomonic of a lesion in the contralateral sub-thalamic nucleus (STN), although recent reports indicate that the STN is involved in only a minority of cases.

3. Medical management has not been successful and the patient is referred for functional neurosurgery. What are the surgical options?

Traditionally, radiofrequency lesioning of the globus pallidus (for dystonia) and the thalamus or globus pallidus (for hemiballismus) have been effective. Recently, deep brain stimulation (DBS) of the same areas has become the preferred treatment in many centres because of its reversibility and the facility to change stimulation settings. Patients for DBS should undergo multidisciplinary evaluation by a neurologist, neurosurgeon, neuropsychologist, and neuropsychiatrist.

4. What is the mechanism of action of deep brain stimulation? What are the possible complications?

The mechanism of action is not fully understood, but the fact that lesioning and high-frequency DBS lead to similar effects suggests that DBS causes inhibition of the stimulated target.

The complications are infection, bleeding, seizures, stroke, and changes to mood, cognition, speech, memory, balance, and vision. As with most neurosurgical procedures, a risk to life should also be mentioned when consent is sought.

The patient undergoes placement of a right globus pallidus internus (GPi) DBS. The electrode position is shown on the fused CT–MRI image (arrow; note that right and left are reversed) and the lateral scout film (note the electrode tip in the basal ganglia—the lead exits the skull through a burrhole and is tunnelled under the scalp through the neck and connected to a battery in the chest wall) (Fig. 63.2).

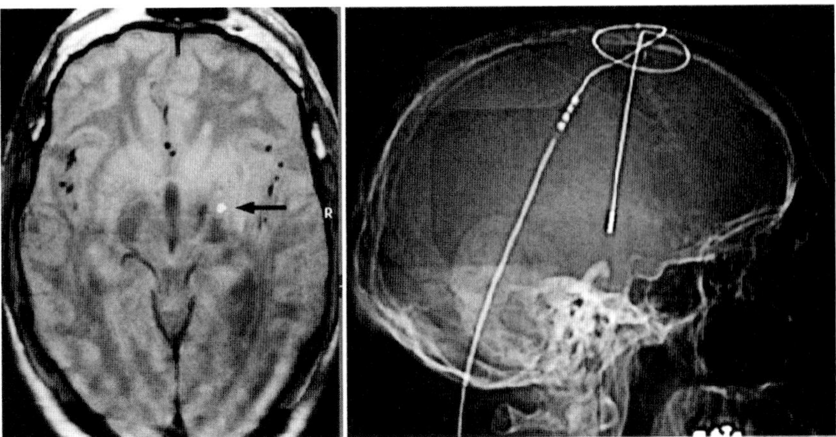

Fig. 63.2 Reproduced with permission from *Mov Disord* 2009 Aug 15; **24**(11): 1697–8. © John Wiley & Sons Inc, 2009.

Question

5. At 2 weeks follow-up, the patient's hemiballismus has settled and his dystonia has improved marginally. What subsequent aftercare should this patient receive?

Answer

5. At 2 weeks follow-up, the patient's hemiballismus has settled and his dystonia has improved marginally. What subsequent aftercare should this patient receive?

After a DBS the patient requires regular follow-up to titrate the stimulator settings to a point where symptomatic control is optimum. The battery needs replacement at periodic intervals, typically 5 years.

Further reading

Alarcón F, Zijlmans JCM, Duenas G, Cevallos N (2004). Post-stroke movement disorders: report of 56 patients. *J Neurol Neurosurg Psychiatry*; **75**: 1568–74.

Kringelbach ML, Jenkinson N, Owen SLF, Aziz TZ (2007). Translational principles of deep brain stimulation. *Nat Rev Neurosci*; **8**: 623–35.

Case 64

A 32-year-old woman with a 10-year history of seizures is referred by her neurologist. The seizures were initially well controlled but have recently increased in frequency. She currently experiences one seizure every 4–5 days despite being on two anticonvulsants. The seizures begin with an odd smell and taste, together with what others describe as a 'glazed look'. She is unresponsive and unaware of events around her for a few minutes, following which she makes a full recovery. She is right-handed and has recently lost her job because of the seizures. She has no other medical history.

Questions

1. What type of seizure is described? How should the patient be investigated?
2. The MRI is shown in Fig. 64.1. What are the findings and the management options?

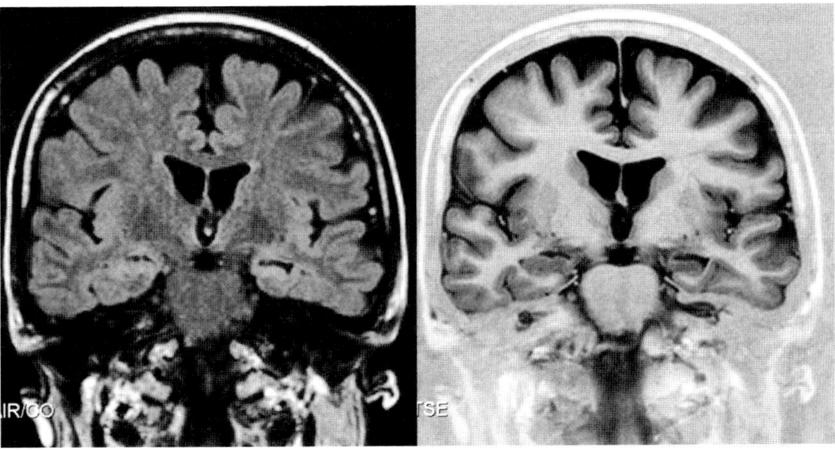

Fig. 64.1

Answers

1. What type of seizure is described? How should the patient be investigated?

This is a complex partial seizure of temporal lobe origin. Partial seizures involve focal symptoms. They are described as complex if consciousness is impaired, and simple if consciousness is preserved through the seizure. Temporal lobe seizures are characterized by stereotyped auditory, gustatory, or olfactory sensations. Patients describe an odd smell or taste, sometimes like burning rubber. There may also be stereotyped motor events.

An MRI is required to exclude an epileptogenic lesion such as a tumour, AVM, or mesial temporal sclerosis (formerly termed hippocampal sclerosis). An EEG is also required to identify and localize abnormal cortical activity. The EEG may be inter-ictal to look for background activity or, if the seizures are sufficiently frequent, intra-ictal with telemetry to simultaneously observe the patient and record the EEG. If scalp EEG fails to identify a source, intracranial recording using subdural or depth electrodes can be performed. This involves a craniotomy to place the electrodes, which are then usually left in place for several days whilst recordings are obtained.

2. The MRI is shown in Fig. 64.1. What are the findings and the management options?

The left hippocampus is smaller than the right on the coronal FLAIR sequence (left image). It is also higher signal. The appearance is diagnostic of mesial temporal sclerosis. The image on the right is an inversion recovery sequence with T_1 weighting. On this scan the small left hippocampus is slightly darker than the right.

This patient has poor seizure control on two anticonvulsants and has a well-defined anatomical abnormality responsible for her seizures. The management options are continued medical therapy or surgery. Surgery involves resection of the medial temporal structures. This procedure offers good prospects of improving seizures due to this condition (approximately 70% success rate), although the chances of achieving a complete cure are slightly lower. Preoperative neuropsychological testing may identify a pre-existing deficit which may be exacerbated or unmasked by surgery. The Wada test is an invasive procedure involving cerebral angiography with selective injection of the ipsilateral internal carotid artery with Sodium Amytal® to temporarily anaesthetize one hemisphere with the patient awake. During this time a neuropsychological assessment is undertaken with a focus on language if the proposed surgery is on the dominant side, as in this case. The extent of language dominance and hence the risk of deficit associated with surgery can then be predicted. The risk of a superior quadrantanopia should also be discussed. Whilst the deficit is not noticed by many patients, in a small minority it is significant enough to affect their ability to hold a driving licence. This is particularly important if patients opt for surgery in the hope of being seizure free and regaining their driving licence.

Further reading

Jehi LE, Silveira DC, Bingaman W, Najm I (2010). Temporal lobe epilepsy surgery failures: predictors of seizure recurrence, yield of reevaluation, and outcome following reoperation. *J Neurosurg*; **113**: 1186–94.

Polkey CE (2004). Clinical outcome of epilepsy surgery. *Curr Opin Neurol*; **17**: 173–8.

Tassi L, Meroni A, Deleo F, *et al.* (2009). Temporal lobe epilepsy: neuropathological and clinical correlations in 243 surgically treated patients. *Epileptic Disord*; **11**: 281–92.

Case 65

A 49-year-old man presented with a 3-week history of a progressive swelling on his forehead. Over the last 2 months his appetite had been reduced and he had lost 4kg in weight. He had previously been well and his medical history was unremarkable. On examination, he was alert and orientated with no neurological deficits. He had a 4cm × 4cm soft fluctuant swelling on his forehead. A CT scan was performed.

Questions

1. The post-contrast scan is shown in Fig. 65.1. Describe the appearances on the scan. What is the differential diagnosis?
2. What is the immediate management of this case? Is there a role for corticosteroids?
3. What are the common causes of this condition? Which is most likely in this case?

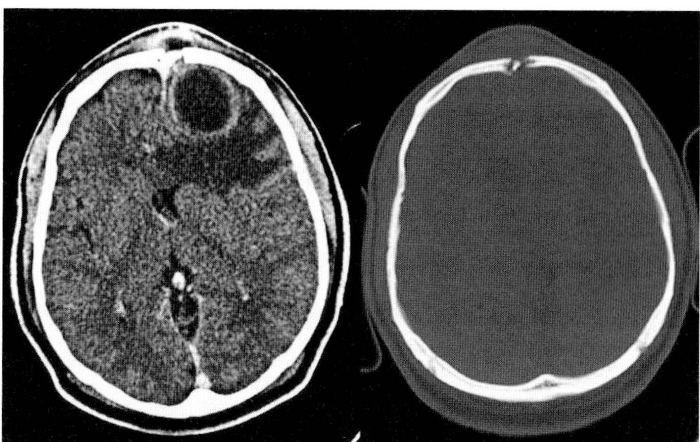

Fig. 65.1

Answers

1. The post-contrast scan is shown in Fig. 65.1. Describe the appearances on the scan (Fig. 65.2) What is the differential diagnosis?

There is a large ring-enhancing lesion in the left frontal lobe (A) with a surrounding area of low density due to oedema (B). There is mass effect with effacement of the frontal horns of the lateral ventricles and subfalcine herniation to the right. The soft tissue swelling is visible overlying the lesion (C). There is a defect in the bone overlying the lesion (D). The bone window illustrates this more clearly, showing breach of the frontal sinus. No other lesions were identified on this CT scan.

The differential diagnosis of a ring-enhancing lesion includes a brain abscess or tumour. Less likely causes include cerebral infarction, resolving haematoma, and radiation necrosis. The clinical presentation of this case (the history, soft tissue mass, and a bone defect over a sinus) makes an abscess most likely, although a tumour is not excluded. Up to 50% of brain abscesses are due to direct spread of infection from air sinuses, and these should be inspected carefully. Other sources of brain abscess are direct inoculation from the ear, trauma, surgery, or meningitis, and haematogenous spread from the teeth, heart (endocarditis), and systemic sepsis.

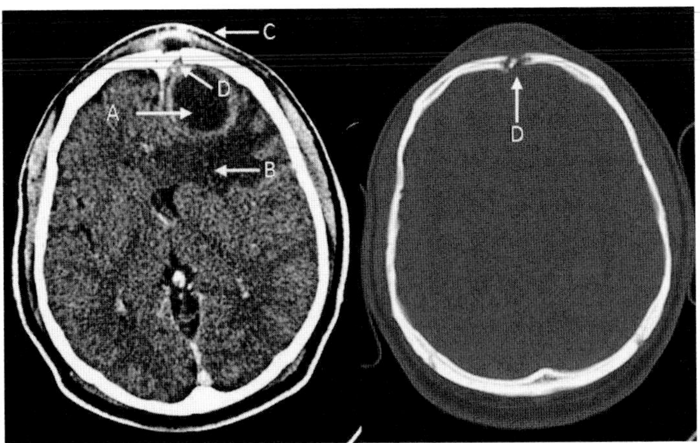

Fig. 65.2

2. What is the immediate management of this case? Is there a role for corticosteroids?

Urgent decompression of the lesion is required in view of the mass effect. A CT scan of the sinuses will be useful preoperatively, as infected sinuses can be washed out during the surgery for the abscess. Anticonvulsants should be commenced because of the highly epileptogenic nature of brain abscesses, and blood cultures should be taken along with routine blood tests, particularly inflammatory markers. Antibiotics should be withheld until the organism is identified unless the patient is septic.

Corticosteroids reduce vasogenic oedema and may improve symptoms associated with intracranial oedema. However, they reduce the rate of capsule formation and slow containment of the abscess. They should not be used in this context unless the mass effect is causing neurological compromise.

3. What are the common causes of this condition? Which is most likely in this case?

Inoculation of the brain may be direct or haematogenous. In this case infection from the sinuses is likely, given involvement of the frontal sinus. The risk of infection is increased in immunocompromised hosts.

Questions

4. What does the bony window CT (Fig. 65.3) show, and how is the forehead lump explained?
5. What is the definitive management?
6. The pus grew *Streptococcus milleri* and the patient was commenced on appropriate antibiotics. What is the duration of antibiotic treatment and subsequent management?
7. What is the typical presentation of epidural abscesses?

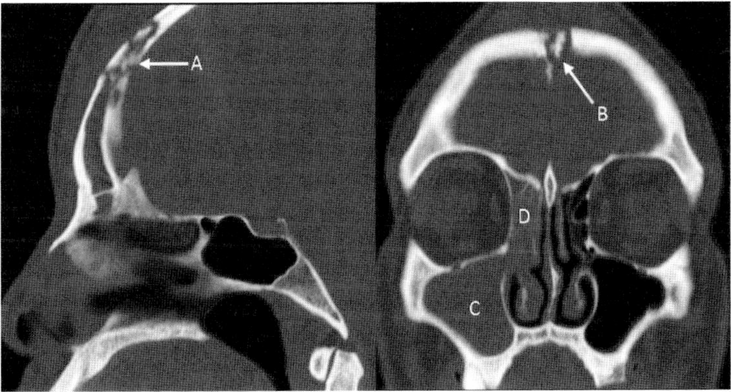

Fig. 65.3

4. What does the bony window CT (Fig. 65.3) show, and how is the forehead lump explained?

On the sagittal view (left) destruction of the frontal bone can be seen, traversing the frontal sinus (A). On the coronal view (right) the destruction due to osteomyelitis of the frontal bone is again noted (B). Opacification of the right maxillary (C) and ethmoid (D) sinuses is also visible. This indicates the presence of fluid or soft tissue, and the most likely cause of this is infection.

Infection has exited the outer table of the frontal bone to form a soft tissue swelling. This is called Potts puffy tumour.

The abscess is likely to have been present for at least 2 weeks as this is the approximate time required for the collagen capsule (represented by ring enhancement) to form. Britt and Enzmann (1983) described the histopathological and radiological appearances of brain abscesses as shown in Table 65.1.

5. What is the definitive management?

The definitive management options are medical (with antibiotics) or surgical (antibiotics plus drainage or excision of abscess). In either case, treatment should start immediately. Medical treatment is only suitable for infection in the cerebritis stage. Once the capsule has formed, antibiotic penetration into the abscess cavity is suboptimal. Medical treatment alone may also be justified if surgery is contraindicated for other reasons.

Surgical treatment allows relief of mass effect and identification of the organism. Needle aspiration can be performed through a burrhole and carries the least operative risk at the expense of a higher rate of recurrence. Craniotomy and excision of the abscess cavity allows a better chance of complete removal and allows additional procedures to be performed, such as removal of osteomyelitic bone. Abscesses close to the ependymal surface of the ventricle are at risk of rupturing into the ventricle, and this event carries a high risk of mortality.

This patient presented at night and underwent burrhole aspiration of the abscess, aspiration of the subcutaneous swelling (found to be pus), and endoscopic sinus surgery with anterior ethmoidectomy, antral washout, and right frontal sinus trephine in a joint procedure with the ENT surgeons.

Table 65.1 Stages of abscess formation

Stage of abscess formation	Histological criteria	Radiological appearance	
		Pre-contrast	**Post-contrast**
Early cerebritis	Area of inflammatory response poorly demarcated from surrounding brain	Irregular area of low density	May or may not show contrast enhancemen Enhancement may be nodular, patchy, or ring-like
Late cerebritis	Fibroblasts appear on margin of developing necrotic centre and lie down a reticulin matrix (the precursor of collagen)	Larger area of low density	Typical ring enhancement Ring is often diffuse and thick, but it may be thin If lesion is small it will appear as solid nodule If lesion is larger, a lucent centre remains
Early capsule formation (2 weeks)	Increase in new blood vessels with migration of additional fibroblasts surrounding necrotic centre Reticulin network surrounds necrotic centre, but is less developed along ventricular surface Mature collagen present in scattered areas of developing capsule	Developing capsule delineated as a possible faint ring surrounding a lower-density necrotic centre Area of low density (oedema) surrounds developing capsule	Ring enhancement May be thinner on ventricular or medial surface
Late capsule formation	A collagen capsule surrounds necrotic centre A zone of gliosis forms around collagen capsule	Capsule visualized as a faint ring	Thin to moderately thick dense ring of contrast enhancement
Healed abscess		Collagen capsule commonly isodense with surrounding brain	May appear as nodular contrast enhancement for 4–10 weeks after completion of antibiotic treatment No contrast enhancement if cured

Britt RH, Enzmann DR (1983). Clinical stages of human brain abscess on serial CT scans after contrast infusion. *J Neurosurg*; **59**: 972–89.

6. The pus grew *Streptococcus milleri* and the patient was commenced on appropriate antibiotics. What is the duration of antibiotic treatment and subsequent management?

A minimum of 6 weeks of intravenous antibiotics is required (see 'Duration of antibiotics in neurosurgery', p. 428). Interval CT scans (usually 1–2 weeks apart) should be performed to check the size of the abscess cavity. Serum inflammatory markers may also be useful. The source of infection needs to be established and additional investigations should be arranged as appropriate (examination of the ears, teeth, and skin, echocardiography, culture of routine specimens). The patient should also have immunological competence testing (e.g. for diabetes and HIV). Continued radiological surveillance is necessary after cessation of antibiotics as radiological resolution can take up to 4 months and contrast enhancement may be present for longer. This patient's abscess recurred after a week and aspiration was repeated. He completed the course of antibiotics and made a good recovery.

7. What is the typical presentation of epidural abscesses?

Spinal abscesses are often difficult to diagnose because they can present in a non-specific manner in patients with multiple comorbidities. Neurological deficits in the limbs with signs of infection should raise suspicion. The presence or absence of meningism can indicate whether the infection is inside or outside the dural sac. The classic symptom triad of an epidural abscess—back pain, fever, and neurological deficit—is only present in a minority of patients.

Further reading

Britt RH, Enzmann DR (1983). Clinical stages of human brain abscess on serial CT scans after contrast infusion. *J Neurosurg*; **59**: 972–89.

Hall WA, Truwit CL (2008). The surgical management of infection involving the cerebrum. *Neurosurgery*; **62** (Suppl 2): 519–30.

Sendi P, Bregenzer T, Zimmerli W (2008). Spinal epidural abscess in clinical practice. *Q J Med*; **101**: 1–12.

A case of a spinal epidural abscess

This 66-year-old man was admitted to hospital with a 3-week history of progressive symptoms, initially of severe diarrhoea and vomiting. This progressed to widespread myalgia and arthralgia. He subsequently became very weak and was eventually his family brought him to hospital as he had been unable to get out of bed for 2 days. On examination he was alert and orientated but tachycardic and pyrexial at 38.5°C. He had symmetrical arm and leg weakness at grade 3/5. He was catheterized because of concerns about sepsis and dehydration and was noted to have preserved catheter sensation. Blood tests showed a white cell count of 18×10^9/L and CRP 297mg/L.

The MRI (Fig. 65.4) shows a diffuse extradural collection throughout the spine (arrows). It is particularly prominent in the lumbar (L1–4) and mid-thoracic

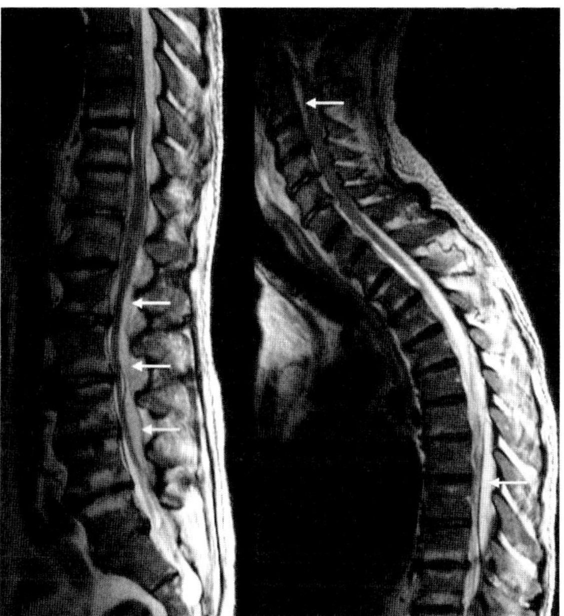

Fig. 65.4

(T5–9) regions where it lies dorsal to the spinal dura and effaces the CSF. In the high cervical spine there is a collection anterior to the dura at the level of C2–4 causing cord compression. He underwent drainage of the cervical, thoracic, and lumbar collections via laminectomies at all three levels. Cultures grew *Staphylococcus aureus*. He was commenced on the appropriate antibiotics and made a gradual improvement over the next 3 weeks, at which point he was able to stand independently and was discharged from hospital for rehabilitation.

Duration of antibiotics in neurosurgery

Table 65.2 lists typical durations of antibiotics for infections encountered in neurosurgery. Individual cases may have specific requirements and local protocols should always be consulted.

Table 65.2 Duration of antibiotics in neurosurgery

Infection	Common source/organisms	Typical duration
Meningitis (following surgical procedure)	*Staph.aureus* Enterobacteriaceae *Pseudomonas*	2 weeks for Gram +ve 3 weeks for Gram –ve
Meningitis (post-traumatic—cranial or spinal)	Nasal cavity *Staph.haemoliticus*, *Staph.warneri*, *Staph.cohnii*, *Staph.epidermidis*, *Strep.pneumonia* Gram –ve bacilli: *E.coli*, *Klebsiella*	Continue 1 week after CSF sterile
Laminectomy wound	*Staph.aureus*	10–14 days
Osteomyelitis of skull	Air sinuses, scalp abscess, penetrating trauma or surgery: *Staph.aureus*, *Staph.epidermidis*, *E.coli* (neonates)	At least 6–12 weeks following surgery
Cerebral abscess	Air sinuses, ear, trauma, surgery, meningitis, haematogenous spread	6 weeks (less if abscess excised completely)
Subdural empyema	Aerobic and anaerobic streptococci (if caused by sinusitis), staphylococci and Gram –ve bacilli	4–6 weeks

Further reading

Tunkel AR, Hartman BJ, Kaplan SL, *et al.* (2004). Practice guidelines for the management of bacterial meningitis. *Clin Infect Dis*; **39**: 1267–84.

van de Beek D, Drake JM, Tunkel AR (2010). Nosocomial bacterial meningitis. *N Engl J Med*; **362**: 146–54.

Case 66

A 38-year-old right-handed woman is referred by her GP with pain in her hands, the right more than the left. It started during her first pregnancy and abated after delivery, but returned during the second pregnancy and did not go away. She describes pain in the lateral aspect of the hand, particularly the thumb and some of the fingers, and she feels the hand has been progressively more numb in recent months.

Questions

1. What are the differential diagnoses, and how do you distinguish them?
2. You suspect carpal tunnel syndrome, but the biceps jerk is dull on the right side. How would you proceed?
3. The nerve conduction tests are shown in Tables 66.1 and 66.2. Can you comment on them? What treatment would you offer the patient?

Table 66.1 Nerve conduction study: sensory summary

Nerve	Side	Stim	Record	LatOn (ms)	LatNPk (ms)	PAmp (μV)	Dist (mm)	CV (m/s)
Median	Right	Digit 2 Wrist	Wrist	2.90	3.53	10.59	126	43.4
Median short seg.	Right	Digit 3 distally	Digit 3 Palm	1.32	1.98	2.71	79	60.0
Median short seg.	Right	Digit 3 distally	Digit 3 Wrist	3.52	4.13	2.85	150	42.7
			Palm–wrist indirect					32.3
Ulnar	Right	Digit 5 Wrist	Wrist	1.77	2.23	8.41	107	60.6
Median	Left	Digit 2 Wrist	Wrist	2.63	3.28	8.86	135	51.3
Median short seg.	Left	Digit 3 distally	Digit 3 Palm	1.35	1.90	5.59	85	63.0
Median short seg.	Left	Digit 3 distally	Digit 3 Wrist	3.32	3.85	7.54	160	48.2
			Palm–wrist indirect					38.1
Ulnar	Left	Digit 5 Wrist	Wrist	1.62	2.13	7.02	107	66.2

Table 66.2 Nerve conduction study: motor summary

Nerve	Side	Stim	Record	LatOn (ms)	Dur (ms)	B-PAmp (mV)	Dist (mm)	CV (m/s)
Median	Right	Wrist	APB	4.23	5.50	13.37		NA
Median	Right	Elbow	APB	8.80	5.67	13.09	260	56.9
Median	Left	Wrist	APB	3.73	5.33	11.16		NA
Median	Left	Elbow	APB	8.13	5.37	11.15	250	56.8

Answers

1. What are the differential diagnoses, and how do you distinguish them?

The two principle neurological causes of lateral hand pain are carpal tunnel syndrome (CTS) and cervical radiculopathy, typically of the C6 dermatome. CTS, or compression of the median nerve behind the flexor retinaculum in the wrist, typically causes pain, paraesthesia, or numbness in the thumb and radial two and a half fingers of the hand, i.e. the index and middle fingers and half the ring finger. The pain may paradoxically radiate up the forearm proximal to the wrist. C6 radiculopathy usually causes pain and paraesthesia in the thumb and index finger. C7 radiculopathy classically affects the middle finger but in practice patients often complain of diffuse hand pain. Nocturnal exacerbation of the symptoms relieved by moving and shaking the hand is strongly suggestive of CTS, as are the exacerbations with pregnancy.

The physical examination may show wasting of the thenar eminence if the condition is long-standing. Tapping over the median nerve in the carpal tunnel (Tinel's test) may reproduce the symptoms. Forced pronation and flexion of the wrist for a period of 30 seconds to reproduce pain (Phalen's sign) suggests CTS. Conversely, the features of C6 radiculopathy should be sought; an absent biceps jerk, sensory symptoms confined to the thumb and index finger, and neck pain or arm pain reproduced by neck extension followed by lateral rotation to the side of the symptoms (Spurling's sign) all suggest C6 root compression.

A final aspect of the examination should involve palpation of the common extensor origin (radial head) during passive pronation–supination to exclude tennis elbow.

2. You suspect carpal tunnel syndrome but the biceps jerk is dull on the right side. How would you proceed?

The diagnostic investigation of choice would be nerve conduction studies to look for a delay in the median nerve at the level of the carpal tunnel. If cervical radiculopathy is suspected an MRI is required.

3. The nerve conduction tests are shown in Tables 66.1 and 66.2. Can you comment on them? What treatment would you offer the patient?

The sensory nerve conduction studies show slowing of the conduction velocity of the median nerve at the wrist on both sides, right more than left, as evidenced by the marked slowing of conduction from distal third digit to wrist, with normal conduction velocity from distal third digit to palm. The lowest conduction velocity is the derived value from palm to wrist, which suggests that this is the location of the lesion. There is a near-normal value bilaterally of the motor studies. This is diagnostic of a predominantly sensory CTS, right more than left.

Given the confirmation of CTS clinically and electrophysiologically, it is reasonable to offer carpal tunnel decompression, in this case on the right side first. If her symptoms improve, the left side can also be done at a later date. The two sides are rarely done at the same time as the period of convalescence is accompanied by the severe inconvenience of having both hands out of use.

Further reading

El Miedany Y, Ashour S, Youssef S, Mehanna A, Meky FA (2008). Clinical diagnosis of carpal tunnel syndrome: old tests-new concepts. *Joint Bone Spine*; **75**: 451–7.

MacDermid JC, Doherty T (2004). Clinical and electrodiagnostic testing of carpal tunnel syndrome: a narrative review. *J Orthop Sports Phys Ther*; **34**: 565–88.

Case 67

A 45-year-old man is referred by his GP with numbness in the medial aspect of the right forearm and hand, principally affecting the little finger. It was intermittent when it began 3 years previously but has become constant and sensation is now almost absent. In recent months he has felt that his right hand is weaker than his left. He is right-handed but has now almost stopped using the hand. There is no diurnal variation or neck pain. He has type 2 diabetes which has been well controlled since diagnosis 5 years previously.

Question

1. What is the differential diagnosis of his symptoms? What would you look for on examination?

Answer

1. What is the differential diagnosis of his symptoms? What would you look for on examination?

According to the distribution of his sensory symptoms, the differential diagnosis is of cervical radiculopathy affecting the C8 nerve root or a lesion of the ulnar nerve. Ulnar nerve lesions most commonly occur at the elbow, but occasionally at the wrist. In both locations the nerve is relatively superficial and contained within a well-defined fascial tunnel, rendering it vulnerable to trauma or entrapment. The third diagnosis to consider is a mononeuritis secondary to diabetes, although this would be unusual in the absence of other complications of diabetes.

Physical examination should allow a clinical diagnosis prior to investigation in such cases. The patient with an ulnar nerve lesion may show wasting of the hypothenar eminence and the lumbricals, giving the hand a clawed and wasted appearance, and making the metacarpal bones more prominent on the dorsum of the hand. If the lesion is at the elbow there may be wasting of the medial flexors of the forearm, particularly flexor carpi ulnaris. The pattern of the sensory disturbance is also important, and splitting of the ring finger, with the sensation preserved on the radial side and reduced on the ulnar side, is suggestive of ulnar nerve pathology. If the nerve is compressed at the elbow, a thickened fascial band may be felt overlying it behind the medial epicondyle. In C8 root compression the small muscles of the hand should be preserved, there may be a depressed triceps jerk, and Spurling's sign may be positive.

Question

2. On the suspicion of ulnar nerve pathology, nerve conduction studies are performed (Tables 67.1 and 67.2). Comment on the results. What treatment would you offer and how would you advise him?

Table 67.1 Nerve conduction study: sensory summary

Nerve	Side	Stim	Record	LatOn (ms)	LatNPk (ms)	P-PAmp (μV)	Dist (mm)	CV (m/s)
Median	Right	Digit 2 Wrist	Wrist	2.40	2.92	8.02	140	58.3
Ulnar	Right	Digit 5 Wrist	Wrist	NR				
Median	Left	Digit 2 Wrist	Wrist	2.18	2.73	8.98	126	57.7
Ulnar	Left	Digit 5 Wrist	Wrist	2.53	3.08	4.30	112	44.2
Radial	Left	Forearm	DorsHandRad	1.95	2.85	19.46	91	46.7
Median short Seg.	Right	Digit 3 distally	Digit 3 Palm	1.68	2.33	5.50	89	52.9
Median short seg.	Right	Digit 3 distally	Digit 3 Wrist	3.10	3.82	4.63	160	51.6
			Palm–Wrist indirect					50.1

Table 67.2 Nerve conduction study: motor summary

Nerve	Side	Stim	Record	LatOn (ms)	Dur (ms)	B-PAmp (mV)	Dist (mm)	CV (m/s)
Median	Right	Wrist	APB	4.27	6.40	7.85		NA
Median	Right	Elbow	APB	9.27	6.27	7.82	265	53.0
Ulnar 1st DIO	Right	Wrist	1st DIO	4.43	5.63	8.49		NA
Ulnar 1st DIO	Right	B.Elbow	1st DIO	9.00	5.87	7.40	210	46.0
Ulnar 1st DIO	Right	A.Elbow	1st DIO	12.30	5.40	5.26	100	30.3
Ulnar 1st DIO	Right	Axilla	1st DIO	13.67	5.50	5.37	80	58.5
Ulnar	Right	Wrist	ADM	3.73	6.37	8.84		NA
Ulnar	Right	B.Elbow	ADM	8.23	6.47	7.51	210	46.7
Ulnar	Right	A.Elbow	ADM	11.67	6.10	4.72	100	29.1
Ulnar	Right	Axilla	ADM	13.13	6.23	4.65	80	54.5
Median	Left	Wrist	APB	3.70	6.40	9.79		NA
Ulnar 1st DIO	Left	Wrist	1st DIO	4.63	4.60	13.84		NA
Ulnar 1st DIO	Left	B.Elbow	1st DIO	8.67	4.97	13.94	215	53.3
Ulnar 1st DIO	Left	A.Elbow	1st DIO	10.73	4.97	13.80	100	48.4
Ulnar 1st DIO	Left	Axilla	1st DIO	12.10	5.03	13.45	80	58.5
Ulnar	Left	Wrist	ADM	3.60	5.83	8.20		NA
Ulnar	Left	B.Elbow	ADM	7.50	6.00	7.51	215	55.1
Ulnar	Left	A.Elbow	ADM	9.57	6.10	7.39	100	48.4
Ulnar	Left	Axilla	ADM	10.80	6.03	7.43	80	64.9

A.Elbow, above elbow; B.Elbow, below elbow.

Answer

3. On the suspicion of ulnar nerve pathology, nerve conduction studies are performed (Tables 67.1 and 67.2). Comment on the results. What treatment would you offer and how would you advise him?

There is a marked slowing of conduction velocity on the right between the above-elbow and below-elbow motor readings of the ulnar nerve. The tests also show an inability to record sensory stimuli in the distal ulnar nerve. This is all consistent with an ulnar nerve lesion at the elbow. This is the most common location of ulnar nerve pathology and is typically an entrapment neuropathy, which is treated by ulnar nerve decompression. This involves a curved longitudinal incision just behind the medial epicondyle to locate the ulnar nerve in the cubital tunnel. The nerve is surgically decompressed along a 5–8 cm length in this canal. The surgery may involve partial removal of the medial epicondyle to allow the nerve to be lifted up and relocated more medially and to prevent it being stretched during elbow flexion after the patient has recovered from the surgery. This is known as transposition of the ulnar nerve, and is performed routinely as part of the operation by some surgeons.

In helping to inform the patient he should be counselled that the aim of surgery is to prevent deterioration rather than to enable full recovery of the hand. This is particularly relevant for this patient for two reasons. First, the severity of the preoperative deficit suggests that complete recovery is unlikely. Secondly, diabetes is an independent predictor of worse outcome after peripheral nerve decompression. This patient opted for surgery, which was performed under general anaesthetic. Six months postoperatively his hand had improved a little but was still very weak.

Further reading

Filippi R, Farag S, Reisch R, Grunert P, Böcher-Schwarz H (2002). Cubital tunnel syndrome. Treatment by decompression without transposition of ulnar nerve. *Minim Invasive Neurosurg*; **45**: 164–8.

Palmer BA, Hughes TB (2010). Cubital tunnel syndrome. *J Hand Surg Am*; **35**: 153–63.

List of cases by diagnosis

Case 1: Chronic subdural haematoma
Case 2: Acute subdural haematoma
Case 3: Extradural haematoma
Case 4: Traumatic head injury
Case 5: Traumatic head injury
Case 6: Depressed skull fracture
Case 7: Penetrating trauma
Case 8: Multiply injured patient with head injury
Case 9: C1 fracture
Case 10: C2 fracture
Case 11: Cervical spine fracture dislocation
Case 12: Dislocated facets
Case 13: Complex cervical spine fracture
Case 14: Thoracolumbar spine fracture
Case 15: Traumatic spinal cord compression
Case 16: Spinal epidural haematoma
Case 17: Subarachnoid haemorrhage
Case 18: Subarachnoid haemorrhage
Case 19: Poor-grade subarachnoid haemorrhage
Case 20: Multiple aneurysms
Case 21: Intracerebral haematoma
Case 22: Ruptured cranial arteriovenous malformation
Case 23: Spinal dural arteriovenous fistula
Case 24: Cavernoma
Case 25: Malignant middle cerebral artery infarction
Case 26: Unruptured aneurysm
Case 27: Recurrent aneurysm and screening for aneurysms
Case 28: Extracranial–intracranial bypass
Case 29: Glioblastoma
Case 30: Recurrent glioblastoma
Case 31: Low-grade glioma
Case 32: Cerebellar tumours in children
Case 33: Meningioma
Case 34: Cerebellar tumour
Case 35: Acoustic neuroma and cerebellopontine angle masses
Case 36: Pineal region tumour
Case 37: Colloid cyst
Case 38: Non-functioning pituitary tumour
Case 39: Functioning pituitary adenoma
Case 40: Pituitary apoplexy
Case 41: Craniopharyngioma
Case 42: Intradural extramedullary tumour
Case 43: Intradural intramedullary tumour
Case 44: Metastatic spinal cord compression
Case 45: Haemangioblastoma
Case 46: Lumbar disc prolapse
Case 47: Cauda equina syndrome
Case 48: Degenerative cervical spine—single level
Case 49: Degenerative cervical spine—multiple levels

Case 50: Degenerative lumbar spine
Case 51: Back pain
Case 52: Spondylolisthesis
Case 53: Normal-pressure hydrocephalus
Case 54: Neonatal hydrocephalus
Case 55: Spina bifida
Case 56: Tethered cord
Case 57: Idiopathic intracranial hypertension
Case 58: Blocked shunt
Case 59: Ventriculitis
Case 60: Over-drainage of shunt
Case 61: Chiari malformation with syringomyelia
Case 62: Trigeminal neuralgia
Case 63: Deep brain stimulation
Case 64: Epilepsy
Case 65: Cerebral abscess
Case 66: Carpal tunnel syndrome
Case 67: Ulnar nerve compression

List of cases by principal clinical features at presentation (case numbers in italics)

Agitation/irritability *3, 4, 5, 32*
Back pain *8, 14, 44, 46, 47, 51, 52*
Confusion/disorientation *1, 4, 5, 6, 22, 37.B*
Conscious level reduction *2, 4, 5, 8, 15, 17, 19, 21, 22, 29, 58, 59*
Eye movement abnormalities *7, 18, 28*
Facial features' changes *39*
Facial pain *62*
Forehead swelling *65*
Gait disturbance/walking problems *1, 23, 32, 34, 43, 51, 53, 56*
Headache *3, 4, 17, 18, 20, 21, 22, 24, 27, 28, 30, 31, 34, 36, 37, 40, 45, 57, 58, 63*
Head circumference abnormality *54, 60*
Hearing loss *35*
Hypertension *21, 25, 37.B, 39, 63*
Fetal anomaly *55*
Limb pain *23, 46, 47, 48, 49, 52, 56, 66*
Libido loss *40*
Limb weakness/movement abnormalities *11, 15, 16, 19, 21, 22, 25, 26, 29, 31, 33, 42, 43, 44, 63, 67*
Nausea/vomiting *3, 17, 18, 20, 21, 27, 32, 36, 37.B, 40, 58*
Neck pain *4, 9, 10, 11, 12, 13, 43, 49*
Papilloedema *36, 57*
Photophobia *27*
Proprioception impairment *23*
Pupillary abnormalities *2, 18, 19, 29*
Seizure *19, 31, 59, 64*
Somatosensory disturbance *11, 12, 16, 23, 42, 44, 47, 48, 49, 50, 61, 66, 67*
Speech disturbance *25, 29, 45*
Urinary disturbance *16, 23, 47, 56*
Visual disurbance *7, 28, 30, 36, 38, 40, 41, 57*
Weight loss *65*

List of cases by aetiological mechanism (case numbers in italics)

Congenital disorders *54, 55, 56, 58, 61*
Cranial trauma *1, 2, 3, 4, 5, 6, 7, 8*
Cyst *37*
Cranial neoplasia *29, 30, 31, 32, 33, 34, 35, 36, 38, 39, 40, 41, 45*
Nerve compression *62, 66, 67*
Infection *59, 65*
Shunt-related problems *58, 59, 60*
Spinal degeneration/disc problems *46, 47, 48, 49, 50, 51, 52*
Spinal neoplasia *42, 43, 44*
Spinal trauma *9, 10, 11, 12, 13, 14, 15*
Idiopathic/unknown *16, 53, 57, 60, 64*
Vascular abnormalities *17, 18, 19, 20, 21, 22, 23, 24, 25, 26, 27, 28, 63*

Index

The index entries appear in word-by-word alphabetical order.
Bold indicates the diagnosis is discussed within the page range.

abdominal breathing 112, 114
abducens (sixth) nerve palsy 141, 205–7, 238, 298
abscess
  cerebral 220–1, **420–6**
  spinal 114, 423, 426, 427
  tumour differentiation 220–1
acetazolamide 379
acoustic neuroma 250–8
acromegaly 279–85
Addisonian crisis 294
adenoma, pituitary 279–85
adrenal insufficiency 288
advance directives 7
agitation, head injury presentation 29, 30, 35, 36, 45
air embolism 33, 262
alcohol intoxication 35, 37, 45, 108, 110
alpha-fetoprotein (AFP) 262
American Spinal Injury Association (ASIA) impairment scale 88–9
anal tone, reduced/absent 84, 309, 310
aneurysms *see* cerebral aneurysms
angiography (cerebral)
  cavernoma 186–8
  circle of Willis 117–18
  haemangioblastoma 316–17
  recurrent aneurysm 201–4
  ruptured cranial arteriovenous malformation 172–4
  spinal dural arteriovenous fistula 180–1, 182–3
  subarachnoid haemorrhage 121, 122–5, 131–2, 134, 142, 147
    multiple aneurysms 150–5
    postoperative deterioration 136, 139
  unruptured aneurysm 205, 208
  vasospasm 139, 142, 147
angioplasty, transluminal 140
anterior communicating artery (ACom) aneurysm 125, 147–8, 152, 197
antibiotic therapy
  cerebral abscess 422, 423, 424–6, 428
  duration in neurosurgery 428
  infected shunt 392
anticoagulation 11–13
  atrial fibrillation 13, 194–5
  reversal of 11
  spinal epidural haematoma risk factor 114
  subdural haematoma management 7, 8
anticonvulsants 37, 40–3, 132, 232, 418, 422; *see also specific drugs*
antidiuretic hormone (ADH) 39
  loss after pituitary surgery 278
  syndrome of inappropriate secretion (SIADH) 38–9
antiplatelet therapy 11, 12, 114
aqueduct stenosis 362–6
arachnoid 24
arachnoid cyst 266
arm
  myotomes 352
  pain 330, 332, 334, 336
  sensory disturbance 330, 332, 434–5
  weakness/movement abnormalities *see* arm weakness/movement abnormalities
  see also hand
arm weakness/movement abnormalities
  cerebral infarction 192
  cranial neoplasm 215, 218, 228, 230, 242, 243
  intracranial haemorrhage 144, 156, 158, 170, 411–14
  spinal abscess 427
  spinal neoplasm 302, 304
  spinal trauma 84, 93, 96, 108
  unruptured aneurysm 199
arteriovenous malformation (AVM)
  anticonvulsant use 43
  cavernoma 184–91
  ruptured cranial 170–5
  spinal dural arteriovenous fistula 176–83
aspirin 11, 12
astrocytomas 40, 232, 260
  anaplastic 306
  pilocytic 235–41
ataxia 358
atlas fracture 69–72
atrial fibrillation 13, 193, 194–5
autoregulation 50
awake neurosurgery 234

back pain
  cauda equina syndrome 324
  lumbar disc prolapse 321, 322, 344–7
  ‘red flags’ 310, 344, 346
  spinal metastases 308, 309, 310
  spinal trauma 103, 114
  spondylolisthesis 348, 350–1

balance problems 246, 248
in child 235–6
balloon occlusion 208
basilar artery aneurysms 125, 197
Battle's sign 50
B-cell lymphoma 233
benign (idiopathic) intracranial hypertension (BHI) 376–82
beta-human chorionic gonadotrophin (β-HCG) 262
bilirubin, in CSF 132, 142
biopsy, brain 232–3
bitemporal hemianopia 290, 292
bladder
innervation 342
problems *see* urinary disturbance/micturition problems
blood pressure management
head injury 46
middle cerebral artery infarction 194
subarachnoid haemorrhage 122, 146
see also hypertension; hypotension
blurred vision 259
bradycardia, spinal cord injury and 88
brain biopsy 232–3
brain herniation 9–10, 167, 195, 422
brain tumours
abscess differentiation 220–1
acoustic neuroma 250–8
anticonvulsant use 40, 42–3
cerebellar tumour 246–9
in child 235–41
craniopharyngioma 290–4
glioblastoma 215–21
glioma (low-grade) 228–33
haemangioblastoma 314–17
meningioma 242–5
pineal region tumour 259–62
brainstem cavernoma 189, 190
brainstem compression 30
brainstem death 272–4
brainstem testing 272–4
Brown–Séquard syndrome 300, 301
burrhole drainage 6, 7, 8, 9, 10

C1 fracture 69–72
C2 fracture 76–82
Canadian Cervical Spine Rule 70
capacity, lack of decision-making 7
carbamazepine 408
cardiorespiratory deterioration, extradural haematoma 30
carotico-ophthalmic aneurysm 205, 206–7
carotid artery injection, angiography 122–3
carotid stenosis 211
carpal tunnel decompression 433
carpal tunnel syndrome (CTS) 332, 336, **429–3**
cauda equina syndrome 323, **324–8**
cavernoma 184–91
cavernous carotid aneurysm 198
cavernous sinus 206–7
central cord syndrome 96, 299, 301
cerebellar haematoma 163–4, 166
cerebellar tumours 246–9, 314–17
in child 235–41
cerebellopontine angle masses 250–8
cerebral abscess 220–1, 420–6
cerebral aneurysms 121–5, 130–8, 146–8
anticonvulsant use 43
Charcot–Bouchard 160
coiling versus clipping 127–8
extracranial–intracranial bypass 208–11
giant proximal intradural internal carotid artery 205–11
multiple 149–55
recurrent 201–4
unruptured 197–8, **199–200, 205–11**
screening for 201, 202
cerebral atrophy 6, 358
cerebral blood flow (CBF) 46, 50
cerebral oedema
cavernoma 186
cerebellar tumour 241, 248
glioblastoma 218, 226
head injury 36–7, 47, 64
types of 216, 218
cerebral perfusion pressure (CPP) 46, 50
cerebral salt wasting (CSW) 38–9, 40
cerebrospinal fluid (CSF)
analysis 388, 391, 393
circulation 360–1
diversion *see* external ventricular drain (EVD); lumbar drain; shunt
hydrocephalus *see* hydrocephalus
leakage 46, 50–1, 169, 284, 404
lumbar puncture *see* lumbar puncture (LP)
metastases 241
cervical central cord syndrome 96
cervical lordosis 332
cervical spine
alignment in 73, 74
C1 fracture 69–72
C2 fracture 76–82
C6 fracture dislocation 84–92
clearing the spine 75, 78
complex fracture 99–102
degenerative 330–3, 334–7
facet dislocation 93–7
immobilization *see* cervical spine immobilization
intradural intramedullary tumour 302–6
traumatic spinal cord contusion 108–11
X-ray interpretation 73–4
cervical spine immobilization 75
cervical spine fracture management 72, 80–2, 91
patient advice 72
raised intracranial pressure concerns and 15, 18, 75
Charcot–Bouchard aneurysms 160

chemotherapy 224, 226
chest X-ray
  cerebellar metastases 246, 248
  multiply injured patient with head injury 60–1, 62
Chiari malformation 368, 370, 371, **399–404**
choriocarcinoma 262
circle of Willis 117–18
claudication 340, 350
claustrophobia, MRI scanning 324, 327
clipping (aneurysm) 123, 124, 136, 146–8
  multiple aneurysms 152–5
  recurrent aneurysms 204
  unruptured aneurysms 197, 208
  versus coiling 127–8
clopidogrel 11, 12, 114
coil embolization 123, 124, 133–4, 148
  multiple aneurysms 152–5
  recurrent aneurysm 201, 204
  unruptured aneurysms 197
  versus clipping 127–8
collapse 144–6, 170, 192, 215, 218
colloid cysts 264–72
coma 144–6
computed tomography (CT) scans
  angiography *see* computed tomography angiography (CTA)
  arteriovenous malformations 170–2, 184–5, 186
  base of skull fracture 45–6, 47, 49, 51
  cerebellar tumour 246–7, 248–9
  cerebral abscess 420, 421–2, 423–4, 426
  cervical spine facet dislocation 94–6
  cervical spine fracture 70–2, 75, 78–82, 87–8, 101–2
  colloid cyst 265–6, 270–2
  deep brain stimulation (DBS) 414–15
  depressed skull fracture 52, 53, 54
  extradural haematoma 23, 26–33
  glioblastoma 216–18, 219
  glioma (low-grade) 228–9, 230
  haemangioblastoma 314, 315, 316
  head injury use guidelines 27
  Kernohan's notch phenomenon 299
  lung cancer staging 312
  malignant middle cerebral artery infarction 192–3, 194, 195–6
  multiply injured patient with head injury 62, 63–4
  neonatal hydrocephalus 362, 363, 364–5
  penetrating head injury 57, 58
  pituitary apoplexy 287–8
  pituitary tumour 275, 276
  right midbrain focal haematoma 411–12
  shunt blockage 383, 386
  shunt overdrainage 394, 395–8
  spinal cord compression 108, 110
  spontaneous intracerebral haemorrhage 156–8, 162–6
  subarachnoid haemorrhage (SAH) 35–7, 120, 123–4, 126, 129, 130
    multiple aneurysms 149–50
    poor-grade 145, 146
    rebleed 135, 136
  subdural effusion 403–4
  subdural haematoma
    acute 16, 17–18, 22–3
    chronic 3, 4, 9, 10
  thoracolumbar spine fracture 104–6
  unruptured aneurysm 199–200
  ventriculitis 387, 388, 389–40
computed tomography angiography (CTA)
  arteriovenous malformation 172–4
  extracranial–intracranial (EC–IC) bypass 209
  multiple aneurysms 150–5
  subarachnoid haemorrhage (SAH) 123–4, 147
  unruptured aneurysm screening 202
confusion 3–4, 31–2, 45, 52, 170, 269
coning 167 *see also* brain herniation
consciousness levels, indications for intubation in reduced 36
consent 7
coordination problems, in child 235–8
corneal reflex 273
cortical sensory loss 244
corticospinal (pyramidal) tract 243, 299, 412
corticosteroids *see* steroid therapy
cortisol 276, 278
cranial nerve palsies
  false localizing signs 298
  see also specific cranial nerves
craniectomy 20
  decompressive 48–50, 192, 195–6
craniopharyngioma 290–4
craniotomy
  abscess excision 424
  aneurysm clipping *see* clipping (aneurysm)
  craniopharyngioma 294
  extradural haematoma 28, 33
  pineal region tumour 262
  subdural haematoma 6, 8, 10, 19
  twist drill 8
cyst, colloid 265–72
cytotoxic (intracellular) oedema 218

deep brain stimulation (DBS) 413, 414–16
deep vein thrombosis (DVT) 13
degenerative cervical spine 330–3, 334–7
degenerative lumbar spine 338–41
delayed cerebral ischaemia (DCI) 138, 139–40
delayed ischaemic neurological deficit (DIND) 139
dementia 358
detrusor instability 342
detrusor-sphincter dyssynergia 342
dexamethasone 10, 241, 248, 298, 306, 312
diabetes insipidus (DI) 278, 294
diabetes mellitus 434–5, 438
diffuse axonal injury (DAI) 64

diplopia 141, 190, 205, 206
disc prolapse
  cauda equina syndrome 324–8
  lumbar 321–3, 324–9
  nerve roots affected by 328–9
discectomy 323, 327–8
  anterior cervical (ACD) 332–3, 337
double vision *see* diplopia
driving
  patient advice 29, 186
  visual disturbance and 190, 418
drowsiness 9, 32, 135–6, 138, 215–16, 219
dura mater 23–4
dural tear 50–1, 340
durotomy 375
dysembryoplastic neuroepithelial tumour (DNET) 40
dysphasia *see* speech disturbance (dysphasia)
dystonia 414–16

ear
  blood-stained discharge 45, 46, 50
  hearing loss 250, 252
elbow, tennis 332, 336
electroencephalography (EEG) 418
electromyography (EMG) studies 337
emboli, unruptured aneurysm and 197
embolization
  ruptured cranial arteriovenous malformation 174–5
  spinal dural arteriovenous fistula 182
  tumour feeding vessels 244, 316–17
  see also coil embolization
embryonal carcinoma 262
empyema, subdural 428
endoscopic third ventriculostomy (ETV) 260, 262, 365, 396
ependymoma 240, **302–6**
epicondylitis 332, 336
epidural abscess 423, 426, 427
epidural haematoma, spontaneous 112–15
epilepsy 40–1, **417–18**
examination, neurological *see* neurological examination
exercise, back pain management 346
external ventricular drain (EVD) 167–8
  colloid cyst 270–1, 272
  indications for 168
  intracerebral haematoma 160, 162, 166
  problems/complications 161–2, 169, 270–1, 272
  ruptured cranial arteriovenous malformation 172, 174, 175
  subarachnoid haemorrhage (SAH) 122, 147
extracranial–intracranial bypass 208–11
extradural haematoma 26–33
  acute spinal 114
  acute subdural haematoma differentiation 16, 19
  meninges structure and pathology 23
extradural tumour 307
extramedullary tumour, intradural 295–8, 307
extubation 22, 46
eye
  care in facial nerve palsy 257
  penetrating injury 57–9
  see also pupillary abnormalities; visual disturbance
eye movement
  abnormalities 57, 129, 130, 238
  assessment of 140–1
eyelid, drooping (ptosis) 129, 130, 138

facet dislocation 93–7
facial nerve monitoring 253, 257
facial nerve palsy 256, 257
facial pain 407–9
facial weakness
  measurement tools 254, 256
  post-acoustic neuroma surgery 254–7
fetal anomaly scanning 365–6
Fisher grading 121, 126, 146
fludrocortisone 40
foramen magnum decompression 402–4
foraminotomy 332–3, 337
fourth (trochlear) nerve palsy 141

gag reflex 273
gait disturbance/walking problems
  cerebellar tumour 246, 248
  in child 235–8
  lumbar disc prolapse 321, 322, 344
  normal pressure hydrocephalus (NPH) 357, 358
  spinal dural arteriovenous fistula 176
  spinal tumour 302
  subdural haematoma 3–4
  tethered cord 372
gamma knife surgery 408
germinomas 260, 262
Glasgow Coma Scale (GCS) 192, 194, 196
glioblastoma 215–21
  glioblastoma multiforme (GBM) 43
  recurrent 222–7
glioma 43, **228–33**, 306
glossopharyngeal neuralgia 410
glucose tolerance test 280–2
grey matter 299
growth hormone 276, 280–2, 284
Guillain–Barré syndrome 302, 304

haemangioblastoma 314–17
haemodilution 140
Hakim's triad 358
halo immobilization/traction 91, 102
hand
  myotomes 352
  pain 429, 432
  sensory disturbance
    cervical spine pathology 84–6, 93, 330–2, 334

Chiari malformation with syringomyelia 399–402
nerve compression 429–32, 434–5
weakness 434–5, 438
Hangman's fracture 80
head circumference, enlarged 362, 364, 394
head injury/traumatic brain injury (TBI)
anticonvulsant use 41, 43
base of skull fracture 45–51
CT scan use guidelines 27
depressed skull fracture 52–6
extradural haematoma 26–33
multiply injured patient with 60–4
penetrating injury 57–9
subarachnoid haemorrhage 35–8
subdural haematoma 15–24
headache
arteriovenous malformation 170, 184, 186
cerebellar tumour 246, 248
colloid cyst 264, 268, 269
extradural haematoma 26, 31, 32
idiopathic intracranial hypertension (IIH) 376, 379
pituitary apoplexy 286
post-foramen magnum decompression 403
right midbrain focal haematoma 411
shunt blockage 383
spontaneous intracerebral haematoma 156
subarachnoid haemorrhage 35, 119, 120, 129, 149, 201
tumour-related 222, 224, 259, 314, 316
unruptured aneurysm presentation 205
hearing loss 250, 252
heart valve prostheses, anticoagulation 3, 7, 8, 12
hemianopia, homonymous 222, 224
hemiballismus 414–16
hemifacial spasm 410
hemiparesis
corticospinal tract interruption 411–12
postoperative deterioration 138, 139
subdural haematoma 19
superficial lobar haemorrhage 166
tumour-related 215–16, 218, 219, 242
see also weakness
hemiplegia 156–8, 192
heparin 12
hepatitis C 112, 114, 115
herniation, brain 9–10, 167, 195, 422
hormonal replacement 275, 277–8
House–Brackmann scale 256
Hunt and Hess grade 146, 147
hydrocephalus
blocked shunt 383–6
cerebellar tumour 248
in child 238–41
cerebrospinal fluid (CSF) circulation and 360–1
colloid cyst 268, 272
craniopharyngioma 294
differentiation of communicating and obstructive 361
fetal anomaly scanning 365–6
haemangioblastoma 316
idiopathic 396
interstitial oedema and 219
myelomeningocoele and 368, 370
neonatal 362–6
normal pressure (NPH) 357–9
pineal region tumour 260
ruptured cranial arteriovenous malformation 172, 175
spontaneous intracerebral haemorrhage 158–62, 166
subarachnoid haemorrhage (SAH) 121, 122, 136, 146, 147
subdural haematoma 22
hydromyelia 371
hypernatraemia 278
hypertension
hypertensive haemorrhage 158, 160, 172
idiopathic intracranial (IIH) 376–82
pituitary tumour 279
subarachnoid haemorrhage 119
in triple-H therapy 140
hyperventilation 48
hypervolaemia 140
hyponatraemia 9, 37–40
hypotension 16, 20, 88

idiopathic intracranial hypertension (IIH) 376–82
incontinence 343, 358
infection
abscess *see* abscess
antibiotic therapy duration 428
external ventricular drain (EVD) 169
VP shunt 387–93
insulin-like growth factor (IGF-1) 280, 281, 282
intensive care unit (ICU)
lack of bed availability 16, 20
subdural haematoma management 16, 19–20
internal capsule 158
internal fixation
cervical spine 82, 91–2
thoracolumbar spine 106
interspinous spacer 341
interstitial oedema 219
intracellular oedema 218
intracerebral haemorrhage
anticonvulsant use 41
myocardial stress in 146
ruptured cranial arteriovenous malformation 170–5
spontaneous 156–67
intracranial haemorrhage (ICH)
anticoagulation and risk of 12–13
anticonvulsant use 43
sudden onset headache differential diagnosis 120
see also specific types of haemorrhage

intracranial pressure (ICP)
  cerebral perfusion pressure (CPP) formula 50
  monitoring 46, 64, 359
  raised *see* raised intracranial pressure (ICP)
intradural tumour
  extramedullary 295–8, 307
  intramedullary 302–6, 307
intramedullary tumour, intradural 302–6, 307
intraparenchymal haemorrhage 224
intraventricular haemorrhage 64
intubation, reduced conscious level indications for 36
irritability 235, 396
ischium, fractured 62

Jefferson's fracture 69–72

Karnofsky score 224, 227
Kernohan–Woltman notch phenomenon 298–9

L3 fracture 103–6
lamellation, spinal cord 300
laminectomy 340–1, 351, 375, 403, 427
  wound infection antibiotic therapy 428
leg pain
  arteriovenous malformation and ascending 176
  cauda equina syndrome 324, 326, 328
  lumbar disc prolapse 321, 322, 323
  tethered cord 372, 374
leg weakness/movement abnormalities
  cerebral artery infarction 192
  intracranial haemorrhage 156–8, 170, 411–12
  neoplasm 215–18, 295, 296, 302–4, 308–10
  spinal abscess 427
  spinal epidural haematoma 112–14
  spinal trauma 84, 89, 108
legal issues, family's views on treatment 7
legs
  myotomes 352–3
  pain *see* leg pain
  sensory disturbance 84–6, 112, 308, 309, 310, 338
    ascending 295, 296, 297
    spinal injury classification 89
  weakness *see* leg weakness/movement abnormalities
levetiracetam 41
libido, loss of 286
lipoma 374–5
local anaesthesia
  awake neurosurgery 234
  nerve root infiltration 337
localizing signs, false 298–9
lordosis, cervical 332
lumbar decompression 340, 351
lumbar disc prolapse 321–3, 324–9, **344–7**
lumbar drain 122, 160
lumbar–peritoneal shunt 379
lumbar puncture (LP)
  coning risk 167
  CSF pressure monitoring 359, 386
  hydrocephalus management 122, 160
  subarachnoid haemorrhage diagnosis 130, 132, 141–2, 150
lumbar spine, degenerative 338–41
lung cancer
  cerebellar metastases 246–9
  spinal metastases 308–12

macrocephaly 362, 364
magnetic resonance imaging (MRI)
  abscess and cerebral tumour differentiation 220–1
  acoustic neuroma 250–2, 254–5, 256
  angiography *see* magnetic resonance angiography (MRA)
  B-cell lymphoma 233
  cauda equina syndrome 324, 325, 327
  cavernoma 186–9
  cerebellar tumour 238–40, 241, 249
  cervical spine fracture dislocation 90
  Chiari malformation 399, 401, 402
  circle of Willis angiogram 117–18
  colloid cyst 267–8
  craniopharyngioma 291, 292
  deep brain stimulation (DBS) 414–15
  degenerative cervical spine 330, 331, 332, 333, 334–5, 336
  degenerative lumbar spine 338–9, 340, 342
  epilepsy 417, 418
  fetal anomaly scanning 366
  glioblastoma 223, 224, 225–6
  glioma (low-grade) 230–2
  haemangioblastoma 314–15, 316
  idiopathic intracranial hypertension (IIH) 376–8
  intradural extramedullary tumour 295, 297
  intradural intramedullary tumour 302–3, 304
  Kernohan's notch phenomenon 299
  lumbar disc prolapse 321, 322–3, 344–5, 346
  lung cancer staging 249
  meningioma 242, 243–4
  metastatic spinal cord compression 311
  normal pressure hydrocephalus 357, 358
  pineal region tumour 259, 260
  pituitary apoplexy 288
  pituitary tumours 277, 282–4
  spectroscopy (MRS) 220
  spinal abscess 427
  spinal dural arteriovenous fistula 178–80, 182–3
  spinal epidural haematoma 112, 113, 114
  spondylolisthesis 348–51
  subarachnoid haemorrhage 142, 154–5
  syringomyelia 399–401, 402
  tethered cord 372–3, 374
  traumatic spinal cord compression 108–9, 110

trigeminal nerve compression 408
unruptured aneurysm 205, 208
magnetic resonance angiography (MRA)
coiled aneurysm follow-up 202
recurrent aneurysm 203–4
spinal dural arteriovenous fistula 180, 181, 182–3
unruptured aneurysm screening 202
mannitol 18
mean arterial pressure (MAP) 50
median nerve
compression *see* carpal tunnel syndrome (CTS)
nerve conduction studies 429–31, 432, 436–7
medulloblastoma 240
melatonin 262
meninges, structure of 23–4
meningioma 43, **242–5**, 252, 260
meningitis
duration of antibiotic therapy 428
prophylaxis in CSF leak 51
shunt-associated 391–3
ventriculitis differentiation 391, 392
metastases
anticonvulsant use 43
cerebellar 246–9
CSF 241
spinal 296, **308–12**
Meyerding classification 348, 351
Miami J collar 72
microvascular decompression 408–9
micturition
normal 342
problems *see* urinary disturbance/micturition problems
middle cerebral artery (MCA)
aneurysms 125, 146–8
multiple 149–55
unruptured 197, **199–200**
malignant infarction 192–8
mobilization
after subdural haematoma surgery 8
problems *see* gait disturbance/walking problems
motor cortex 242, 243–4
motor decline, paediatric 235–6
motor deficit
in acute subdural haematoma 16, 19
fine movements 242
intradural intramedullary tumour 302, 304
ruptured cranial arteriovenous malformation 170
see also hemiparesis; hemiplegia; weakness
motor neuron weakness
upper/lower 301
see also weakness
moyamoya disease 211
multiply injured patient, with head injury 60–4
Murphy's teat 154
mydriasis 129, 130
myelomeningocoele 368–71, 374
myelopathy, spinal dural fistula causation 182
myotomes 352–3

nail gun injury 57–9
nasogastric tube, base of skull fracture use 51
nausea and vomiting
cerebellar tumour in child 235
colloid cyst 269
extradural haematoma 26
pineal region tumour 259
pituitary apoplexy 286
shunt blockage 383
spontaneous intracerebral haematoma 156
subarachnoid haemorrhage 119, 129, 149, 201
subdural haematoma 22, 403–4
neck
pain *see* neck pain
stiffness 403
see also cervical spine
neck pain
cranial trauma 35, 36
degenerative cervical spine 334, 336
spinal trauma 69, 76, 84, 93, 99
spinal tumour 302, 304, 307
needle aspiration, cerebral abscess 424
neonatal hydrocephalus 362–6
nerve conduction tests 429–31, 432, 436–8
nerve roots
cauda equina syndrome 323, **324–8**
local anaesthetic/steroid infiltration 337
prolapsed disc and 328–9
neurofibroma 295–8
neurological examination
in babies 362, 364
myotomes for 352–3
neuropsychological testing, preoperative 418
neurovascular compression syndromes 407–10
NICE guidelines
back pain investigation 346
head injury imaging 27, 54
malignant spinal cord compression 312
nimodipine 121, 139
normal pressure hydrocephalus (NPH) 357–9
nose, blood-stained discharge 45, 46, 50
numbness
ascending 295, 297
see also sensory disturbance

oculomotor (third) nerve palsy 130, 131–3, 141, 197
odontoid peg fracture 76–82
oedema
cerebral *see* cerebral oedema
papilloedema 259, 376, 384
spinal cord 90, 110, 180, 182
ophthalmoplegia 206
optic chiasm 294
optic nerve
transaction of 58
tumour removal complication 294

osmotic therapy 48
osteomyelitis, skull 428
osteophyte fracture 110
ottorhoea 45, 46, 50
oxyhaemoglobin, in CSF 142

paediatrics
  cerebellar tumours 235–41
  craniopharyngioma 290–4
  intradural intramedullary tumour 302–6
  neonatal hydrocephalus 362–6
  neurological examination in babies 362, 364
  overdrainage of shunt 394–8
  spina bifida 368–71
pain
  arm 330, 332, 334, 336
  back *see* back pain
  facial 407–9
  features of spinal cord pathology 300
  hand 429, 432
  head *see* headache
  leg *see* leg pain
  neck *see* neck pain
  radicular 300
  response to painful stimulus 273
papilloedema 259, 376, 384
Parinaud's syndrome 364
PCV chemotherapy 226
pedicle screws/rods 106, 351
pelvic X-rays 60–1, 62
performance status 224, 227
perineal sensory disturbance 324, 326, 328
Phalen's test 332, 336, 432
phenobarbital 42, 43
phenytoin 41–3, 59
photophobia 201
pia 24
pilocytic astrocytoma 235–41
pineal region tumour 259–62
pineoblastoma (pinealoblastoma) 260, 262
pineocytoma (pinealocytoma) 260, 262
pituitary apoplexy 130, 286–9
pituitary hormone screen 276
pituitary tumour
  functioning adenoma 279–85
  non-functioning 275–8
placental alkaline phosphatase (P-ALP) 262
pneumocephalus 51
Pneumovax 51
posterior communicating artery (Pcom) aneurysm 125, 131, 132–4, 152, 197, 201–4
posterior fossa mass lesion 236–8, 248
Potts puffy tumour 424
pregnancy, hand pain 429
preoperative neuropsychological testing 418
primitive neuroectodermal tumour (PNET) 240
prolactin levels 275, 276, 277
promazine 36
proprioception impairment 176, 178
prothrombin complex 11

ptosis 129, 130, 138
pubic rami fractures 62
pulmonary contusions 62
pulmonary embolism (PE) 13
pulsatile tinnitus 410
pupils
  dilation of 129, 130
  overview of disorders 220
  reaction abnormalities 15, 16, 19, 144, 220
  unequal size 215–18, 219, 220
pyramidal (corticospinal) tract 243, 299, 412

quadrantanopia, superior 418

raccoon eyes 50–1
radicular pain 300
radiculopathy, cervical 332, 336, 432, 435
radiofrequency lesioning 414
radiofrequency thermocoagulation 408
radiosurgery 174–5, 190, 191, 244, 253
radiotherapy
  glioblastoma 224, 225
  spinal metastases 312
raised intracranial pressure (ICP)
  bitemporal hemianopia 290, 292
  cerebellar tumour 236, 238, 240, 241
  colloid cyst 272
  external ventricular drain (EVD) blockage 162
  false localizing signs 298
  glioblastoma 219
  head injury 45, 47–50, 64
  ICU management 48, 50
  idiopathic intracranial hypertension (IIH) 376–82
  monitoring 46, 64, 359
  pineal region tumour 259, 260
  subdural haematoma 18
red blood cells, in CSF 393
reflex abnormalities
  brainstem testing 273
  cauda equina syndrome 324, 326
  cervical facet dislocation 95, 96
  spinal claudication 340
  spinal dural arteriovenous fistula 176
  spinal epidural haematoma 112
  spinal tumours 295, 309, 310
respiratory response 273
rhinorrhoea 45, 46, 50
rib fractures 62

sciatica 322, 323
sedation
  agitation management in head injury 36
  weaning from 22, 45, 46
seizures
  anticonvulsant use 40–3, 59
  brain tumour presentation 228
  epilepsy 417–18
  patient advice in risk of 186

seizure threshold lowering factors 228, 230
subarachnoid haemorrhage 144, 146
ventriculitis presentation 387
sellar tumour 43
shear injury 64
shock, spinal 88
shunt
blocked **383–6**
idiopathic intracranial hypertension 379
infection 387–93
movement out of peritoneum 379–82
neonatal hydrocephalus 365
normal pressure hydrocephalus (NPH) 357, 358–9
overdrainage of 394–8
tapping the 384–5
Simpson grade 244, 245
sinuses, cerebral abscess and 422, 423, 424
sixth (abducens) nerve palsy 141, 205–7, 238, 298
skull, osteomyelitis of 428
skull fracture
base of 45–41
depressed 52–6
extradural haematoma 32, 33
skull X-rays 52, 53
sodium valproate 41–2, 43
somatosensory disturbance
arteriovenous malformation 176, 178
ascending 295, 296
cauda equina syndrome 324, 326, 328, 343
Chiari malformation with syringomyelia 399, 402
cortical sensory loss 244
degenerative cervical spine 330, 332
degenerative lumbar spine 338
intradural extramedullary tumour 295, 296, 297
metastatic spinal cord compression 308, 309, 310
spinal cord pathology features 300–1
spinal epidural haematoma 112, 114
spinal trauma 84–6, 93
ulnar nerve compression 434–5
see also specific location of sensory disturbance
somatostatin analogues 284
spastic paraparesis 296
spectrophotometry 132, 142
speech disturbance (dysphasia)
glioblastoma 215–18, 219
haemangioblastoma 314, 316
malignant middle cerebral artery infarction 192, 194
Spetzler, spinal AVM classification 182
Spetzler–Martin scale 175
sphincter disturbance 307
spinal abscess 114, 423, 426, 427
spinal canal stenosis 110
spinal claudication 340
spinal cord, vascular supply 180–1
spinal cord compression 295–8, 300
metastatic 308–12
spinal cord injury
classification 88–9
complete 84–92, 115
spinal cord lesions
micturition problems and 176–8
types of 299–301
spinal cord oedema 90, 110, 180, 182
spinal cord tethering 371, **372–5**
spinal dural arteriovenous fistula 176–83
spinal dysraphism 374
spinal fusion 344, 347, 351
spinal shock 88
spinal stenosis 340–1
spinal tumours
classification and associated symptoms 307
extradural 307
imaging features 114
intradural extramedullary 295–8, 307
intradural intramedullary 302–6, 307
metastases 296
spinal trauma
C1 fracture 69–72
C2 fracture 76–82
C6 fracture dislocation 84–92
clearing the spine 75, 78
complex cervical spine fracture 99–102
facet dislocation 93–7
spontaneous epidural haematoma 112–15
thoracolumbar spine fracture 103–6
spinothalamic tract 299, 402
spondylolisthesis 348–52
Spurling's sign 330, 332, 336, 432, 435
stenting 208
stereotactic biopsy 233
steroid therapy
cerebral abscess 420, 422–3
nerve root infiltration 337
steroid replacement 277–8, 288, 294
traumatic spinal cord compression 110
tumour management 219, 257, 260
see also specific drugs
subarachnoid cisterns 24
subarachnoid haemorrhage (SAH) **35–8, 119–24, 129–38**
anticonvulsant use 41
delayed cerebral ischaemia (DCI) 138, 139–40
family screening in aneurysmal 202
grading of 121, 126–7, 146, 147
multiple aneurysms 149–55
myocardial stress in 146
patterns of bleeding in aneurysmal 125, 154
poor-grade 144–8
subdural effusion 404
subdural empyema 428
subdural haematoma
acute 15–24
chronic 3–13
Kernohan's notch phenomenon 299
overdrainage of shunt and 398
post-foramen magnum decompression 404

superficial lobar haemorrhage 166, 167
sympathetic nervous system, spinal cord injury and 88
syndrome of inappropriate ADH secretion (SIADH) 38–9
syringomyelia 371, **399–404**

temozolomide 224, 226
tennis elbow 332, 336
teratomas 260, 262
tethered cord 371, **372–5**
thiopental 48
third (oculomotor) nerve palsy 130, 131–3, 141, 197
thoracic disc prolapse 296
thoracolumbar spine
  clearing 75
  fracture 103–6
  immobilization 75
thromboembolism, risk of 11, 12, 13
thrombolysis 194
Tinnel's test 332, 336, 432
tinnitus 250
  pulsatile 410
Todd's paresis 230, 232
tonsillar resection 402–3
transfer, of patient 16, 19–20
transient ischaemic attacks (TIAs) 197, 200, 211
transverse ligament 72
traumatic brain injury *see* head injury/traumatic brain injury (TBI)
treatment refusal, family's views 7
trigeminal neuralgia 407–9
triple-H therapy 140
trochlear (IV) nerve palsy 141
tumour markers 261, 262

ulnar nerve
  compression 434–8
  decompression 438
  nerve conduction studies 429–30, 436–8
  transposition of 438
unsteadiness 3–4, 176, 368, 371 *see also* gait disturbance/walking problems
urinary disturbance/micturition problems
  cauda equina syndrome 324, 326, 328, 343
  incontinence 343, 358
  increased output after pituitary surgery 275, 278
  metastatic spinal cord compression 309, 310
  neurosurgery overview 342–3
  normal micturition 342
  spinal dural arteriovenous fistula 176–8
  spinal epidural haematoma 112
  tethered cord 372, 374
  urinary retention/increased residual volume 112, 178, 309, 310, 343

vascular claudication 340
vascular injury, penetrating head injury 58–9
vasodilators, intra-arterial release 140
vasogenic oedema 219, 226, 248
vasospasm
  angiography 139, 147, 152, 154
  delayed cerebral ischaemia (DCI) and 138, 139–40
venous sinuses
  depressed skull fracture over 55–6
  formation of 23, 24
  pineal region tumour surgery and 262
  sagittal sinus tear 32–3
  stenosis 379
venous thromboembolism (VTE) prophylaxis 11–12
ventricular enlargement/ventriculomegaly 358, 360, 385, 390
ventriculitis 387–92
ventriculoperitoneal (VP) shunt 358–9, 365, 371, 379
  blocked 383–6
  infected 387–93
  movement out of peritoneum 379–82
  overdrainage of 394–8
vestibular schwannoma (acoustic **neuroma**) **250–8**
visual disturbances
  bitemporal hemianopia 290, 292
  blurred vision 259
  diplopia 141, 190, 205, 206
  homonymous hemianopia 222, 224
  idiopathic intracranial hypertension 376–9
  oculomotor (third) nerve palsy 130, 131–3, 141, 197
  penetrating eye injury 57, 58
  pituitary apoplexy 286, 288–9
  superior quadrantanopia 418
  temporal visual field defect 275–6
  unruptured aneurysm presentation 197
vitamin K 11
von-Hippel–Lindau disease 316

Wada test 418
walking problems *see* gait disturbance/walking problems
warfarin 3, 7, 11, 12–13
weakness
  arm *see* arm weakness/movement abnormalities
  cauda equina syndrome 324, 326
  cerebral artery infarction 192
  cranial neoplasm 215–18, 228, 230, 242, 243
  facial 254–7
  features of spinal cord pathology 301
  hand 434–5, 438
  intracranial haemorrhage 144, 156–8, 170, 411–14
  leg *see* leg weakness/movement abnormalities
  metastatic spinal cord compression 308, 309, 310
  spinal abscess 427
  spinal epidural haematoma 112–14

spinal neoplasm 295, 296, 302, 304, 308–10
spinal trauma 84, 89, 93, 96, 108
ulnar nerve compression 434–5, 438
unruptured aneurysm 199
see also hemiparesis
white blood cells, in CSF 393
white matter 299
Wiltse–Newman–MacNab classification 348, 351
World Federation of Neurological Surgeons (WFNS) grading 121, 127, 146, 147

xanthochromia 142
X-rays
chest 60–1, 62, 246, 248
pelvis 60–1, 62
skull 52, 54
spine 103–4, 309, 311, 346, 351–2
cervical 69–70, 73–8, 91, 93–4, 99–100, 102
VP shunt 380–1, 382, 383, 385

yolk sac tumour 262